Veterinary Clinical Parasitology

Ninth Edition

Veterinary Clinical Parasitology

Ninth Edition

Anne M. Zajac

Gary A. Conboy

Susan E. Little

Mason V. Reichard

Under the auspices of the **A A V P**
American Association of Veterinary Parasitologists

WILEY Blackwell

This edition first published 2021
© 2021 John Wiley & Sons, Inc.

Edition History
This edition first published 2012 © 2012 by John Wiley & Sons Inc.
First, Second editions, 1948, 1955 © Iowa State College Press
Third, fourth, Fifth, Sixth editions, 1961, 1970, 1978, 1994 © Iowa State University Press
Seventh edition, 2006 © Blackwell Publishing
Eighth edition, 2012 © John Wiley & Sons Inc.

The right of Anne M. Zajac, Gary A. Conboy, Susan E. Little, Mason V. Reichard to be identified as the authors of this work has been asserted in accordance with law.

Registered Office
John Wiley & Sons, Inc., 111 River Street, Hoboken, NJ 07030, USA

Editorial Office
111 River Street, Hoboken, NJ 07030, USA

For details of our global editorial offices, customer services, and more information about Wiley products visit us at www.wiley.com.

Wiley also publishes its books in a variety of electronic formats and by print-on-demand. Some content that appears in standard print versions of this book may not be available in other formats.

Library of Congress Cataloging-in-Publication data applied for

ISBN: 9781119300779 (Paperback)

Cover Design: Wiley
Cover Image: Courtesy of Anne M. Zajac

Set in 10/12pt Times New Roman by SPi Global, Pondicherry, India

Printed in Singapore
M068957_310321

CONTENTS

PREFACE

The first edition of *Veterinary Clinical Parasitology* was published in 1948 and has been used since that time by students, veterinary practitioners and others as an aid in the diagnosis of parasitic infections. Since 1994, it has been published under the auspices of the American Association of Veterinary Parasitology (AAVP) with the proceeds going to support student travel to the AAVP annual meeting. This sponsorship has not only supported development of more than one generation of veterinary parasitologists, but has also involved a community of parasitologists in the production of the book. The relationship with AAVP continues with the 9th edition. Also, as with past editions, this edition focuses on morphologic identification of parasites, which continues to be widely used in veterinary medicine, increasingly in combination with molecular or immunologic techniques.

There are also some new features in the 9th edition. We have added a chapter summarizing information on modern parasiticides. Additionally, preceding the photographs of parasites for each common domestic animal in Chapter 1 there is a table listing current U.S. label-approved treatments for many parasitic infections. We have also added another new chapter called Diagnostic Dilemmas. In this chapter we present challenging clinical scenarios and diagnostic results and allow the reader to make a diagnosis. A discussion of each of these scenarios is available on the accompanying website of the book.

The 9th edition also marks changes in the authorship of *Veterinary Clinical Parasitology*. This is the final edition that will be authored by Dr. Anne Zajac (author since the 6th edition) and Dr. Gary Conboy (author since the 7th edition). Drs. Susan Little and Mason Reichard, who joined as authors for this edition, will guide the book going forward and continue its association with AAVP.

Anne M. Zajac
Gary A. Conboy
Susan E. Little
Mason V. Reichard

ACKNOWLEDGMENTS

As ever, we are very grateful to the members of the American Association of Veterinary Parasitologists (AAVP) and others who have provided material for *Veterinary Clinical Parasitology*. Since the early 1990s appeals for photographs distributed through the AAVP listserv have brought responses from around the world.

We would also like to particularly acknowledge the extensive contributions to this edition of three of our veterinary parasitology colleagues, Dr. Mani Lejeune, Cornell University; Dr. Yoko Nagamori, Zoetis Corporation (formerly of Oklahoma State University); and Dr. Heather Walden, University of Florida, who graciously offered their magnificent photo collections for our use.

Finally, as Anne Zajac and Gary Conboy step away from authorship of *Veterinary Clinical Parasitology* they would like to gratefully acknowledge technical staff who, over many years, have assisted in identification and preparation of clinical samples utilized for photographs in this book. Those individuals include Susan King, Rosemary Cornett, John McInturff, Alex Fox and Diamond McClendon at Virginia Tech and Nicole Murphy, Robert Maloney and Janet Saunders at the University of Prince Edward Island.

Although the source of each figure is credited in the figure legend (with the exception of photos provided by chapter authors), we would also like to list all the contributors here with our deepest thanks:

Mr. Gary Averbeck, College of Veterinary Medicine, University of Minnesota, Minneapolis, MN

Dr. David Baker, School of Veterinary Medicine, Louisiana State University, Baton Rouge, LA

Dr. Byron Blagburn, College of Veterinary Medicine, Auburn University, Auburn, AL

Dr. Katie Boes, Virginia-Maryland College of Veterinary Medicine, Virginia Tech, Blacksburg, VA

Dr. Dwight Bowman, College of Veterinary Medicine, Cornell University, Ithaca, NY

Dr. Erin Burton, University of Minnesota College of Veterinary Medicine, St. Paul, MN

Dr. Lyle Buss, Entomology and Nematology Department, University of Florida, Gainesville, FL

Dr. Katie Clow, Ontario Veterinary College, University of Guelph, Guelph, Ontario, Canada

Dr. George Conder, Pfizer Corporation, Kalamazoo, MI (retired)

Dr. Kathryn Duncan, College of Veterinary Medicine, Oklahoma State University, Stillwater, OK

Dr. Hany M. Elsheikha, School of Veterinary Medicine and Science, University of Nottingham, Loughborough, UK

Dr. James Flowers, College of Veterinary Medicine, North Carolina State University, Raleigh, NC

Dr. Alvin Gajadhar, Centre for Animal Parasitology, CFIA, Saskatoon, Saskatchewan, Canada

Mr. James Gathany, Centers for Disease Control and Prevention, Atlanta, GA

Dr. Ellis C. Greiner, College of Veterinary Medicine, University of Florida, Gainesville, FL (retired)

Ms. Parna Ghosh, College of Veterinary Medicine, Oklahoma State University, Stillwater, OK

Dr. Larry Hammell, Atlantic Veterinary College, University of Prince Edward Island, Charlottetown, PEI, Canada

Dr. Bruce Hammerberg, College of Veterinary Medicine, North Carolina State University, Raleigh, NC

Dr. Patricia Holman, College of Veterinary Medicine and Biomedical Sciences, Texas A&M University, College Station, TX

Dr. Jennifer Ketzis, School of Veterinary Medicine, Ross University, St. Kitts, W.I.

Dr. Manigandan LeJeune, Animal Health Diagnostic Center, Cornell University, Ithaca, NY

Dr. David Lindsay, Virginia-Maryland College of Veterinary Medicine, Virginia Tech, Blacksburg, VA

Ms. Megan Lineberry, College of Veterinary Medicine, Oklahoma State University, Stillwater, OK

Dr. Aaron Lucas, Taylorsville Veterinary Clinic, Mt. Airy, MD

Dr. Eugene Lyons, Department of Veterinary Science, University of Kentucky, Lexington, KY

Dr. Charles Mackenzie, College of Veterinary Medicine, Michigan State University, East Lansing, MI

Dr. Gil Myers, Myers Parasitological Service, Magnolia, TN

Dr. Yoko Nagamori, Zoetis Corp., Stillwater, OK

Dr. Stephen Jones, Lakeside Animal Hospital, Moncks Corner, SC

Dr. Thomas Nolan, School of Veterinary Medicine, University of Pennsylvania, Philadelphia, PA

Dr. Christopher Paddock, Centers for Disease Control and Prevention, Atlanta, GA

Dr. Fernando Paiva, Universidade Federal de Mato Grosso do Sul, Campo Grande, MS, Brazil

Dr. Andrew Peregrine, Ontario Veterinary College, University of Guelph, Guelph, Ontario, Canada

Dr. Sally Pope, Faculty of Veterinary Science, University of Sydney, Sydney, New South Wales, Australia

Dr. Steffan Rehbein, Merial GmbH, Rohrdorf, Germany

Dr. Robert Ridley, College of Veterinary Medicine, Kansas State University, Manhattan, KS

Dr. Meriam Saleh, Virginia-Maryland College of Veterinary Medicine, Virginia Tech, Blacksburg VA

Dr. Nick Sangster, Charles Sturt University, Wagga Wagga, New South Wales, Australia

Dr. Philip Scholl, Porto Alegre, RS, Brazil

Dr. Stephen Smith, Virginia-Maryland College of Veterinary Medicine, Virginia Tech, Blacksburg, VA

Dr. Karen F. Snowden, College of Veterinary Medicine and Biomedical Sciences, Texas A&M University, College Station, TX

Dr. T. Bonner Stewart, School of Veterinary Medicine, Louisiana State University, Baton Rouge, LA

Dr. Bert Stromberg, College of Veterinary Medicine, University of Minnesota, Minneapolis, MN

Ms. Kellee Sundstrom, College of Veterinary Medicine, Oklahoma State University, Stillwater, OK

Dr. Donald B. Thomas, U.S. Department of Agriculture Subtropical Agriculture Research Laboratory, Weslaco, TX

Dr. Donato Traversa, Department of Comparative Biomedical Sciences, Faculty of Veterinary Medicine, Teramo, Italy

Mr. Chris Tucker, Department of Animal Science, University of Arkansas, Fayetteville, AR

Dr. Isabelle Verzberger-Epshtein, NRC Institute of Nutrisciences and Health, Charlottetown, PEI, Canada

Mr. Martin Visser, Merial GmbH, Rohrdorf, Germany

Dr. Heather Walden, College of Veterinary Medicine, University of Florida, Gainesville, FL

Dr. Jerry Weintraub, Agriculture Canada, Lethbridge, Alberta, Canada

Dr. Jeffrey F. Williams, Vanson HaloSource Inc., Redmond, WA

Dr. Roy P. E. Yanong, Tropical Aquaculture Laboratory, University of Florida, Ruskin, FL

Dr. Tom Yazwinski, Department of Animal Science, University of Arkansas, Fayetteville, AR

Dr. Gary Zimmerman, Zimmerman Research, West Montana, Livingston, MT

Dr. Kurt Zimmerman, Virginia-Maryland College of Veterinary Medicine, Virginia Tech, Blacksburg, VA

AUTHORS

Anne M. Zajac, DVM, PhD, Dip. ACVM-Parasitology
Department of Biomedical Sciences and Pathobiology
Virginia-Maryland Regional College of Veterinary Medicine
Virginia Tech
Blacksburg, VA 24061

Gary A. Conboy, DVM, PhD, Dip. ACVM-Parasitology
Department of Pathobiology and Microbiology
Atlantic Veterinary College
University of Prince Edward Island
Charlottetown, Prince Edward Island C1A 4P3
Canada

Susan E. Little, DVM, PhD, Dip. ACVM-Parasitology
Department of Veterinary Pathobiology
College of Veterinary Medicine
Oklahoma State University
Stillwater, OK 74078

Mason V. Reichard, MS, PhD
Department of Veterinary Pathobiology
College of Veterinary Medicine
Oklahoma State University
Stillwater, OK 74078

ABOUT THE COMPANION WEBSITE

This book is accompanied by a companion website:

www.wiley.com/go/zajac/parasitology

- The website includes PowerPoints of all figures from the book for downloading.
- Chapter 8 Diagnostic Dilemma answers.

CHAPTER 1

Fecal Examination for the Diagnosis of Parasitism

The fecal examination for diagnosis of parasitic infections is one of the most common laboratory procedures performed in veterinary practice. Relatively inexpensive and noninvasive, fecal examination can reveal the presence of parasites in several body systems. Parasites inhabiting the digestive system produce eggs, larvae, or cysts that leave the body of the host by way of the feces. Occasionally, even adult helminth parasites may be seen in feces, especially when the host has enteritis. Parasitic worm eggs or larvae from the respiratory system are usually coughed into the pharynx and swallowed, and they too appear in feces. Mange or scab mites may be licked or nibbled from the skin, thus accounting for their appearance in the feces. Many parasitic forms seen in feces have characteristic morphologic features that, when combined with knowledge of the host, are diagnostic for a particular species of parasite. On the other hand, certain parasites produce similar eggs or oocysts, and cannot be identified to the species level (e.g., many of the strongylid-type eggs from livestock). Fecal examination may also reveal to a limited extent the status of digestion, as shown by the presence of undigested muscle, starch, or fat droplets.

COLLECTION OF FECAL SAMPLES

Fecal exams should be conducted on fresh fecal material. If fecal samples are submitted to the laboratory after being in the environment for hours or days, fragile protozoan trophozoites will have died and disappeared. The eggs of some nematodes can hatch within a few days in warm weather, and identification of nematode larvae is far more difficult than recognizing the familiar eggs of common species. Also, free-living nematodes rapidly invade a fecal sample on the ground, and differentiation of hatched parasite larvae from these free-living species can be time-consuming and difficult.

Owners of small animals should be instructed to collect at least several grams of feces immediately after observing defecation. This will ensure the proper identification of the sample with the client's pet (i.e., a sample from a stray animal will not be collected) and that feces rather than vomitus or other material is collected. The limited amount of feces recovered from the rectum on a thermometer or fecal loop should not

Veterinary Clinical Parasitology, Ninth Edition. Anne M. Zajac, Gary A. Conboy, Susan E. Little, and Mason V. Reichard.
© 2021 John Wiley & Sons, Inc. Published 2021 by John Wiley & Sons, Inc.
Companion website: www.wiley.com/go/zajac/parasitology

be relied on for routine parasitologic examination, since many infections that produce only small numbers of eggs will be missed. Owners should be instructed to store fecal samples in the refrigerator if the sample will not be submitted for examination for more than an hour or two after collection.

Feces should be collected directly from the rectum of large animals. This is particularly important when identification of individual animals is needed. Rectal samples are also needed when the sample is to be examined for lungworm larvae or cultured for identification of third-stage larvae, since contaminating free-living nematodes and hatched first-stage larvae of gastrointestinal nematodes may be confused with lungworm larvae. If rectal samples are unavailable, owners should be asked to collect feces immediately after observing defecation. The process of development and hatching of common strongylid eggs can be slowed by refrigeration. Development is also reduced when air is excluded from the sample by placing the collected feces in a plastic bag and evacuating or pressing out the air before sealing the bag.

STORAGE AND SHIPMENT OF FECAL SAMPLES

If collected feces cannot be examined within a few hours, the sample should be refrigerated until it can be tested. Feces should not be frozen, because freezing can distort parasite eggs. If a sample needs to be evaluated for the presence of protozoan trophozoites like *Giardia* and trichomonads, it should be examined within 30 minutes after collection. The trophozoite is the active, feeding form of the parasite and is not adapted to environmental survival; it dies soon after being passed in the feces.

Increasingly, veterinary practitioners in the United States are using reference laboratories for routine diagnostic tests for parasite infection. Specific laboratory instructions for age, storage and transportation of samples to commercial labs should be followed. In general, when fresh fecal material is submitted to another laboratory for examination, it should be packaged with cold packs. In some cases, preservation of samples may be preferred. Helminth eggs can be preserved with a volume of 5%–10% buffered formalin equal to that of the sample. Formalin fixation also inactivates many other infectious organisms that may be present. Special fixatives, such as polyvinyl alcohol (PVA), are required to preserve protozoan trophozoites and are not routinely used in veterinary practices.

Slides prepared from flotation tests do not travel well, even if the coverslip is ringed with nail polish, since hyperosmotic flotation solutions will usually make parasite eggs or larvae unrecognizable within hours of preparing the slide. However, slides from flotation tests can be preserved for several hours to several days by placing them in a refrigerator in a covered container containing moist paper towels to maintain high humidity. It is best to place applicator sticks under the slide to prevent it from becoming too wet.

FECAL EXAM PROCEDURES

Before performing specific tests on the fecal sample, its general appearance should be noted; consistency, color, and the presence of blood or mucus may all be indicative of specific parasitic infections. Hookworm disease in dogs, for example, commonly produces dark, tarry feces, whereas diarrheic feces caused by whipworms may contain excess mucus and frank blood. The presence of adult parasites or tapeworm segments should also be noted.

Fecal Flotation

The technique most commonly used in veterinary medicine for examination of feces is the fecal flotation test. This procedure concentrates parasite eggs and cysts while separating them from much of the sample debris. Fecal flotation is based on the principle that parasite material present in the feces is less dense than the fluid flotation medium and thus will float to the top of the container, where it can be collected for microscopic evaluation. Flotation tests are easy and inexpensive to perform, but in busy practices the choice of flotation solution and test procedure often does not receive much consideration, despite the substantial effect these choices can have on the sensitivity of flotation exams.

Choice and Preparation of Flotation Solutions

Many different substances can be used to make flotation solutions. The higher the specific gravity (SPG) of the flotation solution, the greater the variety of parasite eggs that will float. Additionally, studies have shown that fecal flotation tests recover only a portion of each type of parasite egg/cyst in a sample because of variation in individual eggs, binding to debris, and so on. As SPG increases the portion recovered increases, which is an important consideration when the number of eggs in the sample is low. However, as SPG increases, more debris will also float, and the risk of damage to eggs from the hyperosmotic solution also increases. These factors limit the range of useful flotation solutions to SPG ranging from approximately 1.18 to 1.3. Both salt and sugar flotation solutions are commonly used in veterinary parasitology and provide flotation for common parasites with lower specific gravities than the flotation solution (Table 1.1).

Salt solutions are widely used in flotation procedures. A common flotation solution used in the United States is a commercially available sodium nitrate solution (SPG 1.20). This solution will float common helminth eggs and protozoan cysts. The commercial solution is not a saturated solution of sodium nitrate (SPG 1.33). Slides prepared with any salt solution need to be examined relatively quickly after they are prepared because crystals form as slides dry and parasites may be damaged, making them more difficult to identify.

Zinc sulfate ($ZnSO_4$) solution at a SPG of 1.18–1.2 is another salt flotation solution. It is preferred at SPG 1.18 for recovery of *Giardia*, but recovers a higher proportion of

Table 1.1. **Approximate specific gravity of some common helminth eggs**

Species	Specific gravity
Ancylostoma caninum	1.06[1]
Toxocara canis	1.09[1]
Toxocara cati	1.10[1]
Trichuris vulpis	1.15[1]
Taenia sp.	1.23[1]
Physaloptera	1.24[1]
Parascaris spp.	1.09[2]
Equine strongyles	1.05[2]
Anoplocephala perfoliata	1.06[2]

Sources: From [1]David E., and Lindquist W. 1982. Determination of the specific gravity of certain helminth eggs using sucrose density gradient centrifugation. J. Parasitol. 68:916–919; [2]Norris J., Steuer A. et al. 2018. Determination of the specific gravity of eggs of equine strongylids, *Parascaris* spp., and *Anoplocephala perfoliata*. Vet. Parasitol. 260:45–48.

other parasites at SPG 1.2 and is probably used more frequently at this SPG. It is commercially available and when water is added to the purchased salt solution as directed, the resulting SPG is 1.2.

When detection of *Giardia* is required, a 33% zinc sulfate solution (SPG 1.18) is recommended because it does not cause the same rapid collapse of cysts seen with other flotation solutions and they are more easily recognized in flotation preparations.

Saturated solutions of sodium chloride (SPG 1.20) and magnesium sulfate (Epsom salts, SPG 1.32) are less widely used but can be easily prepared, are inexpensive, and are effective in floating common helminth eggs and protozoan cysts.

None of these salt flotation solutions will reliably float most trematode eggs, some tapeworm eggs, and very dense nematode eggs or larvae.

Another common solution used in routine flotation exams is Sheather's sugar solution (SPG 1.25). Because of its relatively higher SPG, Sheather's solution is also more efficient in recovering helminth eggs than common salt solutions, especially tapeworm and more dense nematode eggs. In addition, it does not distort eggs as rapidly as the salt solutions. Sheather's solution is specifically recommended for recovery of *Cryptosporidium* oocysts in fecal samples, but it does not appear to be as effective as 33% ZnSO$_4$ solution for detection of *Giardia*. Sheather's solution is inexpensive and easy to prepare and is also commercially available in the United States, but it is more viscous and sticky than salt solutions. The advantages and disadvantages of these solutions are shown in Table 1.2 and instructions for preparing them are given below.

Although the SPG of flotation solutions is not often measured in practices, it can be easily determined with an inexpensive hydrometer from a scientific supply company. A hydrometer will last indefinitely and should be considered part of quality control for the veterinary practice laboratory.

Table 1.2. **Comparison of commonly used flotation solutions**

Flotation solution	Specific gravity	Advantages	Disadvantages
Sodium nitrate (NaNO$_3$) Commercial product	1.18–1.2	Floats common helminth and protozoa eggs and cysts	Does not float most fluke and some tapeworm and nematode eggs
Saturated NaNO$_3$	1.33		
Zinc sulfate (ZnSO$_4$)	1.18–1.2	Floats common helminth and protozoa eggs and cysts; preferred for *Giardia* and some lungworm larvae	When used at SPG 1.18 recovers lower proportion of common helminth eggs; does not float most fluke and some some tapeworm and nematode eggs
Saturated sodium chloride (NaCl)	1.2	Floats common helminth and protozoa eggs and cysts	Does not float most fluke and some tapeworm and nematode eggs
Saturated magnesium sulfate (Epsom salts)	1.32	Floats common helminth and protozoa eggs and cysts; higher SPG recovers parasites more efficiently	Higher SPG will float more debris; does not float most fluke and some tapeworm and nematode eggs
Sheather's sugar solution	1.20–1.28	Floats common helminth and protozoa eggs and cysts; higher SPG recovers parasites more efficiently; preferred for *Cryptosporidium* oocysts; generally less damaging than salt solutions	Does not float most fluke and some tapeworm and nematode eggs; creates sticky surfaces

33% ZINC SULFATE SOLUTION (SPG 1.18)

1. Combine 330 g zinc sulfate with water to reach a volume of 1000 mL.
2. Additional water or zinc sulfate can be added to produce an SPG of 1.18. If zinc sulfate solution is used with formalinized feces, the SPG should be increased to 1.20 and a SPG of 1.2 is often preferred for general use.
3. Check the SPG with a hydrometer.

SATURATED SODIUM CHLORIDE (NaCl, SPG 1.2) OR MAGNESIUM SULFATE SOLUTION ($MgSO_4$, SPG 1.32)

1. Add salt to warm tap water until no more salt goes into solution and the excess settles at the bottom of the container.
2. To ensure that the solution is fully saturated, it should be allowed to stand overnight at room temperature. If remaining salt crystals dissolve overnight, more can be added to ensure that the solution is saturated. Table salt contains an anticaking compound that does not dissolve and should not be confused with residual sodium chloride crystals. Pickling salt does not contain this compound.
3. Check the SPG with a hydrometer, recognizing that the SPG of saturated solutions will vary slightly with environmental temperature.

SHEATHER'S SUGAR SOLUTION (SPG 1.2–1.25)

1. Combine 355 mL (12 fl oz) of water and 454 g (1 lb) of granulated sugar (sucrose). Corn syrup and dextrose are not suitable substitutes.
2. Dissolve the sugar in the water by stirring over low or indirect heat (e.g., the top half of a double boiler). If the container is placed on a high direct heat source, the sugar may caramelize instead of dissolving in the water.
3. After the sugar is dissolved and the solution has cooled to room temperature, add 6 mL formaldehyde USP to prevent microbial growth (30 mL of 10% formalin can also be used, with the volume of water reduced to 330 mL).
4. Check the SPG with a hydrometer.

Flotation Procedures

No matter how the flotation procedure is performed, the principle is the same. After mixing the flotation solution and the fecal sample together, the less dense material eventually floats to the top. This process can occur either by letting the mixture sit on the benchtop for a specified time (passive flotation) or by centrifuging the mixture. Centrifugation makes the flotation occur more rapidly and efficiently, regardless of the flotation solution used. Many practitioners like to use convenient commercial flotation kits that provide a container for collection of the sample and performing the test. However, the convenience of the kits is offset by the loss of sensitivity in the fecal exam procedure. A smaller amount of feces is used and the test cannot be centrifuged.

The increased sensitivity of the centrifugation procedure is particularly important in infections where the diagnostic form of the parasite may be present in low numbers (e.g., *Trichuris* and *Giardia* infections in dogs and cats). Centrifugation is also necessary when using 33% $ZnSO_4$ or sugar solution because of the slightly lower SPG of $ZnSO_4$ solution and the high viscosity of sugar solution, both of which retard the flotation process. A veterinary practice that does not centrifuge flotation tests and relies on the traditional benchtop technique substantially reduces the sensitivity of its fecal exams.

CENTRIFUGAL FECAL FLOTATION PROCEDURE

This is the best technique for the standard fecal flotation test regardless of the flotation solution used. It is particularly important to use this procedure with Sheather's sugar and 33% $ZnSO_4$ flotation solutions to ensure that the flotation is effective:

1. Mix 3–5 g (about 1 teaspoonful) of feces with a small amount of flotation solution in a paper or plastic cup. Cat feces and small ruminant pellets, which are sometimes too hard to break up easily, can be ground with a mortar and pestle or allowed to soak in water until they become softer.
    If the sample appears to contain a large amount of fat or mucus, an initial water wash is performed, and water should be used in Step 1. The water wash may be eliminated for most fecal samples of normal appearance.
2. Strain the mixture of feces and flotation solution (or feces and water if a water wash is performed) through a double layer of cheesecloth or gauze. A tea strainer can also be used.
3. Pour the mixture into a 15-mL centrifuge tube. If the rotor on the centrifuge is not angled (i.e., if the tubes hang straight when not spinning), the centrifuge tube can be filled with flotation solution until a reverse meniscus is formed and a coverslip is added (Fig. 1.1). The tube is spun with the coverslip. The centrifugal force generated by the centrifuge will hold the coverslip in place. If the centrifuge has an angled rotor, fill the tube to approximately 10–12 mL (amount that will prevent spilling) and place in the centrifuge.
4. Spin the mixture in a benchtop centrifuge for about 5 minutes at approximately 500–650 × g (650 × g is 2500 rpm on a 4-in. rotor), regardless of whether the feces have been mixed with water or with the flotation solution. If a specific g force and speed setting cannot be determined, spinning the tube at the same speed used to separate serum from blood cells is sufficient.
    If the initial spin is a water wash, the supernatant should be discarded, the sediment resuspended with flotation solution, and Steps 3 and 4 repeated.

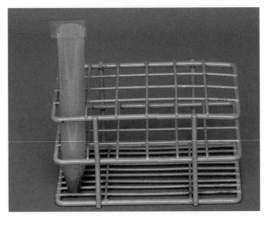

Fig. 1.1 Centrifuge tube filled with flotation solution to the top and coverslip placed in contact with the fluid column.

5. Allow the centrifuge to stop without using the brake. The slight jerking that results from the use of the brake may dislodge parasites from the surface layer. If preferred, the tube can be allowed to sit for an additional 5–10 minutes to maximize recovery of parasite material that may not have completed flotation through the liquid column to the surface.

6. Following centrifugation, there are several ways to harvest the surface layer of fluid containing parasite eggs. If the tube has been spun with the coverslip in place, lift the coverslip off the tube and quickly place it on a microscope slide. When the tube is spun without the coverslip, remove the tube from the centrifuge after spinning and place in a test tube rack. Fill the tube with additional flotation solution to form a reverse meniscus. Place a coverslip on the tube and allow it to sit for an additional 5–10 minutes before removing the coverslip and placing it on a slide.

Alternatively, after the centrifuge comes to a stop, gently touch the surface of the fluid in the tube with a glass rod, microbiologic loop, or base of a small glass tube and then quickly touch the rod to a microscope slide to transfer the drop or two of adhering fluid. This procedure will be less efficient than allowing the tube to stand with a coverslip in place.

BENCHTOP (SIMPLE OR PASSIVE) FLOTATION PROCEDURE

When a centrifugal flotation procedure cannot be performed, sodium nitrate and saturated salt solutions can be used in a benchtop flotation test, although a number of studies have shown that this procedure will detect significantly fewer parasite infections than the centrifugal flotation. This technique is not recommended for 33% $ZnSO_4$ or sugar flotation tests:

1. Mix several grams (a teaspoonful) of feces with the flotation solution in a cup.
2. Strain the mixture through cheesecloth or a tea strainer.
3. Pour into a test tube, pill vial, or container provided in a commercial kit. Add enough mixture or additional flotation fluid until there is a reverse meniscus on the top of the container. Place a coverslip on the fluid drop at the top.
4. Allow the flotation to stand for at least 10 minutes, remove the coverslip, place it on a slide, and examine. If the test is allowed to stand for too long, the salt may crystallize on the edges of the coverslip so that it will not lie flat on the slide.

FLOTATION SLIDES

Fecal flotation slides should be scanned using the 10× objective lens of the microscope (since most microscopes also have an eyepiece magnification of 10×, using the 10× objective gives a total magnification of 100×). Although most helminth eggs can be detected with the 4× objective, protozoan parasites are easily missed and this low power should not be used for scanning. The 40× lens should be used when there is uncertainty about the identity of structures on the slide and for scanning slides for *Cryptosporidium* oocysts. In some practices, to save expense, coverslips are not used. However, slides without coverslips dry out faster, do not have a flat plane of focus, and cannot be examined with the 40× lens, with the result that some parasites will be identified incorrectly or missed entirely.

EGG-COUNTING PROCEDURES (QUANTITATIVE FECAL EXAMS)

Egg-counting techniques are also flotation tests and have several uses in food animals and horses. They can be used to assess the degree to which individual animals or groups are contributing to pasture contaminations with parasites, to assess efficacy of drug treatment (discussed in a later section in this chapter) and, in some cases, to determine relative levels of individual susceptibility to parasite infection.

Egg counts are of limited value in making judgments about the clinical condition of individual animals because many factors affect egg production, including parasite species, individual host immunity, and stage of infection. Also, counts performed on combined samples from a number of animals may not accurately reflect parasitism within that herd.

The easiest quantitative test to perform is the modified McMaster test. This test requires the use of special reusable slides (Fig. 1.2), which can be purchased from several suppliers (including Chalex Corporation, Wallowa, OR [www.vetslides.com]; Focal Point, www.mcmaster.co.za; JA Whitlock & Co., Eastwood, New South Wales, Australia [www.whitlock.com.au]). The capacity of the counting chamber and the number of chambers counted per sample affect the detection level of the test. Saturated salt solutions are usually used as the flotation solution in this test.

As it is most commonly used, the modified McMaster test has a detection level of 25 or 50 eggs per gram (EPG) of feces. This level is acceptable in many situations since parasite control programs do not usually require detection of lower egg numbers. However, the accuracy of the McMaster test is reduced when egg counts are at the lower limits of detection. When egg counts of less than 200 EPG are expected in a group of animals being evaluated (e.g., in adult cattle or camelids) or when it is important to detect low numbers of eggs more accurately (e.g., in fecal egg count reduction tests [FECRTs]), a modification of the test is appropriate. The sensitivity and precision of the McMaster test can be improved by using slides that allow examination of larger quantities of the egg/flotation solution mixture, or by counting additional aliquots of the sample.

Alternatively, other procedures with lower detection limits can be used including the Wisconsin sugar flotation test (double centrifugation procedure) or a modified Stoll egg-counting test. These procedures permit detection of fewer than 10 EPG of fecal material but are more time-consuming to perform. Another procedure, the mini-FLOTAC

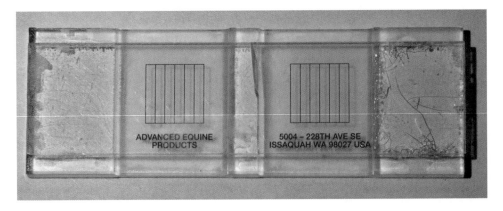

Fig. 1.2   McMaster slide used in the modified McMaster procedure for quantitative egg counts.

test, has been developed in Europe. Several studies have demonstrated greater precision and accuracy of the mini-FLOTAC compared to McMaster and Wisconsin tests but at this time it has limited availability and has been used in the United States primarily in research.

Another commercially available test for determining equine fecal egg counts is Parasight (Lexington, KY [www.parasightsystem.com]). This system provides counts of equine strongyle and *Parascaris* spp. eggs. An equine sample is mixed with reagents and fluorescence-imaging is used with a software counting algorithm to produce a fecal egg count.

Regardless of the procedure used to count parasites, the most important element is consistency. Each step of the procedure should be performed in the same way for every sample.

Modified McMaster test.

1. For ruminants, combine 4 g of fecal material with 56 mL of flotation solution to yield a total volume of 60 mL. The test can also be performed with 2 g of feces and 28 mL of flotation solution when only small amounts of feces are available. For horses, it is standard in the United States to use 4 g of feces and 26 mL of flotation solution. See Note 1 below for modified calculations. Portable electronic scales that weigh in 0.1-g increments are widely available and inexpensive. If a method of weighing feces is not available, adding manure to the measured flotation solution until the final desired volume is reached can also be used (e.g., add manure to 26 mL of fluid to a total volume of 30 mL). This method would be more accurate with horse or cattle manure compared to the pelleted manure of small ruminants or camelids.

2. Mix well and strain through cheesecloth or a tea strainer. The mixture does not have to be strained, but it will be much easier to read the slide if large pieces of debris are removed. An alternative to straining is to use a filter pipette to transfer material to the counting chamber (a pipette with 12 mesh/cm wire mesh at the end is available from JA Whitlock & Co. [www.whitlock.com.au]).

3. Immediately fill each chamber of the McMaster slide with the mixture using a pipette or syringe. The entire chamber must be filled, not just the area under the grid. If large air bubbles are present, remove the fluid and refill.

4. Allow the slide to sit for at least 5 minutes before examining to allow the flotation process to occur. There has been limited investigation of the maximum amount of time slides can be allowed to sit before reading and there is no standard recommendation. Allowing slides to sit for an hour does not seem to alter results.

5. Look at the slide with the 10× lens, focusing on the top layer, which contains the air bubbles. At this level, the lines of the grid will also be in focus. Count eggs, oocysts, and any other parasite stages, in each lane of both chambers. Each type of parasite should be counted separately. In some cases, eggs can be identified to genus or perhaps to species (e.g., *Strongyloides*, *Trichuris*, and *Nematodirus*), whereas others must be counted as a category of parasites (coccidia, strongylid eggs).

To determine the number of parasite EPG of feces, add the counts for both chambers for each parasite. The most commonly used McMaster slides in the United States are calibrated so that the number of eggs counted in a single chamber represents the number present in 0.15 mL of fecal mixture. If both chambers are counted and the results are added, the total represents the number of eggs present in 0.3 mL, which, for example, is 1/200th of a total volume of 60 mL; therefore, the number of eggs counted must be multiplied by 200. However, if a total of 4 g of feces was used in the test, the result must be divided by 4 to yield EPG of feces. Multiplying by 200 and dividing by 4 is equivalent to multiplying the number of eggs counted by 50. Therefore, each egg observed represents 50 EPG in the final count. The same level of detection can be achieved by using 2 g of fecal material and 28 mL of flotation solution. The smaller amount of feces may be preferred when evaluating small lambs or kids.

Additional Notes

1. If a detection level of 25 EPG is desired, the McMaster test should be performed with 4 g of feces and 26 mL of flotation solution (results are then multiplied by 100 and divided by 4 as described earlier). Other combinations of manure and flotation solution can also be used with appropriate calculations using the formula

$$eggs/g = \left[no.eggs\ counted \times (T/V) \right]/F$$

    where T = total volume of feces/flotation solution mixture, V = volume of aliquot examined in slide, and F = grams of feces used.
2. If pelleted feces are very hard, 2–5 mL of water can be added first and left to soften manure for at least an hour. The flotation solution is then added to the softened manure (flotation solution volume reduced by the amount of water used to soften feces).
3. A variety of methods can be used to homogenize feces and liquid. As alternatives to mixing with a tongue blade or other utensil, some laboratories use a mechanical or handheld kitchen mixer to homogenize feces and water/flotation solution. Shaking manure and fluid in a jar with glass beads has also been used, but as previously stated, whatever method is used, it should be consistent across samples.
4. In another procedure for the McMaster test, feces is mixed initially with water, strained, and centrifuged, and the supernatant is discarded. Flotation solution is added to resuspend the sediment and mixed, and the mixture is used to fill the counting chambers. For example, 3 g of feces is mixed with 42 mL of water, strained and the fluid used to fill a 15-mL centrifuge tube, which is then centrifuged at 300–650 × g for 2 minutes. The supernatant is then discarded and flotation solution is added to partially fill the tube, which is either shaken or stirred to resuspend the sediment. Additional flotation solution is added to fill the tube, and the counting chamber is filled. If the eggs in a volume of 0.3 mL are counted, the number of eggs seen is multiplied by 50 to give the number of eggs per g. The EPG can also be calculated using the formula described in Note 1. This procedure is the most effective for reducing debris but increases the time required to perform each test.

Mini-FLOTAC

The Mini-FLOTAC device and the Fill-FLOTAC device, which are used together in the mini-FLOTAC procedure, are available in North America from the University of Georgia. The test should be performed as described in the brochure provided with the test device. This procedure is generally more time-consuming than the basic modified McMaster procedure but is more accurate and precise.

Wisconsin, Cornell-Wisconsin egg-counting test (double centrifugation procedure).

The Wisconsin egg-counting test or double centrifugation flotation test is used to quantitate eggs when low EPG are expected. Unlike the McMaster test, where eggs are counted in an aliquot of the mixture of feces and flotation solution, the Wisconsin test preparation collects eggs from the entire fecal sample/flotation solution mixture. Because it is time-consuming and difficult to accurately count numerous eggs on a slide with no grid this test is not suited to many circumstances where a quantitative count is needed. Any flotation solution can be used in this test:

1. Combine 1–5 g feces and 12–15 mL of water in a cup. Mix and strain into another cup, rinsing first cup with 2–3 mL of water and straining, pressing the liquid through. Pour into a 15 mL centrifuge tube.
2. Centrifuge (properly balanced) at 300–650 × g for 5–10 minutes.
3. After spinning, discard the supernatant and resuspend the pellet in flotation solution.
4. Either spin the tube with a coverslip in place or allow additional incubation after spinning as described for the centrifugal flotation procedure.
5. Remove the coverslip and place on a glass slide.
6. Examine with the 10× objective lens.
7. Count and record the number of each type of parasite egg/cyst seen, systematically scanning the slide and counting eggs or cysts of each parasite species or group separately. Care must be taken to ensure that each microscope field on the coverslip is examined once but only once so that no eggs are missed or counted twice.
   This technique allows the quantification of less than 1 EPG of feces.

Additional Notes

1. If desired, the initial water wash can be omitted and the sample can be mixed directly with flotation solution and then centrifuged.
2. Alternatively, 22 mL of flotation solution is mixed with 5 g of feces, and the resulting mixture is divided between two tubes. This modification increases the accuracy of the procedure.

Modified Stoll test.

There are many modifications for the Stoll test, depending on the level of detection desired. Like the McMaster test, the modified Stoll egg-counting procedure is based on determining the number of eggs present in an aliquot of the prepared feces/flotation solution mixture. Any of the fecal flotation solutions can be used in this procedure.

1. Combine 5 g of feces and 20 mL of water in a cup.
2. Mix into a slurry and transfer 1 mL of the mixture to a centrifuge tube. If the mixture is not strained, a widemouthed or mesh-covered filter pipette is needed to transfer the mixture.
3. Fill the tube with flotation solution.

4. Place the tube in the centrifuge and add flotation solution until a slight inverse meniscus is formed.
5. Place a coverslip on top of the tube. It should contact the mixture without causing any to overflow.
6. Centrifuge (properly balanced) at 300–650 × g for 10 minutes.
7. Remove the coverslip and place on a glass slide.
8. Examine with the 10× objective lens.
9. Count and record the number of each type of parasite egg/cyst seen, systematically scanning the slide and counting eggs or cysts of each parasite species or group separately. Care must be taken to ensure that each microscope field on the coverslip is examined once but only once so that no eggs are missed or counted twice.

In this test, all the eggs present in 1 mL of the feces/flotation solution mixture were counted following centrifugation. This represents 1/25 of the volume of the mixture so the number of eggs counted multiplied by 25 represents the total number of eggs present, but this must be divided by 5 (grams of feces used) to yield EPG. In this situation, the multiplication factor is 5 and the minimum sensitivity of the test is 5 EPG. If the volume of fluid added to feces in the first step is 45 mL, the final multiplying factor would be 10.

For additional information on quantitative egg-counting procedures, see references by Verocai et al. (2020), Neilsen and Reinemeyer (2018), Taylor et al. (2015), Coles et al. (2006), and the Ministry of Agriculture, Fisheries and Foods (1986).

Additional Procedures for Fecal Examination

The following procedures are used for identification of specific parasitic infections.

Direct Smear and Stained Fecal Smears

The direct smear is used to identify protozoan trophozoites (*Giardia*, trichomonads, amoebae, etc.) or other structures that float poorly or are readily distorted by flotation solutions. Because very little fecal material is used, the sensitivity of this test is low. It is not recommended for routine fecal examinations:

1. Mix a very small amount of feces with a drop of saline on a microscope slide to produce a layer through which newsprint can be read. Saline should be used because water will destroy protozoan trophozoites.
2. Use a coverslip to push large particles of debris to the side and place the coverslip on the slide. Examine with 10× and 40× magnification. The 100× lens (oil immersion) cannot be used effectively with fecal smears.
3. If the fecal layer is too thick, it will be impossible to see small, colorless protozoa moving in the field. Movement is the principal characteristic that allows recognition of trophozoites in fresh fecal smears. A drop of Lugol's iodine will enhance the internal structures of protozoan cysts but will also kill trophozoites present. To maximize the use of this test, it is best to look at an unstained smear before adding iodine.

Fecal smears can also be stained for identification of intestinal protozoa. Several stains can be used for identification of *Cryptosporidium*, including Ziehl–Neelsen,

Kinyoun, carbol-fuchsin, and Giemsa stains. Trichrome stain is widely used in human medicine for detection of *Giardia* cysts. In general, however, stains are not used extensively in veterinary practices and are not required for the identification of parasitic organisms. For details on performing these stains, a standard text on human parasitologic diagnosis should be consulted.

Fecal Sedimentation

A sedimentation procedure is used to isolate eggs of flukes, acanthocephalans, and some tapeworms and nematodes whose eggs do not float readily in common flotation solutions. In the simple sedimentation test, tap water is combined with feces and allowed to settle briefly before the supernatant is removed. This allows the removal of fine particulate material, but unlike the flotation exam, sedimentation tests have only limited concentrating ability. Fat and mucus can be removed from the fecal sample if a centrifugal sedimentation exam is performed using ethyl acetate. Unfortunately, ethyl acetate is toxic and very flammable. It should be stored in a flameproof cabinet and used only in well-ventilated areas. An alternative to ethyl acetate is Hemo-De, available through Fischer Scientific (www.fischerscientific.com), which is generally regarded as a safe compound and appears to give equivalent results in a centrifugal sedimentation procedure (see Neimester et al. 1987).

The Flukefinder® is a commercially available apparatus for performing sedimentation tests in the laboratory. It utilizes several screens to rapidly remove fecal debris. This device is very useful in practices conducting routine fecal examinations for flukes. Information on the Flukefinder can be obtained at www.flukefinder.com.

SIMPLE SEDIMENTATION TEST

1. Mix about 100 mL of water with about 10 g of feces, strain, and place in a beaker or other container.
2. Allow mixture to sit for 1 hour and then decant the supernatant.
3. Add more water, mix, and repeat the sedimentation procedure.
4. Stir remaining mixture and place a few drops on a microscope slide. If desired, add one drop of 0.1% methylene blue. The methylene blue will stain the background debris blue but will not stain fluke eggs, which will stand out with a yellowish brown color.
5. Coverslip and scan the slide using the 10× objective lens.

A smaller amount of feces and water can be used, placed in a test tube, and left to sit for 3–5 minutes between decantation steps. Addition of a drop of dishwashing soap to the water used in the test helps to free eggs from surrounding debris.

CENTRIFUGAL SEDIMENTATION TEST

1. Mix 1 g of feces with about 10 mL of 10% buffered formalin or water. Pour mixture into a 15-mL centrifuge tube (with cap) until it is one-half to three-quarters full.
2. Add ethyl acetate (see earlier discussion on safety) or Hemo-De until the tube is almost full. Because organic solvents may dissolve some plastic centrifuge tubes, it is recommended that glass or polypropylene tubes be used for performing this test.
3. Cap and shake the tube approximately 50 times.

4. Centrifuge for 3–5 minutes at about $500 \times g$ (as for centrifugal flotation procedure).

5. When the tube is removed from the centrifuge, it will have three layers: (1) an upper layer containing ethyl acetate, fat, and debris; (2) a middle layer containing formalin or water and fine particulate matter; and (3) a bottom layer of sediment. Using an applicator stick, loosen the top debris plug that sticks to the sides of the tube, then decant the supernatant, leaving only the bottom sediment.

6. Resuspend the sediment in a few drops of water or formalin, place one or two drops of the sediment on a slide, coverslip, and examine with the 10× microscope objective.

Baermann Test

The Baermann test is used to isolate larvae from fecal samples and is employed most often to diagnose lungworm infections. *It is very important that the fecal sample be fresh.* If feces of a grazing animal are being examined and an old sample is used, strongylid or *Strongyloides* eggs may have hatched, or free-living nematodes may have invaded the sample, making nematode identification much more difficult. In small-animal samples, hookworm eggs may hatch very quickly and can be confused with lungworm or *Strongyloides* larvae. Coprophagy and hunting can also result in larvae of spurious parasites being present in Baermann test preparations. For discussion of identification of nematode larvae see the section in this chapter: "Identification of nematode larvae recovered with fecal flotation or Baermann procedures."

A further consideration for using a Baermann test in diagnosis is that metastrongyloid lungworms typically show erratic larval shedding patterns. Dramatic day-to-day variation in larval shedding increases the chance of false negative Baermann fecal examination results. Therefore, a single negative Baermann result is weak evidence for ruling-out lungworm infection in an animal showing signs of respiratory disease. Detection sensitivity is increased by doing multiple (at least 3) Baermann examinations.

A Baermann test requires equipment to hold the fecal sample in water so that larvae can migrate out and be collected. This can now be most easily accomplished with the use of a plastic wine glass with a hollow stem. In the absence of disposable wine glasses, the original Baermann apparatus can be used. This consists of a funnel clamped to a metal stand. A short piece of tubing with a clamp is attached to the end of the funnel. Larvae in feces placed either in the bowl of the wine glass or in the funnel migrate out of the sample and fall down into the hollow stem or the tubing above the clamp, where they can be easily collected (Fig. 1.3):

1. Place at least 10 g of feces in a piece of double-layer cheesecloth. Gather the cheesecloth around the sample so that it is fully enclosed. Use a rubber band to fasten the cheesecloth, and pass through the rubber band two applicator sticks, a pencil or other object that will rest on the edges of the glass or funnel and suspend the sample. Alternatively, place the sample on a suspended piece of wire mesh or sieve.

2. Fill the funnel or wine glass with lukewarm water. Make sure that the corners of the cheesecloth do not hang over the edge of the funnel or glass, because they will act as wicks for the water.

3. Allow the sample to sit for at least 8 hours, preferably overnight.

4. If using the disposable plastic glass, remove the fecal sample and collect the material at the bottom of the hollow stem using a Pasteur or transfer pipette or syringe.

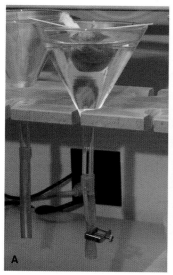
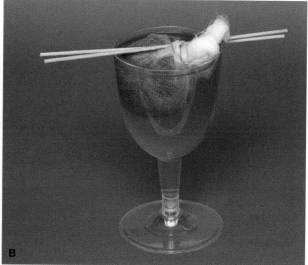

Fig. 1.3   (A) The traditional Baermann apparatus consisting of a suspended funnel with clamped tubing attached. For diagnostic testing of fecal samples, it is much more convenient to perform the Baermann exam with a disposable plastic wine glass (B).

Transfer some of the fluid to a microscope slide, coverslip, and examine with the 4× or 10× objective lens.

5. If using the funnel, release the clamp and collect the first 10 mL of fluid into a centrifuge tube. Spin as for a flotation exam, discard the supernatant, and examine the sediment. Alternatively, the very steady handed can carefully loosen the clamp and collect the first three or four drops onto a microscope slide.

Immunologic and Molecular Methods of Parasite Diagnosis

Immunologic methods have been important in the diagnosis of blood and tissue parasites for many years, and they are now being used increasingly for identification of specific parasites in fecal samples. Molecular diagnostic methods are also now being applied to detection of parasites in fecal samples. Although these techniques cannot currently replace morphologic exam of feces as a routine screening procedure for all parasites, they are useful for specific diagnosis of protozoan and helminth parasites that are detected in feces. For the discussion of these procedures, see Chapter 4.

QUALITY CONTROL FOR FECAL EXAM PROCEDURES

Although the concept of quality control is not often applied to fecal exams, attention to both equipment and training will help ensure that fecal exams are consistently done correctly:

1. Keep microscopes in good repair. Objective lenses and eyepieces should be routinely cleaned with lens cleaner and lens paper. Have microscopes professionally cleaned and checked every few years.

2. Check the SPG of flotation solutions with a hydrometer when first prepared to ensure that they will recover parasites effectively. If a batch of solution is used over an extended period, SPG should be checked at least monthly.
3. Use an ocular micrometer (see section on microscope calibration later in this chapter) to measure structures seen on fecal exams. If possible, recalibrate the microscope at regular intervals.
4. Make sure that personnel performing the fecal exams are adequately trained. It is not unusual for untrained assistants to be given rudimentary instruction on performing flotation tests and then be assigned to do them. Under these circumstances, it is hardly surprising that air bubbles are identified as coccidia and that smaller parasites are missed entirely.
5. As a check on the diagnostic accuracy of in-clinic fecal exams, periodically submit duplicate portions of fecal samples to a diagnostic laboratory. Both negative and positive samples should be submitted.

USE OF THE MICROSCOPE

There are several points to remember in using the compound microscope to examine preparations for parasites:

1. Use the 10× objective lens of the microscope for scanning slides. This will provide a total magnification of 100× since most microscope eyepieces contain an additional 10× lens. Start in one corner and systematically scan the entire slide. The 40× objective lens (400× total magnification with eyepiece) is useful for closer examination or for looking for very small organisms such as *Giardia* or *Cryptosporidium*. The 100× (oil immersion) lens should not be used for flotation preparations. Not only is it likely that flotation solution will contact the lens and possibly damage it, but the pressure of the lens on the coverslip will create currents in the fluid on the slide, keeping everything in motion and making examination of structures difficult.
2. Most parasite eggs and larvae have little or no color and do not stand out well, so it is important to maximize the contrast between the parasites and their backgrounds. If a microscope has a substage condenser it can be used to increase contrast by adjustment of the condenser diaphragm or placement of the condenser in a low position. Even when a substage condenser is not available, reducing the intensity of light projected on the slide is generally advisable, either by decreasing the microscope rheostat setting or by reducing the aperture of the iris diaphragm. A higher power used for close examination will, of course, require an increased amount of light.
3. When reading a slide, it is helpful to focus up and down with the fine focus to change somewhat the plane of focus. Frequently, worm eggs will be at a slightly different level than protozoan cysts or oocysts, and a small manipulation of the fine focus may make structures more readily visible (Figs. 1.4–1.6).

Microscope Calibration

The ability to measure the size of parasitic organisms and structures is very helpful when identifying unusual parasites or where different organisms are similar in appearance but differ in size. For measurements, a micrometer disc, also known as a reticle

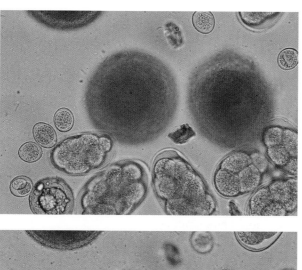

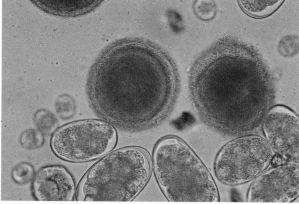

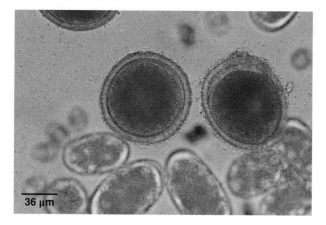

Figs 1.4–1.6 The importance of small changes in the microscope focus can be seen in these three photos of the same field in a canine fecal flotation test. In each case, a slight manipulation of the fine focus brings a different parasite into clearer view (first *Cystoisospora* oocysts, then hookworm eggs, and finally *Toxocara* eggs) since each egg or oocyst type may be present on a slightly different level.

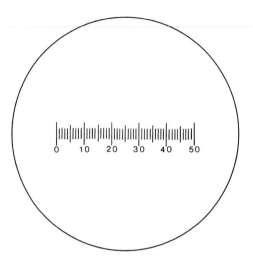

Fig. 1.7 A typical ocular micrometer of 50 divisions. The divisions have no meaning until calibrated against a stage micrometer.

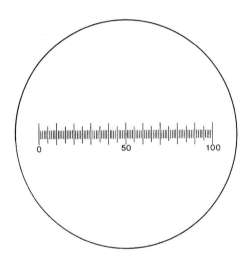

Fig. 1.8 A typical stage micrometer of 1 mm total length. Each division represents 10 μm.

(Fig. 1.7), is inserted into the ocular tube of the microscope and calibrated against a known reference in the form of a stage micrometer (Fig. 1.8). Each objective lens of the microscope must be individually calibrated with the ocular lens/micrometer combination to be used, and the calibrations should be posted close to the microscope for easy reference. The calibration will be accurate only for that particular microscope ocular and objective combination. Even if each lens is not calibrated with the stage micrometer, the ocular grid will provide a consistent reference against which to compare objects seen in fecal samples. These ocular micrometer discs and stage micrometers are not expensive and can be purchased from scientific catalogs that include microscope equipment.

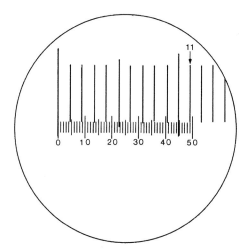

Fig. 1.9   Appearance at 40× of an ocular micrometer being calibrated with a 10 μm/division stage micrometer. Note the conjunction of line 11 of the stage micrometer with line 49 of the ocular micrometer.

Calibration of the 40× objective illustrates the procedure for calibration of the micrometer:

1. To calibrate the 40× objective, place the stage micrometer on the stage of the microscope and focus until the lines are sharp. In the example (Fig. 1.9), the stage micrometer is 1 mm (1000 μm) long and is divided into 100 parts; thus, each small division of the stage micrometer represents 10 μm.
2. Superimpose any convenient numbered line of the ocular micrometer (usually the 0 mark) on a convenient line of the stage micrometer (the first large line in the example). The field should now resemble Figure 1.9.
3. Find the two lines that are exactly superimposed. In the example, line 49 of the ocular micrometer falls exactly on line 11 of the stage micrometer. Thus, 49 divisions of the unknown ocular micrometer represent 11 divisions, each 10 μm in length, for a total of 110 μm. To complete the calibration, divide 110 μm by 49 divisions, resulting in a calibration factor of 2.24 μm per division for the ocular micrometer in the example.
4. Repeat this procedure for each objective lens to be calibrated on the microscope.

To use the calibrated microscope, superimpose the ocular micrometer scale on an egg or cyst and count the number of divisions subtended by the specimen, for example, 12. Multiply 12 by the calibration factor (2.24 for the 40 × lens in the example; 12 × 2.24 = 26.88 μm, the size of the object measured).

PSEUDOPARASITES AND SPURIOUS PARASITES

Fecal samples may contain deceptive "pseudoparasites" and "spurious parasites." Pseudoparasites are ingested objects that resemble parasite forms; these include pollen grains, plant hairs, grain mites, mold spores, and a variety of harmless plant and animal debris (Figs. 1.10–1.15). "Spurious parasites" are parasite eggs or cysts from one species of host that may be found in the feces of a scavenger or predator host as the result of coprophagy or predation (Figs. 1.16-1.18). One of the best ways to avoid

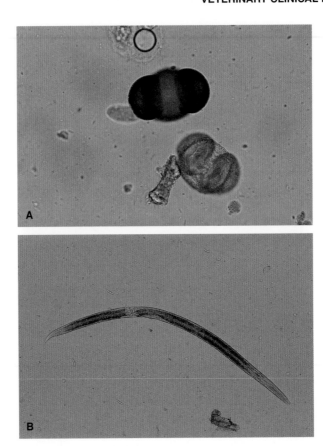

Fig. 1.10   Examples of pseudoparasites. (A) Pine pollen is a common pseudoparasite found in fecal samples of many animals (400×). (B) Adult free-living nematodes are also commonly found in fecal samples collected from the ground. These nematodes can rapidly invade fecal material. The presence of adults and variation in size and morphology (indicating different stages of the life cycle) are helpful in distinguishing these worms from parasite larvae.

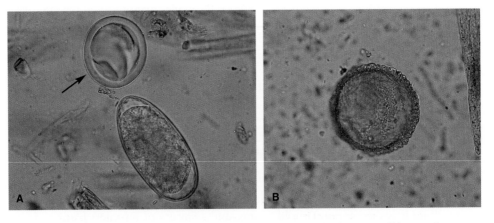

Fig. 1.11   Examples of pseudoparasites. (A) In this ovine fecal sample, both a strongylid egg and a pseudoparasite (*arrow*) are present. Characteristics helpful in the recognition of pseudoparasites are lack of clear internal structure and discontinuities in the outer layer. (B) Pseudoparasite, probably a pollen grain (400×).

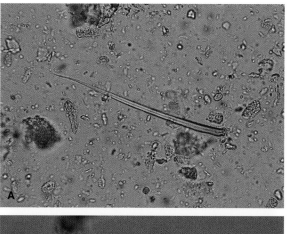
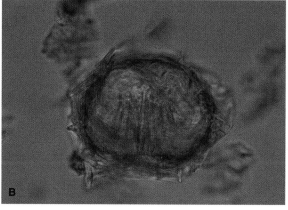

Fig. 1.12   Examples of pseudoparasites. (A) Insect hair from the feces of an insectivorous bird. Insect and plant hairs may be confused with worms but have no internal structure. (B) This artifact in ruminant feces appears to have structures resembling the hooks of a tapeworm embryo, but there is no distinct embryo and the outer layer is poorly defined with projections that are variable in size and shape (40×).

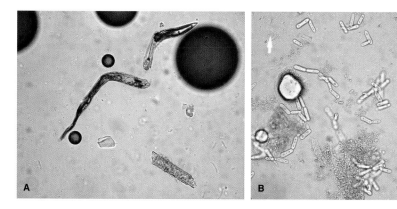

Fig. 1.13   Examples of pseudoparasites. (A) Plant hairs and other fibrous material can resemble nematode larvae. They can be present in a variety of shapes and colors, but can usually be easily differentiated from nematodes because they lack clear internal structures like a digestive tract. Also, while one end is tapered, the other end often looks as though it has been broken off another structure. (B) This photo shows *Saccharomycopsis guttulatus*, a nonpathogenic yeast common in rabbits and seen occasionally in dogs (400×).

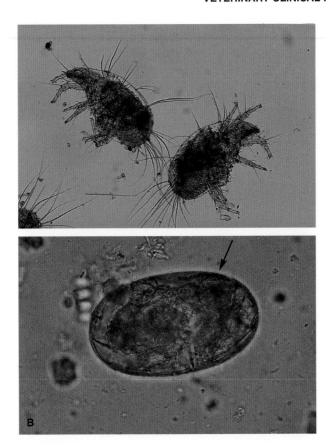

Fig. 1.14   Examples of pseudoparasites. (A) Free-living mites that contaminate animal feed can be found in fecal flotation procedures. Unlike many parasitic mites, free-living species lack specialized structures on their legs (suckers etc.) for adhering to the host. (B) Eggs from free-living mites will also float in flotation solution. They are usually very large (>100 μm). Developing legs of the mite can sometimes be seen inside the egg (*arrow*).

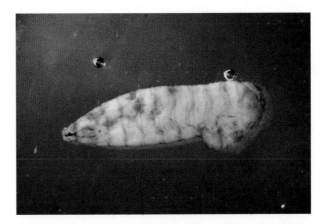

Fig. 1.15   Examples of pseudoparasites. Among the most common pseudoparasites found in feces are insect larvae, which may still be alive and moving when presented. Insect larvae may be ingested in food or, in the case of fly maggots, like the one shown here, eggs that are laid on the feces hatch rapidly in hot weather. Spiracles are present on the posterior (right) end of the segmented larva.

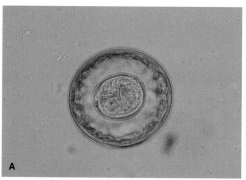
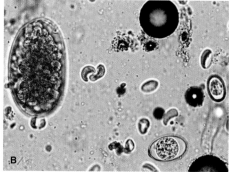

Fig. 1.16   Spurious parasites are parasite eggs or cysts from another host that are acquired through predation or coprophagy and have merely passed through the digestive tract of the animal being tested. (A) Tapeworm egg found in a fecal sample from a calf. Although the configuration of hooks inside this egg clearly identifies it as a tapeworm, it is most likely a rodent or bird tapeworm egg. (B) Spurious parasites are common in samples from dogs that ingest fecal material. Eggs of livestock strongylid species can be found in feces of manure-eating dogs. Ruminant and equine strongylid eggs look like canine hookworm eggs but are larger and ruminant coccidia can usually be differentiated from dog and cat species based on size and shape.

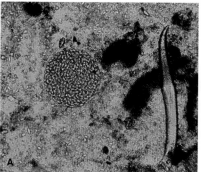
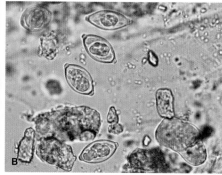

Fig. 1.17   Examples of spurious parasites. (A) Large cyst of *Monocystis*, a protozoan parasite of earthworms found in the feces of a snake that feeds on earthworms (100×). (B) Individual *Monocystis* oocysts that have been freed from a large cyst like the one shown in Figure 1.17A. These individual *Monocystis* oocysts are common pseudoparasites (400×). Photo B courtesy of Dr. Yoko Nagamori, College of Veterinary Medicine, Oklahoma State University.

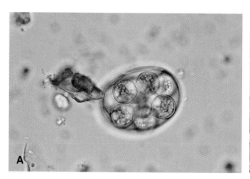
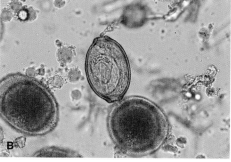

Fig. 1.18   Examples of spurious parasites. (A) *Adelina* sp. oocyst in a canine fecal sample. The oocysts of this genus are coccidia of insects and oligochetes and contain eight sporocysts. (B) Feline fecal sample containing two eggs from a feline parasite (*Toxocara*) and a single egg of a spurious parasite, *Trichosomoides*, a rodent parasite that is present as a result of hunting activity. Photos courtesy of Dr. Manigandan Lejeune, Animal Health Diagnostic Center, Cornell University.

misidentifying these pseudo- and spurious parasites is to appreciate the variety of parasites that normally infect a host species. If a fecal sample contains a possible pseudoparasite or spurious parasite, it is best to repeat the examination with another sample collected at a later time. To limit opportunities for coprophagy or predation leading to ingestion of additional pseudo- and spurious parasites, small animals (dogs and cats) should be confined or leash walked only for 2–3 days prior to collection of the second sample.

IDENTIFICATION OF NEMATODE LARVAE RECOVERED WITH FECAL FLOTATION OR BAERMANN PROCEDURES

Nematode larvae are passed in the feces of animals infected with various species of lungworms (*Aelurostrongylus abstrusus, Angiostrongylus vasorum, Crenosoma vulpis, Dictyocaulus* spp., *Filaroides hirthi, Muellerius capillaris, Oslerus osleri, Protostrongylus* spp., and others) or the intestinal threadworm, *Strongyloides stercoralis*. Accurate identification of nematode larvae detected on fecal flotation or Baermann tests tends to be a challenge for the veterinary laboratory diagnostician. In many cases where larvae are detected on fecal flotation, the damage due to the effects of high SPG flotation media obscures the larval morphology to the point that identification is not possible (Fig. 1.19). Therefore, the Baermann technique is the preferred method to recover first-stage nematode larvae from feces except in the case of *O. osleri* or *F. hirthi* infection in dogs (Figs. 1.94, 1.95). The Baermann technique is effective in recovering larvae that are vigorous and able to move out of the fecal matter. The larvae present in feces of dogs infected with *Oslerus* and *Filaroides* are sluggish and unable to migrate out of the feces. Therefore, zinc sulfate centrifugal flotation is the recommended method for the detection of larvae in the feces of dogs infected with these lungworms.

A further complication in larval identification may occur when there is a loss of sample integrity due to improper collection. Fecal samples that are not collected immediately after deposit on the ground may be invaded by free-living soil or plant parasitic nematodes. The challenge of sorting out these nematodes from the true parasitic ones is

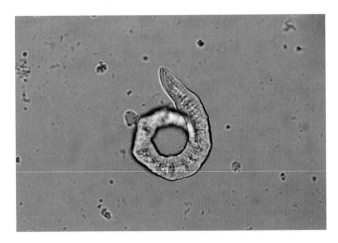

Fig. 1.19   Larva detected on fecal flotation from a dog infected with lungworm. The larva is damaged due to the osmotic pressure of the high specific gravity flotation fluid. Loss of morphologic detail to this degree prevents specific identification.

beyond the training and experience of most veterinary laboratory diagnosticians. In addition, hookworm, strongyle, or trichostrongyle eggs, if present in feces, can develop and hatch in a short time under warm conditions, resulting in the detection of larvae that will be difficult to distinguish from those parasites normally passed as larvae in the feces. In small-animal practice where pet owners collect the fecal sample, the clients must be given guidance as to the requirements for a proper fecal sample. In the case of dogs, clients should be instructed to collect the fecal sample immediately after deposit and place it in an airtight, leakproof container. If submission to the veterinarian cannot occur within several hours of collection, the sample should be refrigerated at 4°C. In the case of cats, the litter pan should be cleaned and the next fecal sample observed in the pan should be collected and handled as above. Ruminant or horse samples should be collected from the rectum. If clients are collecting samples from the ground, they should be instructed to avoid collection of the portion of manure in direct contact with the soil. Lastly, a further complication in test evaluation can be the presence of spurious parasites acquired through predation or coprophagy.

The first question in the decision tree when evaluating nematode larvae is: parasite or free-living? Parasite larvae range in size from 150 to 400 μm and their simple anatomy consists of a mouth opening leading to a buccal tube, esophagus, intestine, and anus. There may also be a discernable genital primordium. Free-living/soil/plant nematodes often occur in multiple life stages (from egg to adult), and size measurements are highly variable. The presence of adult female (eggs in the uterus, vaginal opening—Fig. 1.20) or adult male (spicules—Fig. 1.21) worms or the presence of an oral stylet in the buccal tube (Fig. 1.22) indicates that the sample may have been invaded by free-living nematodes. Unfortunately, *Strongyloides* spp. have a free-living generation that will develop if the sample is incubated and therefore are also a possibility when adult stages are recovered in a fecal sample. Detection of adult worms in the sample is an indication that the animal should be resampled and a fresh fecal sample should be submitted.

Another source of potential confusion in identifying larvae in feces is particularly common in coprophagic dogs, and can also occur in dogs or cats that are allowed to

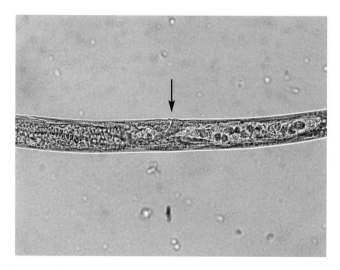

Fig. 1.20 Vaginal opening (*arrow*) of a free-living adult female nematode recovered from the feces of a dog. The feces were left on the ground long enough prior to collection to allow free-living soil nematodes to invade the sample.

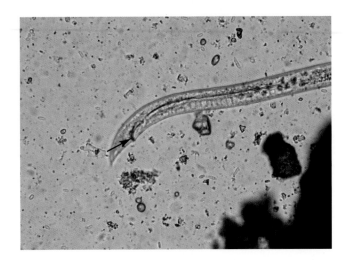

Fig. 1.21   Tail of an adult male free-living nematode recovered from an improperly collected fecal sample of a dog. Note the chitinized spicules (*arrow*) at the cloacal opening.

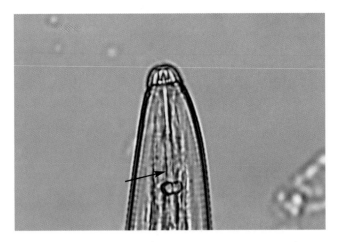

Fig. 1.22   Anterior end of a plant parasitic nematode recovered from an improperly collected fecal sample of a dog. Note the oral stylet (*arrow*) in the buccal chamber. The stylet is a daggerlike structure used in the feeding process to pierce plant roots. No parasitic first-stage larvae have this structure.

hunt. First-stage larvae present in feces or a prey animal will pass through the gastrointestinal tract intact. Depending on the timing of ingestion, the larvae may still be vigourously motile when recovered as a spurious parasite on Baermann examination. Reports of *Aelurostrongylus abstrusus* infection in the dog have all been based on detection of L1 in feces and are most likely false positive due to the ingestion of cat feces. Familiarity with common lungworms of other species will be helpful in recognizing the possibility of spurious parasitism.

Detection of larvae on microscopic examination of a slide prepared from a Baermann test is facilitated by the eye-catching vigorous motion of the larvae. However, once detected, a careful evaluation of the morphologic features is not possible in actively motile larvae. Therefore, it is necessary to kill them in a way that does not damage the morphology. Larvae are best killed by adding a drop of dilute Lugol's iodine (the color of weak tea) to the edge of the coverslip. The iodine will be slowly drawn across the

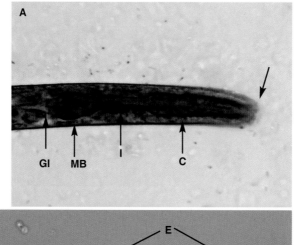

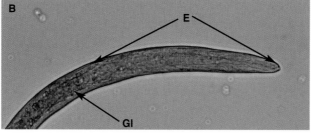

Fig. 1.23 (A) Anterior end of a first-stage larva of *Strongyloides stercoralis* recovered from the feces of a dog. This larva has been killed and stained with dilute iodine. The rhabditiform esophagus is well defined and obvious. Note the short buccal tube (*arrow*) and the rhabditiform esophagus made up of the corpus (C), isthmus (I), and muscular bulb (MB). Also note the distinct border demarcating the end of the esophagus and the start of the intestine (GI). (B) Anterior end of an iodine-stained first-stage larva of *Crenosoma vulpis* recovered from the feces of a dog. Note the poorly defined esophagus (E). It is difficult to discern the demarcation between the end of the esophagus and the start of the intestine (GI).

coverslip resulting in the death of the larvae. Alternatively, the larvae can be heat killed by passing the coverslip over the flame of a Bunsen burner to effect (several to many times). Larvae recovered on fecal flotation may or may not be already dead. Fecal flotation slides should be viewed as quickly as possible since the larval damage due to osmotic pressure will progressively worsen over time. Differentiation of the various parasitic nematode first-stage larvae is based on overall size and the morphology of the esophagus and tail. First-stage larvae of intestinal parasites (i.e., *S. stercoralis* or hookworm–strongyle–trichostrongyle eggs that have hatched) can be differentiated from the numerous lungworm larvae based on the presence of a distinct rhabditiform esophagus (Figs. 1.23A, 1.24, and 1.26). The rhabditiform esophagus consists of an anterior corpus that narrows to an isthmus and then ends in a muscular bulb. The rhabditiform esophagus is sharply delineated and well defined with an obvious sharp demarcation between the end of the esophagus and the beginning of the intestine. The overall length of the rhabditiform esophagus is less than 25% of the total length of the larvae (Fig. 1.24). In contrast, the esophagus of the lungworm larvae tends to be less well defined and longer, making up about 33%–50% of the total length of the larvae (Figs. 1.23B and 1.25). The relatively short buccal tube differentiates the larvae of *Strongyloides* (Fig. 1.23A) from those of hookworms–strongyles–trichostrongyles, which have a long buccal tube (Fig. 1.26).

Differentiation of the various lungworm larvae is based on tail morphology. In dogs, larvae with a straight tail and lacking a rhabditiform esophagus are *Crenosoma vulpis* (see

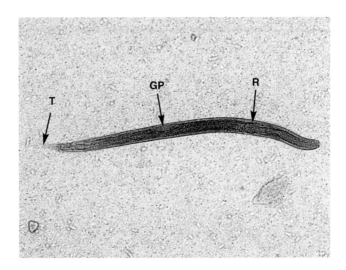

Fig. 1.24 *Strongyloides stercoralis* first-stage larvae recovered from the feces of a dog (Lugol's iodine stained and killed). Note the rhabditiform esophagus (R), prominent genital primordium (GP), and the straight tail (T). The rhabditiform esophagus makes up about 25% of the total length of the larvae.

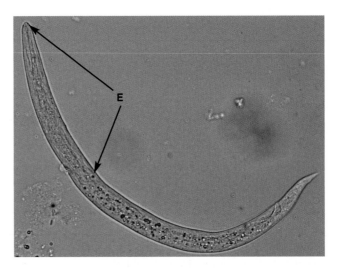

Fig. 1.25 *Crenosoma vulpis* first-stage larva recovered from the feces of a dog. Note the indistinct poorly defined esophagus (E). The esophagus makes up about 33%–50% of the total length of the larvae in metastrongyloid lungworms.

Figs. 1.25 and 1.92). Larvae that have a kinked S-shaped tail but lack a dorsal spine are either *Oslerus osleri* or *Filaroides hirthi* (see Figs. 1.94 and 1.95). Larvae with a kinked tail and a dorsal spine are *Angiostrongylus vasorum* (see Fig. 1.93). In cats, larvae with a kinked tail and a dorsal spine are *Aelurostrongylus abstrusus* (see Figs. 1.90 and 1.91).

There should be only a single species of nematode lungworm larva, *Dictyocaulus viviparus* (see Fig. 1.151), recovered in properly collected fresh feces of cattle. The larvae have an abundance of visible food granules and a straight tail. The same situation occurs with the horse, although infection with *Dictyocaulus arnfieldi* (see Fig. 1.176, 1.177) is patent in donkeys, but only rarely in horses. In small ruminants, there are two larvae with

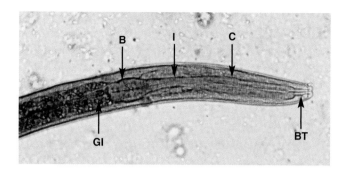

Fig. 1.26 Anterior end of a first-stage larva of a hookworm, *Uncinaria stenocephala*, recovered from an improperly collected fecal sample of a dog. This larva has been killed and stained with dilute iodine. As with *Strongyloides*, note the corpus (C), isthmus (I), and muscular bulb (B) of the rhabditiform esophagus and the intestine (GI). In contrast to *Strongyloides*, note the long buccal tube (BT).

straight tails, one with an abundance of visible food granules (*Dictyocaulus filaria*) (see Fig. 1.152) and the other without (*Protostrongylus rufescens*) (see Figs. 1.149 and 1.150). Another lungworm, *Muellerius capillaris*, produces larvae with a kinked tail and dorsal spine (see Figs. 1.146 and 1.147). *Cystocaulus* and *Neostrongylus* are small ruminant lungworms that are found in parts of Europe and Asia. The tails of their larvae have additional spines that can be used to differentiate them from *Muellerius* larvae.

TECHNIQUES FOR EVALUATION OF STRONGYLID NEMATODES IN GRAZING ANIMALS

Grazing animals are infected with a variety of species of strongylid nematodes, which produce eggs that are not easily differentiated. In veterinary practices, it is usually unnecessary to identify individual species because treatment and control are generally directed to the entire group of nematodes rather than to a single species. If identification of the strongylid genera present in an animal or group of animals is needed, the simplest method for identification is culture of eggs to the third larval stage. In ruminants, these larvae can then be identified to parasite genus. In horses, this technique can be used to differentiate large and small strongyle larvae and identify some genera specifically. Currently, researchers are developing protocols for identification of parasite genera using molecular techniques (polymerase chain reaction [PCR]), and these procedures are now becoming commercially available.

Fecal Culture

1. Fresh feces from cattle or horses should be thoroughly mixed and moistened with water if dry. Feces should not be wet, only moist. Larvae do not survive well in very wet fecal material. If feces are very soft or liquid, peat moss or vermiculite can be added to create a more suitable consistency. Sheep and goat pellets can be cultured as they are, without breaking them up. Rectal fecal samples are preferred for culture to prevent contamination with free-living nematodes.
2. Place feces in a cup or jar in a layer several centimeters deep. The container should have a loose cover that does not prevent air circulation but will deter flies and reduce

desiccation. The culture can be kept at room temperature for 10–20 days or at 27°C for 7 days. Daily stirring of the culture will inhibit mold growth and circulate oxygen for the developing larvae. Additional water can be added if feces begin to dry out.

3. Following the culture period, harvest larvae with the Baermann test described previously. Alternative containers and methods for harvest of larvae can be found in Bowman (2014), Taylor et al. (2015), and other textbooks of veterinary parasitology.

Identification of Ruminant and Camelid Third-Stage Larvae

To identify larvae, place a drop or two of liquid containing larvae from the Baermann procedure on a microscope slide. Add an equal amount of Lugol's iodine. The iodine will kill and stain the larvae so that they can be examined closely.

Larvae recovered from ruminant fecal material can be most easily identified by a combination of morphology and size. The shape of the head and the shape of the tail and of the sheath extending beyond the tail at the posterior end of the larva are important characteristics, and both should be evaluated on each larva before an identification is made. The sheath is the retained cuticle of the second larval stage and provides larvae with increased protection from environmental conditions. Measurements of total larval and sheath length are helpful as well (Table 1.3), but sizes often overlap between genera and size characteristics can be affected by culture conditions and age of larvae. Consequently, measurements alone should not be used to identify larvae.

Table 1.3. Morphologic characteristics of infective third-stage strongylid larvae of domestic ruminants

Genus	Overall length (µm)	Anus to tip of sheath (µm)	End of tail to tip of sheath (µm)	Other characteristics
Trichostrongylus				Head rounded; tail of sheath short; tail may have one or two tuberosities
Sheep	622–796	76–118	21–40	
Cattle	619–762	83–107	25–39	
Ostertagia				Head squared; tail of sheath shorter in sheep
Sheep	797–910	92–130	30–60	
Cattle	784–928	126–170	55–75	
Haemonchus				Head rounded; sheath tail medium length, offset
Sheep	650–751	119–146	65–78	
Cattle	749–866	158–193	87–119	
Cooperia				Head squared with two refractile oval bodies at anterior end of the esophagus; medium-length sheath tail tapering to fine point
Sheep	711–924	97–150	35–82	
Cattle	666–976	109–190	47–111	
Nematodirus				Broad, rounded head; intestine with eight cells; tail notched and lobed; long thin sheath tail
Sheep	922–1118	310–350	250–290	
Cattle	1095–1142	296–347	207–266	
Bunostomum				Small larva with rounded head; long thin sheath tail
Sheep	514–678	153–183	85–115	
Cattle	500–583	129–158	59–83	
Oesophagostomum				Rounded head; long thin sheath tail; 16–24 triangular intestinal cells
Sheep	771–923	193–235	125–160	
Cattle	726–857	209–257	134–182	
Chabertia				Rounded head; long thin sheath tail; 24–32 rectangular intestinal cells
Sheep	710–789	175–220	110–150	

Sources: Bowman (2014) and Ministry of Agriculture, Fisheries and Food (1986).

Relative proportions of parasite genera in larval cultures cannot be used to predict numbers of adult worms in the gastrointestinal tract. For example, *Haemonchus contortus* is highly prolific and may dominate in small ruminant fecal cultures, even when adult parasites of other genera are present in substantial numbers. Figures 1.27–1.37 show morphologic characteristics of common third-stage larvae of small ruminants and cattle.

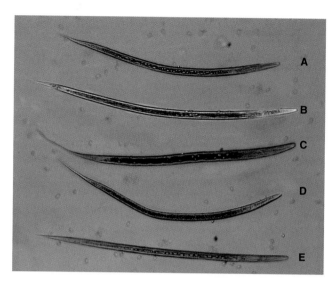

Fig. 1.27   Third-stage larvae of common small ruminant strongylid genera collected from fecal culture. This photo shows the relative size relationships among the larvae. The following photographs show the details and the anterior and posterior ends of the individual larvae. *Nematodirus* spp. larvae are usually not encountered in cultures and are not illustrated here. They are bigger in total length and have a longer tail sheath than other larvae. (A) *Trichostrongylus*, (B) *Teladorsagia*, (C) *Oesophagostomum/Chabertia*, (D) *Haemonchus*, and (E) *Cooperia*. Photo courtesy of Dr. Tom Yazwinski and Mr. Chris Tucker, Department of Animal Science, University of Arkansas, Fayetteville, AR.

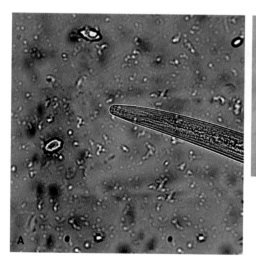
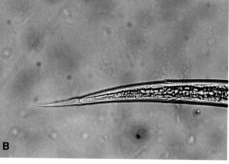

Fig. 1.28   *Trichostrongylus* larva from sheep, head (A) and tail sheath (B). The head of *Trichostrongylus* larvae is tapered and the tail sheath is short. The tail may end in one or two tuberosities. Photo courtesy of Dr. Tom Yazwinski and Mr. Chris Tucker, Department of Animal Science, University of Arkansas, Fayetteville, AR.

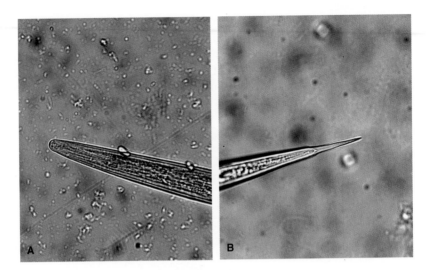

Fig. 1.29   Ovine *Teladorsagia* head (A) and tail sheath (B). *Teladorsagia* can easily be confused with *Trichostrongylus*, but *Teladorsagia* is generally larger and the head is squared, not tapered. The sheath of the tail of *Teladorsagia* is short. Photo courtesy of Dr. Tom Yazwinski and Mr. Chris Tucker, Department ofAnimal Science, University of Arkansas, Fayetteville, AR.

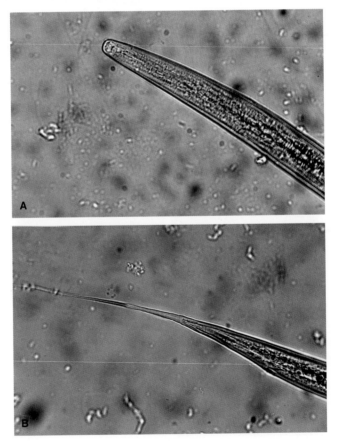

Fig. 1.30   *Oesophagostomum/Chabertia* head (A) and tail sheath (B). The larvae of these two genera are not easily distinguishable, but they are not difficult to differentiate from other genera. The tail sheath is long and filamentous, and the head is broad and rounded. Photo courtesy of Dr. Tom Yazwinski and Mr. Chris Tucker, Department of Animal Science, University of Arkansas, Fayetteville, AR.

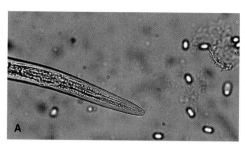
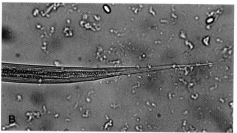

Fig. 1.31   *Haemonchus* head (A) and tail sheath (B). The larvae of *Haemonchus* have the most narrowly rounded head of the common larvae. The tail sheath is medium in length and often has a slight kink at the end of the tail. Photo courtesy of Dr. Tom Yazwinski and Mr. Chris Tucker, Department of Animal Science, University of Arkansas, Fayetteville, AR.

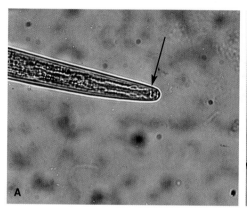
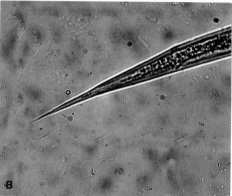

Fig. 1.32   *Cooperia* from a sheep, head (A) and tail sheath (B). *Cooperia* third-stage larvae are distinguished by a pair of refractile bodies (*arrow*) present in a squared head. These bodies are difficult to photograph but easy to appreciate under the microscope. The sheath of the tail is medium in length and tapering or finely pointed. Photo courtesy of Dr. Tom Yazwinski and Mr. Chris Tucker, Department of Animal Science, University of Arkansas, Fayetteville, AR.

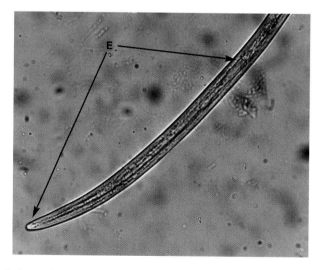

Fig. 1.33   *Strongyloides papillosus* is a nematode of ruminants that is unrelated to the important strongylid nematodes. Infective third-stage larvae of *Strongyloides* may be present in larval cultures. They do not have a sheath and the esophagus is very long (E). Additionally, free-living nematodes may be numerous in cultures contaminated with soil. For information on identifying free-living nematodes, see the section on identifying larval nematodes in fecal samples. Photo courtesy of Dr. Tom Yazwinski and Mr. Chris Tucker, Department of Animal Science, University of Arkansas, Fayetteville, AR.

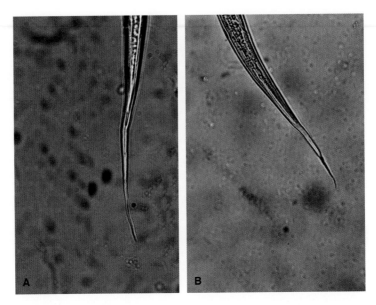

Fig. 1.34   Third-stage *Cooperia* larvae from cattle. Several species of *Cooperia* infect ruminants, and the length of the tail sheath is variable. *Cooperia oncophora* (A) produces larvae with a longer tail sheath than other species of the genus (B). Photo courtesy of Dr. Tom Yazwinski and Mr. Chris Tucker, Department of Animal Science, University of Arkansas, Fayetteville, AR.

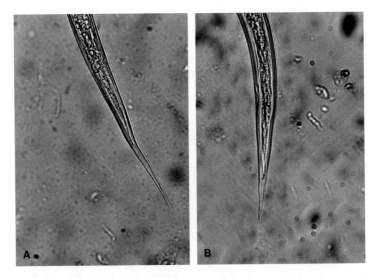

Fig. 1.35   Tail sheath of *Ostertagia* (A) and *Trichostrongylus* (B). Both genera have a short tail sheath, but *Ostertagia* has a blunter head. Photo courtesy of Dr. Tom Yazwinski and Mr. Chris Tucker, Department of Animal Science, University of Arkansas, Fayetteville, AR.

Additional information on identification of ruminant third-stage larvae can be found at the website of the RVC/FAO Guide to Veterinary Diagnostic Parasitology: www.rvc.ac.uk/review/Parasitology/Index/Index.htm and in van Wyk and Mayhew (2013).

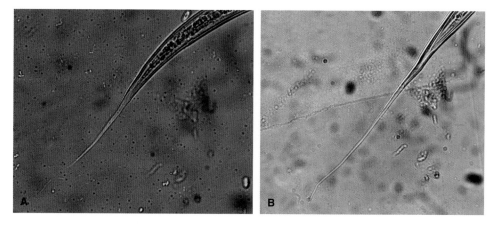

Fig. 1.36 Tail sheath of *Haemonchus* (A) and *Oesophagostomum* (B) from cattle. The tail sheaths of the parasites occurring in cattle are similar to those in sheep. Photo courtesy of Dr. Tom Yazwinski and Mr. Chris Tucker, Department of Animal Science, University of Arkansas, Fayetteville, AR.

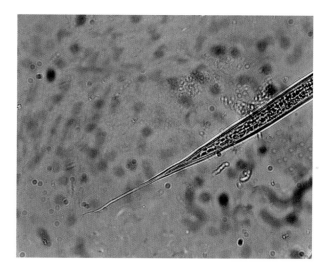

Fig. 1.37 Tail sheath of *Bunostomum*. Species of this ruminant hookworm infect both cattle and sheep. The third-stage larva is smaller than those of other genera and has a thin tail sheath. Photo courtesy of Dr. Tom Yazwinski and Mr. Chris Tucker, Department of Animal Science, University of Arkansas, Fayetteville, AR.

Identification of Third-Stage Larvae of Equine Strongyles

Horses are infected with over 30 species of strongylid parasites, but only a few can be identified on the basis of the third-stage larva. Most of the small strongyle species can only be identified as cyathostomin parasites from the infective larval stage (Fig. 1.38 and Table 1.4). The posterior portion of the sheath of horse strongyle larvae is very long and filamentous, making these larvae easily recognizable as infective parasite larvae. The number of intestinal cells in these larvae is variable and is useful in identification.

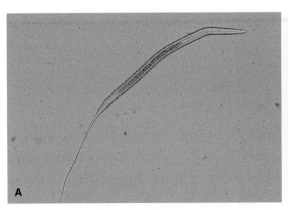
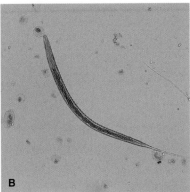

Fig. 1.38   Infective third-stage larvae of both large and small equine strongyles have a very long filamentous extension of the sheath. (A) The larvae of small strongyles (cyathostomes) have eight intestinal cells, which can be easily counted in the larva shown here. (B) Larvae of large strongyle species have more than eight intestinal cells, like this *Strongylus vulgaris* larva with at least 28 cells.

Table 1.4.   **Morphologic characteristics of infective third-stage strongylid larvae of horses**

Genus	Characteristics
Strongyloides	Sheath absent; esophagus almost half the length of the body
Trichostrongylus axei	Tail of sheath short, not filamentous
Most small strongyles (Cyathostominae)	Long filamentous sheath; eight triangular intestinal cells
Gyalocephalus (small strongyle)	Long filamentous sheath; 12 rectangular intestinal cells
Oesophagodontus (small strongyle)	Large larva; long filamentous sheath; 16 triangular intestinal cells
Posteriostomum (small strongyle)	Long filamentous sheath; 16 roughly rectangular intestinal cells
Strongylus equinus (large strongyle)	Long, thin larva with filamentous sheath; 16 poorly defined rectangular intestinal cells
Triodontophorus (large strongyle)	Medium-length and broad larva with filamentous sheath; 18–20 well-defined rectangular intestinal cells
Strongylus edentatus (large strongyle)	Smaller larvae with filamentous sheath; 18–20 poorly defined and elongated intestinal cells
Strongylus vulgaris (large strongyle)	Large larvae with filamentous sheath; short esophagus; 28–32 well-defined, rectangular intestinal cells

Source: Adapted from Ministry of Agriculture, Fisheries and Food (1986).

Fecal Egg Count Reduction Test (FECRT)

One of the principal uses of quantitative egg counts is the evaluation of drug efficacy. Anthelmintic resistance in strongylid nematodes of horses, small ruminants, and cattle is rapidly increasing worldwide. The only technique for evaluating drug efficacy that can be conducted by veterinary practitioners in all host species is the FECRT. In this procedure, the percentage reduction in strongylid fecal egg counts following treatment is calculated to evaluate the efficacy of the product. This test has also been used to evaluate resistance to anthelmintics in equine *Parascaris* spp. infections.

The World Association for the Advancement of Veterinary Parasitology (WAAVP) is an international organization that assembles expert opinion and has issued recommendations for testing and evaluating antiparasiticide efficacy. Updated recommendations for evaluating drug resistance are expected in the near future. Some general principles for conducting FECRT are presented here. For additional details in conducting these tests several recent publications can be consulted: Kaplan R. M. 2020. Biology, epidemiology, diagnosis, and management of anthelmintic resistance in gastrointestinal nematodes of livestock. Vet. Clin. North Am. Food Anim. Pract. 36:17–30, and American Association of Equine Practitioners. Internal Parasite Control Guidelines, updated 2019; https://aaep.org/guidelines/parasite-control-guidelines.

Although there is some variation in protocols for conducting FECRT, the following general principles are presented followed by comments specific to host species.

Test Groups and Selection of Animals

An accurate FECRT requires adequate animal numbers. In cases where owners wish to test very small flocks or herds, it is important to be cautious in interpretation of results. For ruminants 15 animals are preferred, but at least 10 should be used for each drug to be tested. For horses, where herd sizes are often low, at least six horses per group is recommended. Where only one or two animals are available an impression of drug efficacy can be obtained following treatment, but it should not be considered a reliable or accurate FECRT. In very large herds, 10% of the total population is adequate.

All animals used in the FECRT should have adequate egg counts to allow reductions to be determined accurately. For sheep, lambs of 3–6 months of age and cattle less than 16 months are the best candidates for a FECRT. Goats of all ages can generally be used. It is best if animals used in the test are similar in age and management. Fecal egg counts in adult cattle usually are too low to be used in an FECRT. It will be helpful to perform the FECRT at the time of year when fecal egg counts are expected to be the highest, based on epidemiology of the parasites in a region.

As a general guideline, the modified McMaster test can be used when the average FEC is 500 EPG with a group size of 10 or 250 EPG with a group size of 20. If average egg counts fall below this level, an alternative test for quantifying parasite eggs must be used to provide an accurate picture of drug efficacy. Alternatives include decreasing the detection limit of the modified McMaster test by using larger sample aliquots (e.g., using larger counting chambers available from several companies,) or using other tests with a lower detection limit (mini-FLOTAC, Stoll, or Wisconsin tests; see section on "Egg-Counting Procedures [Quantitative Fecal Exams]").

An alternative procedure for conducting a FECRT using composite fecal samples is described in Kaplan (2020).

Test Drugs and Collection of Posttreatment Samples

Once the test group or groups of animals have been established with a pretreatment fecal egg count, each animal should be individually weighed and treated with the test drug at the manufacturer's recommended dose.

On farms where individual animals cannot be weighed, the fecal egg count reduction (FECR) can be approximated by treating all animals with the drug dose for the estimated heaviest animal in the group. The results, however, will not be entirely accurate because some animals will be receiving more than the recommended dose, which may be temporarily effective against worms resistant to the recommended dose. This will lead to an overestimation of drug efficacy.

The optimum time following treatment for collection of posttreatment samples varies with the test drug because of variable effects on larval stages and temporary sterilizing effects on adult parasites. For ruminants, the following intervals are recommended:

- benzimidazoles, levamisole, or pyrantel 10–14 days,
- ivermectin and other avermectins 14–17 days,
- moxidectin 17–21 days.

For convenience in both ruminants and horses, a standard period of 14 days before collection of the posttreatment samples is often recommended.

Interpretation of Results

The % FECR is calculated using arithmetic group means in the following formula:

$$\%FECR = ([\text{pretreatment FEC} - \text{posttreatment FEC}]/\text{pretreatment FEC}) \times 100$$

When small groups of animals are used, individuals with particularly high fecal egg counts can dramatically skew the FECR when group means are used in the calculation. In these cases (e.g., in small groups of horses), it is best to calculate individual FECR using the above formula and then average the individual FECR to obtain a group average.

The FECRT can also be conducted by comparing mean posttreatment EPG in a group of untreated animals with that of a group of treated animals. This procedure is used less often than the comparison of pre- and posttreatment samples of individuals in the same group of animals because more animals are needed and pretreatment egg counts must be similar in the two groups. The formula for calculating FECR is altered accordingly when treatment and control groups are used:

$$\%FECR = ([\text{control FEC} - \text{treatment FEC}]/\text{control FEC}) \times 100$$

If no resistance is present, and the test is administered correctly, anthelmintics in ruminants can reliably decrease fecal egg counts by >95%. For horses, reductions in fecal egg counts when no resistance is present should be >95% for benzimidazoles, >98% for ivermectin and moxidectin, and >90% for pyrantel.

The FECR obtained when testing a group of animals gives an indication of drug efficacy, but is not equivalent to the proportion of the adult worm population that is removed by treatment. For example, if the percentage reduction is 10%, a large proportion of worms in the animals are probably resistant. If the reduction is 80%, the proportion of resistant worms is much smaller, but still significant. To further evaluate which worm genera are resistant in ruminants, the nematode eggs present in both pre- and posttreatment fecal samples can be identified by larval culture (see earlier) or PCR. In horses, drug resistance is most often present in small strongyles (cyathostomins), which cannot be readily differentiated to species based on morphology.

IDENTIFICATION OF ADULT WORMS

Tapeworm segments and adult gastrointestinal nematodes may occasionally be passed in feces and presented for identification by concerned owners. Segments of common tapeworms can usually be readily identified to the level of genus by shape and identification of eggs in the segments (see Figs. 1.99, 1.102, 1.105, 1.106, and 1.154 for photographs of common tapeworm segments), but nematode parasites may be more difficult to identify. When preserving nematodes for further identification, it is helpful to place them first in tap water and refrigerate the container for several hours. This will relax the worms and make them easier to examine. After relaxation, the worms can be placed in 70% ethanol or 10% buffered formalin. Ethanol, but not formalin, allows later identification with molecular assays. While not optimum preservatives for all helminths, these chemicals are readily available to most veterinarians.

The most common nematodes presented by pet owners are the ascarids (roundworms; see Fig. 1.72). These large, stout-bodied worms are common in feces and vomitus of kittens and puppies. Horse owners might also see equine ascarids that are up to 50 cm (about 20 in.) in length. Smaller nematodes present in equine manure may be the large and small strongyles or pinworms (*Oxyuris*). Larval or adult horse strongyles may be red or cream in color and no more than about 2–4 cm in length (see Fig. 1.168). *Oxyuris*, the equine pinworm, can reach 15 cm, and the females have distinctive long, thin tails (see Fig. 1.174). Nematodes are most likely to be seen in diarrheic feces or following treatment.

Specific identification of adult nematodes is usually based on morphologic variations of the outer layer, or cuticle, of the worms. Microscopic examination of the mouthparts and accessory sexual structures may be required. To enhance visualization of these structures, the worm can be mounted in a clearing solution, which dissolves the soft tissue, leaving only the cuticle. If the worm is large, the areas of diagnostic importance (usually the anterior and posterior ends) can be cut off and mounted in a few drops of the clearing solution. Procedures for making Hoyer's and lactophenol solutions are given below, but they are not usually prepared in veterinary practices because they require either controlled or hazardous substances. Both are commercially available.

Depending on the parasite species, accurate worm identification may require the evaluation of subtle morphologic characteristics that will be unfamiliar to most practicing veterinarians. When specific parasite identification is needed, worms should be submitted to a parasitologist for examination.

Hoyer's Solution

Hoyer's solution also provides a permanent mounting medium for specimens, although the clearing process will continue until eventually internal structures will no longer be visible:

- 30 g gum arabic;
- 16 mL glycerol;
- 200 g chloral hydrate;
- 50 mL distilled water.

Dissolve the gum arabic in water with gentle heat. Add the chloral hydrate, then the glycerol.

Lactophenol

- 20 mL glycerin, pure;
- 10 mL lactic acid;
- 10 mL phenol crystals, melted;
- 10 mL distilled water.

  Combine all ingredients.

PARASITES OF DOMESTIC ANIMALS

The following photographs in this chapter illustrate the diagnostic stages found in feces of a wide variety of both common and some uncommon parasites of major domestic species. Because an appreciation of relative sizes of parasite eggs, cysts, and oocysts, is very helpful in identification, a line drawing precedes sections showing parasites of common mammalian hosts (Figs. 1.39, 1.40, 1.121, 1.122, 1.162, 1.180). Generally, photographs of eggs and cysts were taken using the high-dry (40×) objective, although some photographs using the 10× objective are included to show relative sizes of eggs and cysts.

The figures in which each parasite appears are listed after the name. They may include figures in other sections where more than one parasite is illustrated.

An effort has been made to minimize taxonomic information while still permitting an appreciation of the larger groups to which each individual species belongs. For more specific taxonomic information, a textbook of veterinary parasitology should be consulted.

Also at the beginning of the sections for dogs and cats, ruminants, horses, and swine are tables showing common U.S. label approved products for treatment of a number of parasitic infections. Label dose and withdrawal information should always be consulted before treatment of animals with parasiticides.

Dogs and Cats

Helminth Eggs, Larvae and Protozoan Cysts
found in freshly voided feces of the
Dog, Wolf, Coyote and Fox

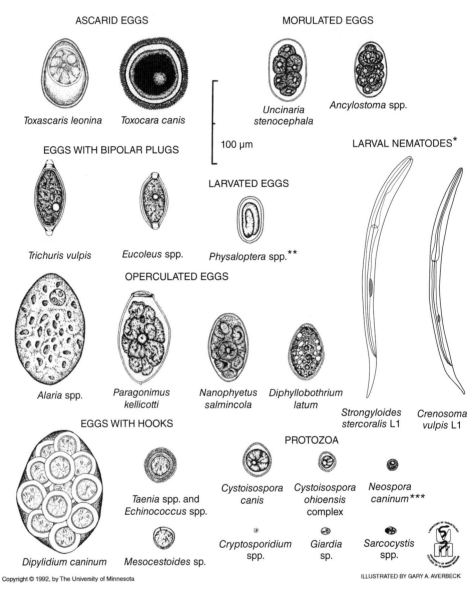

ILLUSTRATED BY GARY A. AVERBECK

Fig. 1.39   Parasites found in canine feces. Figure courtesy of Dr. Bert Stromberg and Mr. Gary Averbeck, College of Veterinary Medicine, University of Minnesota, Minneapolis, MN.
*Differentiate from other larvae that could be present in canine feces, including *Filaroides, Oslerus* and *Angiostrongylus.*
**Spirocerca lupi*, which is common in many parts of the world, has a larvated egg similar in appearance to *Physlaoptera*, but more elongated.
***Oocysts of *Hammondia heydorni* are similar in appearance to *Neospora.*

Helminth Eggs, Larvae and Protozoan Cysts
found in freshly voided feces of
Cats

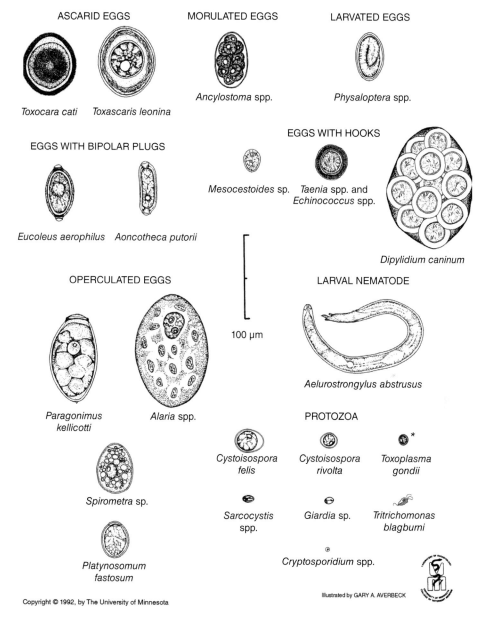

ASCARID EGGS

Toxocara cati   Toxascaris leonina

MORULATED EGGS

Ancylostoma spp.

LARVATED EGGS

Physaloptera spp.

EGGS WITH BIPOLAR PLUGS

Eucoleus aerophilus   Aoncotheca putorii

Mesocestoides sp.

EGGS WITH HOOKS

Taenia spp. and
Echinococcus spp.

Dipylidium caninum

OPERCULATED EGGS

100 µm

LARVAL NEMATODE

Aelurostrongylus abstrusus

Paragonimus
kellicotti

Alaria spp.

Spirometra sp.

Platynosomum
fastosum

PROTOZOA

Cystoisospora
felis

Cystoisospora
rivolta

Toxoplasma
gondii *

Sarcocystis
spp.

Giardia sp.

Tritrichomonas
blagburni

Cryptosporidium spp.

Illustrated by GARY A. AVERBECK

Fig. 1.40   Figure courtesy of Dr. Bert Stromberg and Mr. Gary Averbeck, College of Veterinary Medicine, University of Minnesota, Minneapolis, MN.
*Oocysts of *Hammondia hammondi* and *Besnoitia* spp. are similar in appearance to *Toxoplasma* oocysts.

DOGS AND CATS

Table 1.5.   **Representative treatments for selected parasites of dogs**

Parasite	Effective treatments	Dose and administration route
Cystoisospora spp.	[a]Ponazuril, [a]toltrazuril	10–30 mg/kg orally q 24 h × 1–3 d
	[b]Sulfadimethoxine	Administer according to label directions
Giardia sp.	[a]Febantel	30 mg/kg q 24 h × [c]3 d (combined with praziquantel and pyrantel); avoid in pregnant animals
	[a]Fenbendazole	50 mg/kg orally q 24 h × [c]3 d
Ancylostoma spp. *Toxascaris leonina* *Toxocara canis* *Uncinaria stenocephala*	Febantel, fenbendazole, [d]milbemycin oxime, transdermal moxidectin, pyrantel pamoate	Administer according to label directions
Trichuris vulpis	Febantel, fenbendazole, milbemycin oxime, transdermal moxidectin	Administer according to label directions
Eucoleus spp.	[a]Milbemycin oxime, [a]transdermal moxidectin	Extralabel use of label dose of transdermal moxidectin or elevated dose (2 mg/kg) of milbemycin oxime
Physaloptera spp.	[a]Pyrantel pamoate	20 mg/kg, repeat q 14 d until clinical signs resolve
Spirocerca lupi	[a,e]Doramectin	0.4 mg/kg subcutaneously q 7 d × 12 weeks
Strongyloides stercoralis	[a]Fenbendazole [a,e]Ivermectin	50 mg/kg fenbendazole orally q 24 h × 5 d, repeat in 4 weeks; 0.2 mg/kg ivermectin subcutaneously, repeat in 2 weeks
Dipylidium caninum *Taenia* spp. *Echinococcus* spp.	[f]Epsiprantel, [g]fenbendazole, praziquantel	Administer according to label directions
Mesocestoides spp. *Alaria* spp.	[a]Praziquantel	Effective against intestinal stages when administered according to label directions
Diphyllobothrium latum *Spirometra* spp.	[a]Praziquantel	Administer elevated dose (25 mg/kg) for 2 consecutive days
Heterobilharzia americana *Paragonimus kellicotti*	[a]Fenbendazole [a]Praziquantel	50 mg/kg orally for 10–14 days 25 mg/kg every 8 hours for 2–3 days
Nanophyetus salmincola	[a]Praziquantel	20–30 mg/kg once

[a] Extralabel use supported by published data.
[b] Label-approved for treating dogs with bacterial enteritis associated with coccidiosis.
[c] Longer courses of treatment may be necessary in some patients.
[d] Monthly products are label-approved against *Ancylostoma* spp., *Toxocara canis*, and *Toxascaris leonina*, but not *Uncinaria stenocephala*.
[e] Extralabel use of high-dose cattle products can be fatal in dogs; establish MDR1 status prior to treatment.
[f] Not label-approved against *Echinococcus* spp.
[g] Only effective against *Taenia* spp., not *D. caninum* or *Echinococcus* spp.
Additional information on parasite treatments can be found in Chapter 7.

Table 1.6. **Representative treatments for selected parasites of cats**

Parasite	Effective treatments	Dose, route, and regimen
Cystoisospora spp.	[a]Ponazuril, [a]toltrazuril	10–30 mg/kg orally q 24 h × 1–3 d
	[a]Sulfadimethoxine	Administer according to label directions
Tritrichomonas blagburni	[a]Ronidazole	30–50 mg/kg orally q 12 h × 14 d; use with caution due to safety concerns
Giardia sp.	[a]Febantel	30 mg/kg × [b]3 d (combined with praziquantel and pyrantel); avoid in pregnant animals
	[a]Fenbendazole	50 mg/kg orally q 24 h × [b]3 d
Ancylostoma spp. *Toxocara cati*	Emodepside, eprinomectin, [c]ivermectin, milbemycin oxime, pyrantel pamoate, transdermal moxidectin, selamectin	Administer according to label directions
Strongyloides spp.	[a]Fenbendazole [a,d]Ivermectin	50 mg/kg fenbendazole orally q 24 h × 5 d, repeat in 4 weeks; 0.2 mg/kg ivermectin subcutaneously, repeat in 2 weeks
Aelurostrongylus abstrusus	[a]Transdermal moxidectin	Administer according to label directions
Dipylidium caninum *Taenia* spp. *Echinococcus* spp.	[e]Epsiprantel, praziquantel	Administer according to label directions
Mesocestoides spp. *Alaria* spp.	[a]Praziquantel	Effective against intestinal stages when administered according to label directions
Diphyllobothrium latum *Spirometra* spp.	[a]Praziquantel	Administer elevated dose (25 mg/kg) for 2 consecutive days
Paragonimus kellicotti	[a]Fenbendazole [a]Praziquantel	50 mg/kg orally for 10–14 days 25 mg/kg every 8 hours for 2–3 days
Platynosomum concinnum	[a]Praziquantel	25 mg/kg every 8 hours for 2–3 days

[a] Extralabel use supported by published data.
[b] Longer courses of treatment may be necessary in some patients.
[c] Monthly product is only label-approved against *Ancylostoma* spp., not *Toxocara cati*.
[d] Extralabel use of high-dose cattle products can be fatal in cats; use with particular caution in young or debilitated patients.
[e] Not label-approved against *Echinococcus* spp.
Additional information on parasite treatments can be found in Chapter 7.

Protozoan Parasites

Parasite: ***Cystoisospora (Isospora)* spp.** (Figs. 1.4–1.6, 1.41–1.45, 1.47, 1.70, 1.78, 1.101)

Common name: Coccidia.

Taxonomy: Protozoa (coccidia). Several host-specific species are found in the dog (*C. canis, C. ohioensis, C. neorivolta, C. burrowsi*) and cat (*C. felis, C. rivolta*).

Geographic Distribution: Worldwide.

Location in Host: Small intestine, cecum, and colon.

Life Cycle: Cats and dogs are infected by ingestion of sporulated oocysts or infected transport hosts (often rodents, but also including rabbits, ruminants, birds, and other prey animals). Following development in the final host, oocysts are passed in feces and undergo sporulation in the environment.

Laboratory Diagnosis: Oocysts are detected by fecal flotation examination. Oocysts have smooth, clear cyst walls, are elliptical in shape, and contain a single, round cell (sporoblast) when freshly passed. The oocysts of *C. ohioensis, C. burrowsi,* and *C. neorivolta* are not morphologically distinguishable and are referred to as the *C. ohioensis* complex.

Size:	*C. canis, C. felis*	38–51 × 27–39 μm
	Other *Cystoisospora* spp.	17–27 × 15–24 μm

Clinical Importance: These are the organisms typically referred to as "coccidia" of dogs and cats, although other parasites also fall into this taxonomic group. Oocysts can be found in the feces of many clinically normal young dogs and cats. Clinical coccidiosis most often occurs in puppies and kittens, often in association with weaning, change of owner, or other stress factors. Signs include diarrhea, abdominal pain, anorexia, and weight loss. In severe cases, bloody diarrhea and anemia may occur. Respiratory and neurologic signs have also been reported in some animals. Clinical disease has been difficult to reproduce in experimental infections.

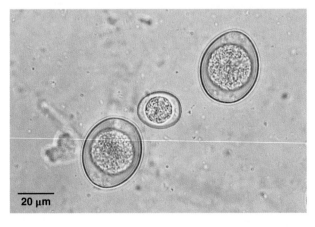

Fig. 1.41   Dog and cat coccidia species produce oocysts of different sizes. This figure shows *C. canis* (larger oocysts) and an oocyst of the *C. ohioensis* complex (smaller oocyst). Photo courtesy of Dr. David Lindsay, Virginia-Maryland College of Veterinary Medicine, Virginia Tech, Blacksburg, VA.

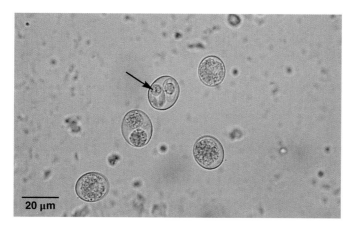

Fig. 1.42 *Cystoisospora* oocysts usually require a minimum of 1–2 days to become infective for the next host (sporulated). In warm conditions, oocysts undergo the first cell division soon after being passed in the feces. In the two-cell stage, they may be mistaken for sporulated oocysts. In this fecal sample, a sporulated oocyst (*arrow*) is adjacent to one in the two-cell stage.

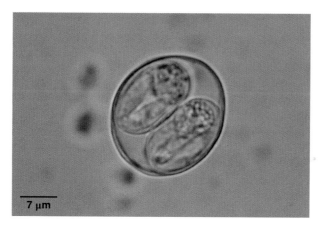

Fig. 1.43 A sporulated *Cystoisospora* oocyst contains two sporocysts, each containing four sporozoites. The two sporocysts can be seen in this oocyst, although only two of the four sporozoites can be visualized in each sporocyst. A large, round residual body is also present in each sporocyst.

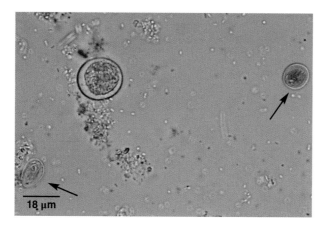

Fig. 1.44 *Cystoisospora* oocyst and two iodine-stained *Giardia* cysts (*arrows*) in a canine fecal sample. Photo courtesy of Dr. Robert Ridley, College of Veterinary Medicine, Kansas State University, Manhattan, KS.

Parasite: ***Toxoplasma gondii, Neospora caninum*** (Fig. 1.47)

Taxonomy: Protozoa (coccidia).

Geographic Distribution: Worldwide.

Location in Host: Intestine and other tissues of cats and other felids (*Toxoplasma*) and dogs and other canids (*Neospora*).

Life Cycle: *Toxoplasma* is transmitted to cats by ingestion of cysts containing bradyzoites in tissues of intermediate hosts. Prenatal and transmammary transmission as well as direct transmission through ingestion of sporulated oocysts can also occur. Transmission of *Neospora* in dogs appears to be similar to *Toxoplasma* transmission.

Laboratory Diagnosis: Oocysts are detected in feces by centrifugal or simple flotation techniques. However, very few oocysts of *Neospora* appear to be produced in infected dogs. Immunodiagnostic tests are available to identify current and past exposure to *Toxoplasma* in cats but are usually not positive until after fecal passage of oocysts has ceased. Dogs can also be tested for antibody to *Neospora*. The small, spherical-shaped oocysts of the two genera are morphologically identical, have a clear smooth cyst wall, and contain a single round sporoblast. Some other coccidia genera, including *Hammondia*, produce similar oocysts, which precludes definitive identification of *Toxoplasma* or *Neospora* on the basis of oocyst presence alone.

Size: 11–14 × 9–11 μm

Clinical Importance: *Toxoplasma* infections in cats are generally well tolerated. Clinical disease (ocular, respiratory, etc.) can occur in cats, especially young or immunosuppressed animals. Toxoplasmosis is an important zoonotic disease with especially serious consequences in pregnant women and the immunosuppressed. Congenital *Neospora* infection can result in severe central nervous system disease in dogs. *Neospora* infection is also an important cause of abortion in the bovine intermediate host.

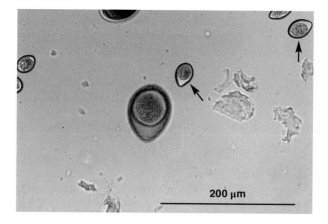

200 μm

Fig. 1.45 *Cystoisospora canis* oocysts in this canine fecal sample (arrows) are similar to the larger *Toxascaris leonina* egg (also Fig. 1.65), but the oocysts are smaller and lack the membranous appearance of the inside of the shell seen in *Toxascaris* eggs.

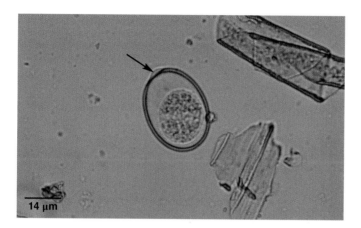

14 μm

Fig. 1.46 *Eimeria* spp. oocysts are sometimes seen in dog and cat feces. *Eimeria* does not infect these hosts, but oocysts consumed as a result of predation or coprophagy will pass unharmed through the gastrointestinal tract and may be misidentified as *Cystoisospora*. Many (but not all) *Eimeria* oocysts have a knob at one end called the micropyle cap (*arrow*), whereas *Cystoisospora* spp. lack a cap. If this cap is present, an oocyst in dog or cat feces can be identified as a "spurious parasite."

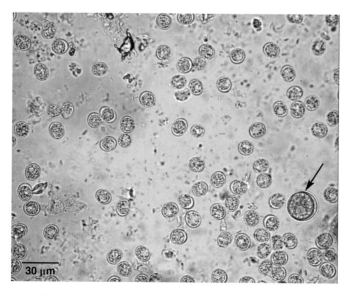

30 μm

Fig. 1.47 *Neospora* and *Toxoplasma* oocysts are similar to common *Cystoisospora* spp., but they are smaller. The oocysts of these two coccidia genera are similar in appearance and also cannot be distinguished from oocysts of *Hammondia*, another coccidia genus of small animals. This photo of a feline fecal sample also shows an oocyst of *C. rivolta* (*arrow*).

Parasite: **Sarcocystis spp.** (Figs. 1.48 and 1.49)

Taxonomy: Protozoa (coccidia). A number of species infect dogs or cats, each with a specific intermediate host.

Geographic Distribution: Worldwide.

Location in Host: Small intestine of dogs and cats.

Life Cycle: Cat and dog definitive hosts are infected by ingesting intermediate host tissue containing sarcocysts. Sexual reproduction in dogs or cats leads to formation of oocysts that sporulate while still in the intestinal tract.

Laboratory Diagnosis: Oocysts form within the gastrointestinal tract of dogs and cats. The oocyst wall breaks down in the gut, and small, ellipsoidal sporulated sporocysts are released in the feces. They are detected by centrifugal or simple flotation techniques.

Size: $7–22 \times 3–15$ μm

Clinical Importance: *Sarcocystis* is generally nonpathogenic in the definitive host, although some species can cause severe disease in the intermediate host (cattle, sheep, pigs, horses).

Parasite: **Cryptosporidium spp.** (Fig. 1.50)

Taxonomy: Protozoa (coccidia). *Cryptosporidium felis* and *C. canis* appear to be the primary species infecting cats and dogs, respectively.

Geographic Distribution: Worldwide.

Location in Host: Small intestine.

Life Cycle: These parasites have a direct life cycle. Cats and dogs are infected following ingestion of oocysts, which are infective as soon as they are passed in the feces. Following asexual and sexual multiplication of the organism in the intestine, oocysts are produced and exit the host in the feces.

Laboratory Diagnosis: Small oocysts in the feces are detected by use of acid-fast or other stains of fecal smears, Sheather's sugar flotation test, fecal antigen tests, or molecular diagnostic procedures. Oocysts of *C. parvum* and *C. canis* are morphologically indistinguishable, while *C. felis* oocysts are smaller than those of the other two species.

Size:	*C. felis*	$3.5–5$ μm in diameter
	C. parvum, C. canis	7×5 μm

Clinical Importance: Cryptosporidiosis has been reported as an uncommon cause of chronic diarrhea in cats. Affected cats are often immunosuppressed by other causes. Although implicated in rare instances, *Cryptosporidium* infections in dogs and cats do not appear to be a significant source of zoonotic exposure for humans.

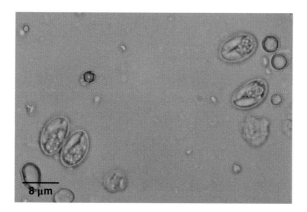

Fig. 1.48   *Sarcocystis* sporocysts are smaller than typical coccidia oocysts and have a smooth, clear cyst wall. Each sporocyst contains four banana-shaped sporozoites. Photo courtesy of Dr. Robert Ridley, College of Veterinary Medicine, Kansas State University, Manhattan, KS.

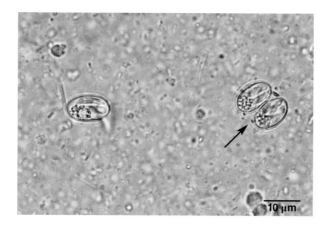

Fig. 1.49   *Sarcocystis* sporulates in the intestines and the oocyst wall usually ruptures before exiting the body so that only sporocysts are seen. Rarely, intact *Sarcocystis* oocysts are present (*arrow*). The 2 sporocysts appear to be surrounded by a thin membrane. Figure courtesy of Dr. Yoko Nagamori, College of Veterinary Medicine, Oklahoma State University, Stillwater, OK.

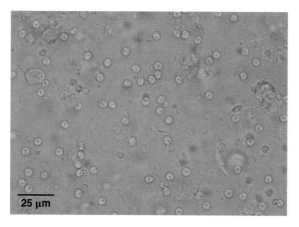

Fig. 1.50   *Cryptosporidium* sp. in a sugar flotation preparation. The oocysts of *C. canis* and *C. felis* are difficult to distinguish by microscopic techniques; *C. felis* oocysts are slightly smaller in size. *Cryptosporidum* oocysts can also be detected with acid-fast stains and immunodiagnostic tests.

Parasite: **Trichomonads** (Figs. 1.51 and 1.52)

Taxonomy: Protozoa (flagellate). Species identification of these organisms in dogs and cats is currently under investigation. *Tritrichomonas blagburni* has recently been identified as a species of feline trichomonad.

Geographic Distribution: Probably worldwide.

Location in Host: Large intestine of cats and dogs.

Life Cycle: Very little is known about transmission. Infection is probably by direct contact since no environmentally resistant cyst stage is known to occur.

Laboratory Diagnosis: The presence of trophozoites can be detected in direct saline smears of fresh feces. Flotation solutions will destroy trophozoites. Trichomonad organisms can be confused with *Giardia* but have an undulating membrane and lack the facelike appearance of *Giardia*. For detection of *T. blagburni* in the United States, the InPouch™ TF-Feline culture system, similar to the method used for bovine *T. foetus* infections in cattle (see Chapter 2), can be used. Commercial PCR tests are also available.

Size: 6–11 × 3–4 μm

Clinical Importance: Cases of chronic diarrhea in cats have been associated with feline *T. blagburni* infection; however, most trichomonad infections are generally considered to be of limited pathogenicity.

Parasite: *Giardia duodenalis* (= *G. intestinalis*, *G. lamblia*, *G. canis*, *G. cati*, etc.) (Figs. 1.44, 1.53–1.59)

Taxonomy: Protozoa (flagellate). Species number and nomenclature are under investigation. Molecular analysis is used to allocate isolates into assemblages. Most isolates from dogs belong to Assemblages C and D, and most cat isolates to Assemblage F.

Geographic Distribution: Worldwide.

Location in Host: Small intestine of dogs, cats, many other animals, and humans.

Life Cycle: Dogs and cats are infected by ingesting cysts in the environment. Trophozoites are stimulated under certain conditions to encyst and are passed from the host in feces.

Laboratory Diagnosis: The preferred flotation procedure for cyst detection is centrifugal flotation with 33% $ZnSO_4$ solution; other flotation solutions may cause rapid distortion. To improve sensitivity of testing, centrifugal flotation combined with a *Giardia* fecal antigen test is recommended. Trophozoites are infrequently seen in a direct saline smear of fresh diarrheic feces or duodenoscopic aspirates. Examination for trophozoites should occur within 30 minutes of collection or refrigeration. Commercial PCR and indirect fluorescent antibody (IFA) tests are also available.

Size: Cyst   9–13 × 7–9 μm
          Trophozoite   12–17 × 7–10 μm

Clinical Importance: *Giardia* is a common parasite of small animals. Many infections are asymptomatic, but acute, chronic, or intermittent diarrhea may occur, particularly in young dogs and cats. Although a low-risk zoonosis, cats and dogs are infrequently infected with assemblages associated with humans.

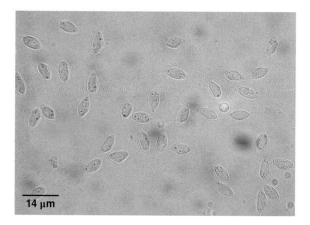

Fig. 1.51 Trichomonad parasites in dogs and cats have a distinctive undulating membrane. In fresh saline smears, they are most easily confused with *Giardia* trophozoites, but trichomonads lack the facelike appearance and the concave ventral surface of *Giardia*. In addition, the movement of *Giardia* trophozoites is usually described as "leaflike," while trichomonads movement is more jerky.

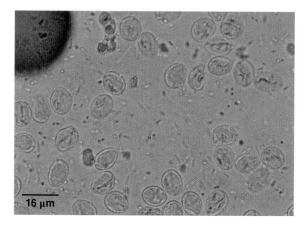

Fig. 1.52 Stained fecal smear of a trichomonad organism showing the anterior flagella and part of the undulating membrane (*arrow*).

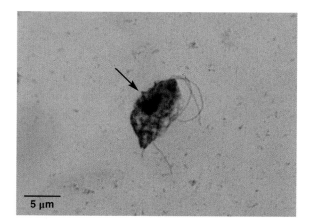

Fig. 1.53 *Giardia* cysts recovered with 33% ZnSO$_4$ centrifugal flotation. Cysts are elliptical with a thin, smooth cyst wall and contain two to four nuclei, two slender, linear intracytoplasmic flagella, and two thick, comma-shaped median bodies.

DOGS AND CATS

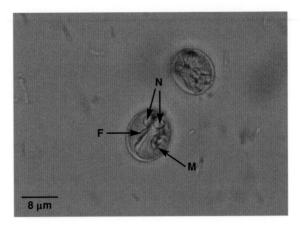

Fig. 1.54   A drop of Lugol's iodine may be added to a flotation preparation to stain *Giardia* cysts and make internal structures more prominent. Two nuclei (N), intracytoplasmic flagella (F), and median bodies (M) can be seen in the cyst shown here.

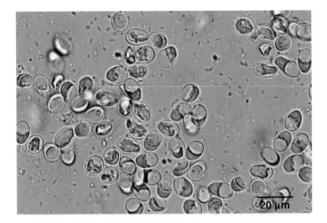

Fig. 1.55   *Giardia* cysts undergo osmotic damage when exposed to high specific gravity. With time, increasing numbers of cysts appear vacuolated, with a characteristic half-moon shape. Plant pollen and yeast cells that mimic *Giardia* cysts do not undergo this same artifact change.

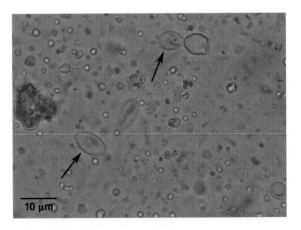

Fig. 1.56   The structures most often confused with *Giardia* cysts are yeast (*arrows*), which may be found in diarrheic feces in large numbers. Yeast are commonly slightly smaller than *Giardia* cysts and lack the complex internal structure seen in *Giardia* cysts.

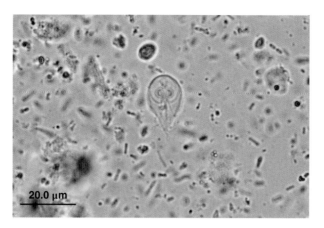

Fig. 1.57 *Giardia* trophozoite in a direct saline smear. Trophozoites are bilaterally symmetrical and pyriform shaped with two nuclei, eight flagella, two rodlike median bodies, and a ventral, concave, adhesive disk that gives them a clown face.

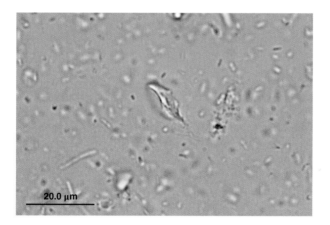

Fig. 1.58 Unstained *Giardia* trophozoite in a direct saline smear. The concave sucking disc is distinctive on the lateral view. Live trophozoites have a characteristic wobbling motion when swimming (often described as looking like a falling leaf) and are easily kept in the microscopic field of view.

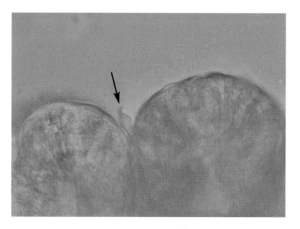

Fig. 1.59 *Giardia* trophozoite (*arrow*) associated with a portion of mucosa in a duodenal aspirate. Aspirates should be examined within 30 minutes of collection, before the fragile trophozoites die.

Helminth Parasites

Parasite: *Ancylostoma* **spp.,** *Uncinaria stenocephala* (Figs. 1.4–1.6, 1.60, 1.61, 1.70, 1.71, 1.76)

Common name: Hookworm.

Taxonomy: Nematodes (order Strongylida).

Geographic Distribution:

Ancylostoma caninum (dogs) and *A. tubaeformae* (cats): worldwide.
A. braziliense (dogs and cats): tropical and subtropical distribution; in the United States found primarily in the Gulf Coast region.
A. ceylanicum (dogs and cats): various parts of Asia.
Uncinaria stenocephala (dogs, rarely cats): primarily cooler northern temperate regions, including the northern United States, Canada, and Europe.

Location in Host: Small intestine of dogs and cats and wild canids and felids.

Life Cycle: Transmission of *A. caninum* to dogs occurs by transmammary transmission and direct skin penetration by infective larvae, ingestion of infective larvae from the environment or in paratenic hosts. Transmission of *U. stenocephala* occurs by ingestion of infective larvae or paratenic hosts, direct skin penetration is rare. Cats can be infected with hookworms either by skin penetration, by ingestion of infective larvae, or in paratenic hosts (rodents). Adult hookworms produce eggs that exit the host in the feces.

Laboratory Diagnosis: Eggs are detected using centrifugal or simple flotation techniques. *Ancylostoma* and *Uncinaria* eggs are morphologically identical, with an elliptical shape and smooth shell wall containing a grapelike cluster of cells (morula). However, they differ in size.

Size:	*Ancylostoma* spp.	52–79 × 28–58 μm
	U. stenocephala	71–92 × 35–58 μm

Clinical Importance: *Ancylostoma caninum* is common in North America. In heavy infections, particularly in puppies, the blood-feeding behavior of hookworms can cause fatal anemia. Peracute, acute, and chronic disease syndromes may occur. *Ancylostoma braziliense* and *A. caninum* may cause cutaneous larva migrans and, rarely, eosinophilic enteritis in humans. *Ancylostoma* infections in cats are less common than in dogs. Many feline infections are subclinical, but heavy infections causing anemia and weight loss can be fatal. *Uncinaria stenocephala* is less pathogenic than *A. caninum*.

DOGS AND CATS

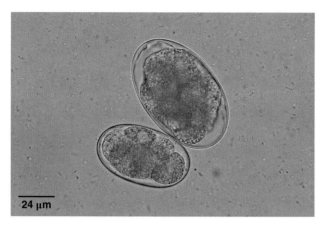

Fig. 1.60   Although *Ancylostoma* is the most common genus of hookworm in the United States, slightly larger *Uncinaria* eggs may also be seen in canine feces, and mixed infections can occur, as shown here.

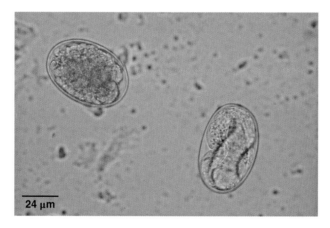

Fig. 1.61   *Ancylostoma tubaeforme* larvated and undeveloped eggs from a cat. The egg on the right contains a developed first-stage larva; the egg on the left is undifferentiated. Hookworm eggs exposed to warm temperatures for several hours rapidly develop to the larvated stage and hatch.

Parasite: *Mammomonogamus* **spp.** (Figs. 1.62, 1.76)

Taxonomy: Nematode (order Strongylida).

Geographic Distribution: Caribbean, Asia.

Location in Host: Nares and nasopharynx primarily.

Life Cycle: The life cycle has not been completely described. Infection probably follows ingestion of infective larvae.

Laboratory Diagnosis: Centrifugal fecal flotation with solutions of ≥1.25 SPG will detect eggs. Mucus surrounding eggs in nasal discharge samples may inhibit flotation. Mucus can be removed by pretreatment with 5% potassium hydroxide followed by repeated sedimentation in water.

Size: 90–133 × 54–88 µm

Clinical Significance: Asymptomatic infection in cats. Human cases have been reported.

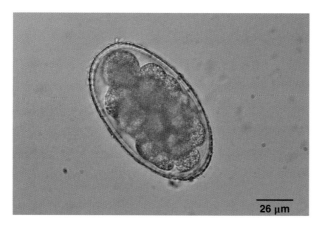

Fig. 1.62   Egg of *Mammomonogamus* from a cat. This egg is most likely to be seen in cats from Caribbean islands or parts of Asia. The shell wall has subtle striations and is slightly thicker than that of a hookworm egg. Photo courtesy of Dr. Jennifer Ketzis, School of Veterinary Medicine, Ross University, St. Kitts, W.I.

Parasite: **Toxocara spp.** (Figs. 1.4–1.6, 1.18, 1.63–1.65, 1.67–1.74, 1.101, 1.103, 1.109)

        Common name: Roundworm.

Taxonomy: Nematode (order Ascaridida).

Geographic Distribution: Worldwide.

Location in Host: Small intestine of dogs (*T. canis*) and cats (*T. cati*).

Life Cycle: Single-celled eggs pass from the host in the feces and develop to the infective stage in the environment. Dogs acquire infections of *T. canis* by transplacental and transmammary transmission or by the ingestion of larvated eggs or paratenic hosts (rodents). Cats acquire *T. cati* infection by ingestion of larvated eggs or paratenic hosts. Transmammary transmission may also occur in some circumstances.

Laboratory Diagnosis: Eggs are detected using centrifugal or simple flotation examination techniques. *Toxocara* eggs have a dark, round, single-celled embryo contained in a thick shell wall. Eggs of the two species may be difficult to differentiate. *Toxocara canis* tends to be subspherical, and *T. cati* tends to be elliptical in shape.

Size:	*T. canis*	85–90 × 75 μm
	T. cati	71–75 × 61–65 μm

Clinical Importance: *Toxocara* is an important pathogen in puppies and kittens. Stillbirths, neonatal deaths (*T. canis*), or chronic ill-thrift (*T. canis*, *T. cati*) can occur in infected animals. Adult dogs and cats are much less likely to have symptomatic infections. Additionally, both species have zoonotic importance as causes of visceral and ocular larva migrans, particularly in children.

Parasite: **Toxascaris leonina** (Figs. 1.45, 1.65, 1.73, 1.74)

        Common name: Roundworm.

Taxonomy: Nematode (order Ascaridida).

Geographic Distribution: Worldwide.

Location in Host: Small intestine of dogs, cats, wild canids and felids.

Life Cycle: The life cycle is similar to that of *Toxocara* spp., although there is no transmammary or transplacental infection. Dogs and cats are infected following ingestion of larvated eggs or animals with encysted larvae in their tissues (rodents, rabbits).

Laboratory Diagnosis: Eggs are detected using centrifugal or simple flotation fecal examination techniques. *Toxascaris* eggs are elliptical with a thick, smooth outer shell wall containing a light-colored, single-celled embryo. The internal surface of the shell wall appears rough or wavy due to the vitelline membrane.

        Size: 75–85 × 60–75 μm

Clinical Importance: *Toxascaris* is much less common in dogs and cats than *Toxocara* and is considered to be of minor clinical significance.

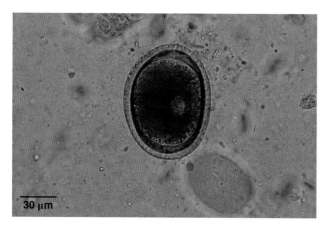

Fig. 1.63   *Toxocara* eggs are typical ascarid eggs with a thick shell. They contain a single cell when first passed in host feces.

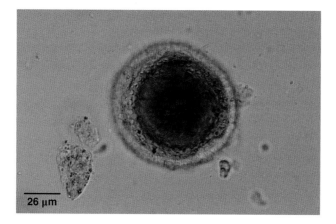

Fig. 1.64   When the microscope is focused on the surface of a *Toxocara* egg, the rough, pitted shell-wall surface has a golf-ball-like appearance.

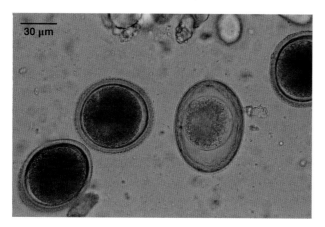

Fig. 1.65   *Toxascaris leonina* egg and *Toxocara cati* eggs. Note the dark single-cell embryo and rough mammillated (pitted) outer shell-wall surface of the *Toxocara* egg contrasted to the lighter appearance of the embryo and to the smooth outer shell-wall surface of the *Toxascaris* egg.

Parasite: ***Baylisascaris procyonis*** (Figs. 1.66–1.68, 1.74)

Common name: Raccoon roundworm.

Taxonomy: Nematode (order Ascaridida).

Geographic Distribution: Parts of North America and Europe.

Location in Host: Small intestine of raccoons and occasionally dogs.

Life Cycle: Raccoons are infected by ingestion of infective eggs or paratenic hosts (rodents, rabbits, birds). Routes of infection in dogs are presumed to be the same. Dogs may also pass *Baylisascaris* eggs following coprophagy.

Laboratory Diagnosis: Eggs are detected by simple or centrifugal fecal flotation examination. Eggs are thick walled, elliptical in shape, and contain a single, large, round-celled embryo. The eggs are often covered with a brown proteinaceous substance and have a fine granular shell-wall surface.

Size: 63–75 × 53–60 µm

Clinical Importance: Infection is well tolerated in the raccoon definitive host. Severe central nervous system or ocular disease can result when birds, rabbits, rodents, marsupials, and humans ingest infective *B. procyonis* eggs. Infections in dogs may result in either patent adult worms in the small intestine or larval tissue migration causing central nervous system disease.

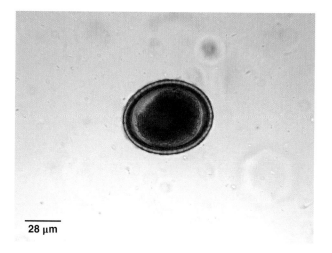

28 μm

Fig. 1.66 *Baylisascaris procyonis* egg in feces of a naturally infected dog. Usually, *Baylisascaris* eggs are brown due to the presence of a protein coat (see Fig. 1.67). When lacking the protein coat, *Baylisascaris* eggs are easily misidentified as *Toxocara* eggs. *Baylisascaris* eggs can be differentiated from those of *Toxocara* based on their smaller size and granular shell-wall surface rather than the pitted surface of *Toxocara*.

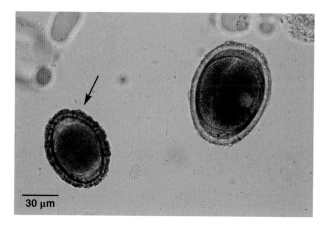

30 μm

Fig. 1.67 *Toxocara canis* egg and *Baylisascaris procyonis* egg (*arrow*). Eggs of *B. procyonis* appear in the feces of dogs due to either patent infections or coprophagy. The larger *Toxocara* egg (85–90 × 75 μm) has a rough, pitted, outer shell-wall surface. The *B. procyonis* egg is smaller, has a finely granular shell-wall surface, and may be brown in color. *Baylisacaris* eggs are easily misidentified as *Toxocara* in canine fecal exams. Mistakes can be minimized with the use of an ocular micrometer to measure egg size.

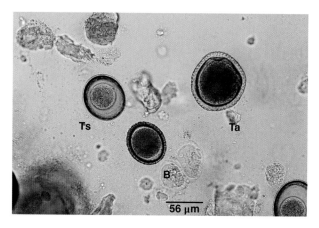

Ts

Ta

B

56 μm

Fig. 1.68 *Toxocara* (Ta), *Toxascaris* (Ts) and *Baylisascaris* (B) eggs in a canine fecal sample. *Toxascaris* eggs have a smooth outer layer on the egg shell in contrast to the other two species.

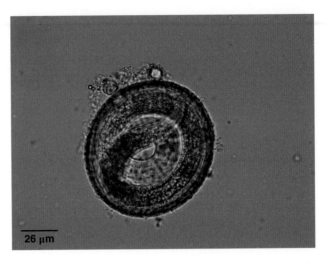

26 µm

Fig. 1.69   *Toxocara* and other ascarids typically require several weeks of development in the environment before an infective larva forms, although initial larval development can occur in a few days in hot weather.

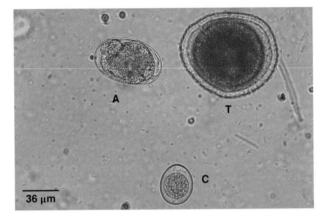

36 µm

Fig. 1.70   Canine fecal sample containing *Toxocara canis* (T) and *Ancylostoma* (A) eggs and a *Cystoisospora* oocyst (C).

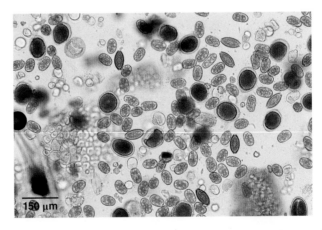

150 µm

Fig. 1.71   *Toxocara*, *Ancylostoma*, and *Trichuris* eggs in a canine fecal sample. These are the most common intestinal helminths encountered in dogs. Photo courtesy of Dr. Robert Ridley, College of Veterinary Medicine, Kansas State University, Manhattan, KS.

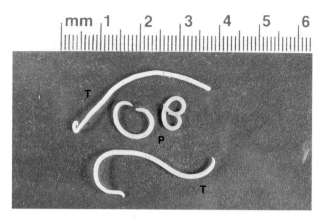

Fig. 1.72   Ascarids are often passed in the feces or vomitus of dogs and cats, particularly in young or recently dewormed animals. They are the only large, thick-bodied nematodes commonly seen by owners. Rarely, the stomach worm *Physaloptera* is present in vomitus. It usually assumes a C shape when passed out of the host. Two specimens each of *Toxocara* (T) and *Physaloptera* (P) are shown here.

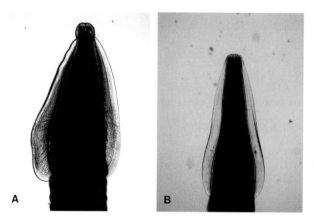

Fig. 1.73   The morphology of the anterior end of small animal ascarids can be used to differentiate species. The anterior end of adult *Toxocara cati* has an "arrowhead" appearance due to the cervical alae (winglike expansions of the cuticle). Adult specimens of *Toxocara cati* (A) recovered from the feces or vomitus of cats can be differentiated from *Toxascaris leonina* (B), which has less prominent cervical alae.

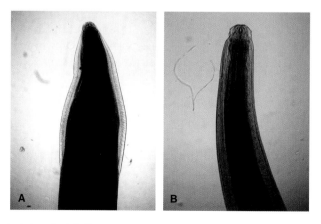

Fig. 1.74   The cervical alae of adult *Toxocara canis* (A) are similar in appearance to those of *Toxascaris leonina*. In contrast to the other ascarids infecting dogs (*Toxocara, Toxascaris*), adult *Baylisascaris* (B) lack visible cervical alae.

DOGS AND CATS

Parasite: **_Trichuris vulpis_** (Figs. 1.71, 1.75, 1.76, 1.78, 1.79, 1.116)

Common name: Whipworm.

Taxonomy: Nematode (order Enoplida).

Geographic Distribution: Worldwide. _Trichuris felis_ (_serrata_, _campanula_) occurs in cats in South America, Caribbean, semi-tropical United States (Florida), Australia.

Location in Host: Cecum and large intestine.

Life Cycle: Dogs are infected by ingesting infective eggs in the environment. Eggs are produced by adult worms in the large bowel and, after leaving the host in the feces, develop to the infective stage in the environment.

Laboratory Diagnosis: Eggs are best detected by centrifugal flotation and less effectively by simple flotation examination of feces. Eggs are typically symmetrical about the bipolar plugs, barrel-shaped, and brown. The shell-wall surface is smooth.

Size: 72–90 × 32–40 μm

Clinical Importance: Heavy infection in dogs can cause weight loss, unthriftiness, and profuse diarrhea that may be bloody. Resultant electrolyte imbalance can mimic endocrine disease. Infection with feline whipworm is considered rare, although on some Caribbean islands prevalence is high. Clinical signs are often absent.

Parasite: **_Eucoleus_ (= _Capillaria_) _aerophilus_, _E. boehmi_** (Figs. 1.77–1.81, 1.101)

Common name: Fox lungworm (_E. aerophilus_).

Taxonomy: Nematode (order Enoplida).

Geographic Distribution: _Eucoleus aerophilus_ is found worldwide; _E. boehmi_ has been reported from North and South America and Europe.

Location in Host: Trachea, bronchi, and bronchioles of dogs, cats, and foxes (_E. aerophilus_). Epithelium of nasal turbinates and sinuses of dogs and wild canids (_E. boehmi_).

Life Cycle: The definitive host is probably infected by ingestion of eggs containing infective larvae, although an earthworm intermediate host may be involved.

Laboratory Diagnosis: Eggs are detected by fecal flotation tests or in tracheal or nasal mucus samples. The eggs are clear to golden (_E. boehmi_) or brownish green (_E. aerophilus_), are bipolar plugged, tend to be asymmetrical in shape, and contain a multicelled embryo.

Size: _E. aerophilus_   58–79 × 29–40 μm

E. boehmi   54–60 × 30–35 μm

Clinical Importance: _Eucoleus aerophilus_ infections in dogs and cats are usually subclinical; in some cases, chronic cough occurs. It is an important pathogen of farmed foxes. _Eucoleus boehmi_ infections are usually subclinical. Clinical signs include sneezing and a mucopurulent nasal discharge that may contain blood.

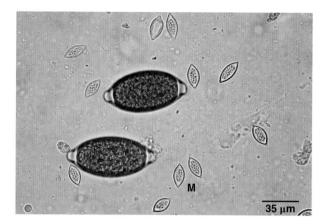

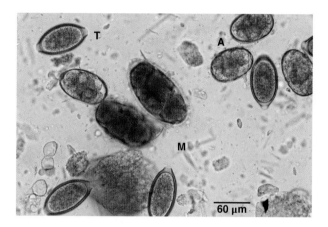

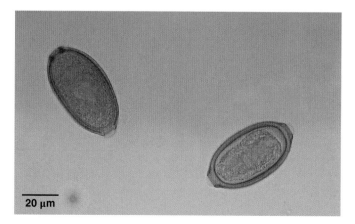

Fig. 1.75   The egg of *Trichuris vulpis* with its prominent bipolar plugs is one of the most common found in canine feces. Capillarid species also produce eggs with polar plugs. Also shown in this photo are *Monocystis* cysts (M), a spurious protozoan parasite of earthworms. Although cysts are similar in shape to whipworm eggs, they are far too small to be confused with helminth eggs. Photo courtesy of Dr. Manigandan Lejeune, Animal Health Diagnostic Center, Cornell University, Ithaca, NY.

Fig. 1.76   Feline fecal sample containing eggs of *Ancylostoma* (A), *Mammomonogamus* (M), and *Trichuris* (T). While feline *Trichuris* eggs are similar to those of *T. vulpis*, they are generally smaller. Photo courtesy of Dr. Jennifer Ketzis, School of Veterinary Medicine, Ross University, St. Kitts, W.I.

Fig. 1.77   *Eucoleus* eggs are passed in the undifferentiated one- or two-celled stage. *Eucoleus boehmi* (*right*) and *E. aerophilus* (*left*) eggs are similar in appearance, although in fresh feces, eggs of *E. boehmi* already contain a morula (cluster of cells) that does not completely fill the interior of the egg. Differences in the eggshell can also be used to differentiate the species (see Figs. 1.80 and 1.81). Photo courtesy of Dr. Robert Ridley, College of Veterinary Medicine, Kansas State University, Manhattan, KS.

Parasite: *Aonchotheca (= Capillaria) putorii* (Fig. 1.82)

Taxonomy: Nematode (order Enoplida).

Geographic Distribution: North America, Europe, and New Zealand,

Location in Host: Small intestine and stomach of cats, raccoons, foxes, and wild felids and mustelids.

Life Cycle: Definitive hosts are infected following ingestion of larvated eggs. Adults develop in the gastrointestinal tract and produce eggs that are passed in the feces.

Laboratory Diagnosis: Eggs are detected by centrifugal or simple flotation tests. The yellow-gray eggs are asymmetrical about the bipolar plugs. The sides of the eggs tend to be parallel. The shell-wall surface has a network of deep longitudinal ridges.

Size: 56–72 × 23–32 µm

Clinical Importance: Infections in cats are usually subclinical and are uncommon in North America. Gastritis with vomiting can occur. Hemorrhagic enteritis can occur in mink.

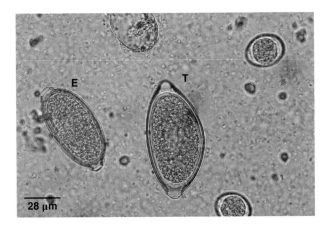

Fig. 1.78   The only canine parasite eggs that could be mistaken for whipworm eggs belong to the capillarid parasites *Eucoleus* and *Aonchotheca*. *Trichuris vulpis* eggs (T) are larger, have a smooth-walled shell, and are usually browner than capillarid eggs (E). In cats, *Trichuris* eggs are smaller, and other characteristics should be used to differentiate them from capillarids. *Cystoisospora* oocysts are also present in this sample.

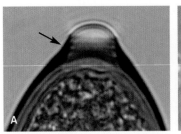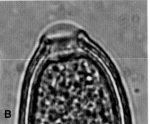

Fig. 1.79   Portion of a *Trichuris vulpis* egg (A) demonstrating the ridges seen in the bipolar plug (*arrow*). Capillarid eggs (B) lack ridges on the plugs. Capillarid eggs are also smaller than whipworm eggs and their bipolar plugs often appear asymmetrical.

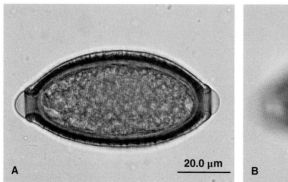
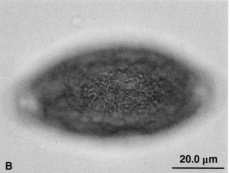

Fig. 1.80   Examination of the surface of the shell wall of small-animal capillarid eggs can be used in making a specific identification. The images on this page were taken with an oil immersion lens (100×). However, even with the high-dry objective (40×) of the microscope differences in the surface of the egg can be seen. The surface of the *Eucoleus aerophilus* egg (A) has a network of interconnecting ridges (B).

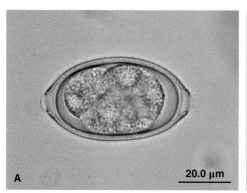
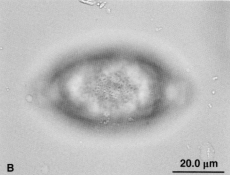

Fig. 1.81   In addition to having a morula that does not fill the interior of the egg, the surface of *Eucoleus boehmi* eggs (A) is pitted, resulting in a stippled appearance (B).

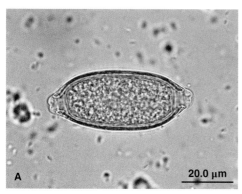
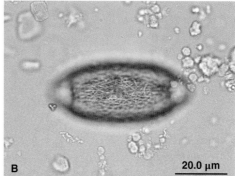

Fig. 1.82   Eggs of *Aonchotheca putorii* are similar to those of other capillarids (A), but in contrast to the ridges of the *Eucoleus aerophilus* egg, the shell surface of *A. putorii* consists of a network of deep longitudinal ridges (B).

Parasite: **Physaloptera spp.** (Figs. 1.72, 1.83, 1.84)

Taxonomy: Nematode (order Spirurida). Several species have been described (*P. praeputialis*, *P. felidis*, *P. pseudopraeputialis*, *P. rara*, *P. canis*).

Geographic Distribution: Worldwide.

Location in Host: Stomach of dogs, cats, and various wild animals.

Life Cycle: Cockroach, beetle, or cricket intermediate hosts ingest eggs shed in feces of wild animals, dogs or cats. The definitive host is infected by ingesting the insect intermediate host or a paratenic host (reptiles and possibly other animals).

Laboratory Diagnosis: Eggs of this group of nematodes are not reliably detected by fecal flotation due to their density. *Physaloptera* eggs are best detected by fecal sedimentation. The eggs are clear and elliptical, have a smooth shell wall, and contain a larva coiled inside.

   Size: 42–53 × 29–35 µm

Clinical Importance: Infections may result in clinical signs of vomiting and anorexia.

Parasite: **Spirocerca lupi** (Fig. 1.85)

        Common name: Esophageal worm.

Taxonomy: Nematode (order Spirurida).

Geographic Distribution: Worldwide but primarily in warmer regions.

Location in Host: Adults are found in the wall of the esophagus, stomach, and, rarely, aorta of dogs, wild canids, and various other wild animals.

Life Cycle: Dung beetle intermediate hosts ingest eggs in feces. The definitive host is infected by ingesting the insect intermediate host or a paratenic host (rodents, other mammals, birds, reptiles).

Laboratory Diagnosis: Eggs are best detected by fecal sedimentation or (less reliably) by fecal flotation. The eggs are narrow, ellipsoidal, and cylindrical; have a smooth, clear shell wall; and contain a fully developed larva coiled inside.

   Size: 30–38 × 11–15 µm

Clinical Importance: Infections are often subclinical. The most common clinical signs are dysphagia and regurgitation, but aortic stenosis, aneurysm, esophageal rupture, or obstruction, cachexia, and esophageal sarcomas may occur. *Spirocerca* infection is uncommon in the United States.

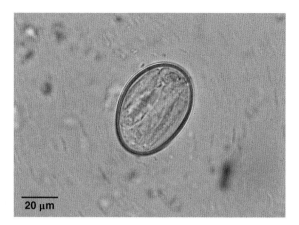

Fig. 1.83   *Physaloptera* eggs do not float consistently in routine flotation exams. The eggs are larger and less elongated than those of *Spirocerca* (Fig. 1.85). *Physaloptera* eggs are smaller and have a thicker shell than larvated hookworm eggs, with which they might be confused. Photo courtesy of Dr. Robert Ridley, College of Veterinary Medicine, Kansas State University, Manhattan, KS.

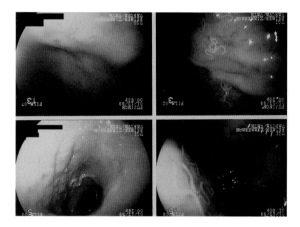

Fig. 1.84   Adult *Physaloptera* may be seen with gastroscopy in cases where routine fecal flotation does not detect the parasite eggs. Several worms can be seen on the surface of this canine stomach. Photo courtesy of Dr. Michael Leib, Virginia-Maryland Regional College of Veterinary Medicine, Virginia Tech, Blacksburg, VA.

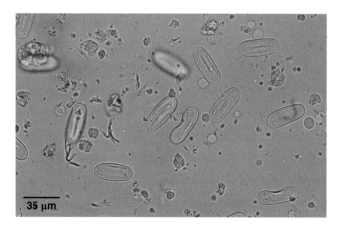

Fig. 1.85   *Spirocerca* eggs do not float consistently in common flotation solutions. These larvated eggs are more elongated than *Physaloptera* eggs. Photo courtesy of Dr. Isabelle Verzberger-Epshtein, NRC Institute for Nutrisciences and Health, Charlottetown, PEI, Canada.

Parasite: ***Strongyloides stercoralis*** (Figs. 1.23, 1.24, 1.86–1.89)

Common name: Intestinal threadworm.

Taxonomy: Nematode (order Rhabditida).

Geographic Distribution: Worldwide.

Location in Host: Adult females live in the canine small intestine.

Life Cycle: *Strongyloides* parthenogenetic females in the small intestine release larvae that may develop into infective parasitic larvae or, alternatively, may undergo a single free-living cycle of maturation and reproduction before infective parasitic larvae are formed. Infection of the host from the environment is primarily through skin penetration. Transmammary transmission may also occur if the dog is newly infected during lactation.

Laboratory Diagnosis: First-stage larvae may be identified in fresh feces using a Baermann test. *Strongyloides* larvae do not have the modifications of the tail seen in most lungworm larvae. They closely resemble hatched hookworm larvae or free-living nematodes that may be present in fecal samples that have been allowed to sit for a period of time prior to collection (see section on identification of nematode larvae collected by Baermann exam, which is at the beginning of this chapter). If identification of the first-stage larvae is uncertain, larvae in the feces can be cultured for a few days, and the third-stage larvae can be identified.

Size: 150–390 μm in fresh feces. *Strongyloides* larvae can grow quickly in the environment and their size increases before the molt to the second larval stage. This results in a large size range for the larvae. In addition, the size range may be increased by the mistaken identification and measurement of larger second-stage larvae.

Clinical Importance: Infections may be subclinical, but heavy infection can produce respiratory signs from migrating larvae as well as enteritis associated with adults. *Strongyloides stercoralis* also infects humans and may produce severe and even fatal infections in immunocompromised humans. The degree to which canine strains infect humans is unclear, but because of the seriousness of some human cases, infection in dogs should be considered a zoonosis.

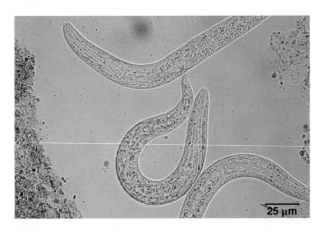

Fig. 1.86   *Strongyloides* larvae must be differentiated from hatched hookworm larvae and free-living nematodes. Photo courtesy of Dr. Yoko Nagamori, College of Veterinary Medicine, Oklahoma State University, Stillwater, OK.

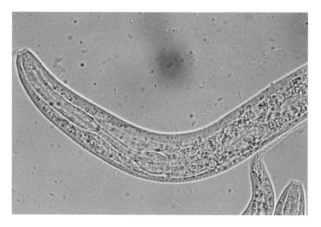

Fig. 1.87 First-stage larvae of *Strongyloides stercoralis* have a well-defined rhabditiform esophagus, a characteristic shared by first-stage hookworm larvae and free-living nematodes, but not seen in canine lungworm larvae. Photo courtesy of Dr. Yoko Nagamori, College of Veterinary Medicine, Oklahoma State University, Stillwater, OK.

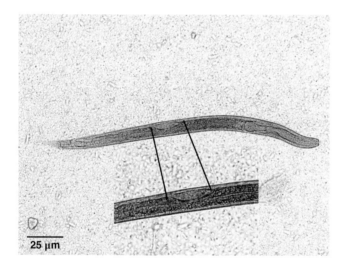

Fig. 1.88 Iodine-stained *Strongyloides* first-stage larva. The prominent genital rudiment (*inset*) and a straight tail lacking accessory spines are helpful in identifying first-stage *Strongyloides* larvae.

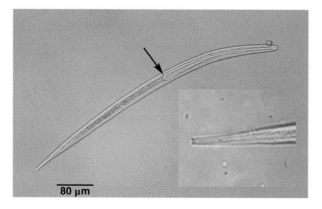

Fig. 1.89 To confirm identification of *S. stercoralis*, the fecal sample can be cultured for 2–4 days and examined for third-stage larvae, which have a distinctively long esophagus *(arrow indicates junction of esophagus and intestine)* and a double-pronged tail tip (inset). Photo courtesy of Dr. Yoko Nagamori, College of Veterinary Medicine, Oklahoma State University, Stillwater, OK.

Parasite: ***Aelurostrongylus abstrusus*** (Figs. 1.90 and 1.91)

Taxonomy: Nematode (order Strongylida).

Geographic Distribution: Worldwide.

Location in Host: Lung parenchyma (terminal respiratory bronchioles, alveolar ducts) of cats. Reports of canine infection based on fecal examination are most likely spurious parasitism due to coprophagy.

Life Cycle: First-stage larvae are released in the airways, coughed up, swallowed, and passed out in the feces. Cats are infected by ingesting a snail or slug intermediate host or paratenic hosts (rodents, birds).

Laboratory Diagnosis: First-stage larvae are detected in feces using the Baermann technique (most reliable) or by $ZnSO_4$ centrifugal flotation. The first-stage larval tail has a severe kink (S-shaped curve) and a dorsal spine.

   Size: 360–400 × 15–20 μm

Clinical Importance: Infrequently diagnosed; infected animals may suffer signs of chronic cough and anorexia. Heavy infection may be fatal.

Parasite: ***Crenosoma vulpis*** (Figs. 1.25, 1.92)

Taxonomy: Nematode (order Strongylida).

Geographic Distribution: Northeastern North America and Europe.

Location in Host: Bronchioles, bronchi, and trachea of dogs, foxes, and various wild carnivores.

Life Cycle: Canid definitive hosts are infected by ingestion of slug/terrestrial snail intermediate hosts containing third-stage larvae. Larvae produced in the respiratory system by adult worms are coughed up, swallowed, and passed from the host in feces.

Laboratory Diagnosis: Detection of first-stage larvae in feces using the Baermann technique (most reliable) or by $ZnSO_4$ centrifugal fecal flotation. First-stage larvae tend to assume a C shape when they are killed by gentle heat or iodine. The terminus of the tail has a slight deflection but does not show the kink and spine seen in other nematode lungworms.

   Size: 264–340 × 16–22 μm

Clinical Importance: *Crenosoma vulpis* infection in dogs produces a nonfatal chronic cough. Canine infection is generally rare in North America, except in the Atlantic Canadian provinces, where crenosomosis is a frequent cause of chronic respiratory disease.

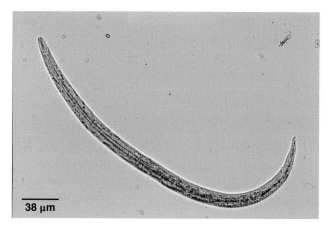

38 μm

Fig. 1.90 *Aelurostrongylus* larva in a feline fecal sample. Larvae have the distinctive S-shaped kink at the end of the tail that is typical of many members of this group of lungworms. These larvae also show a subterminal spine (Fig. 1.91).

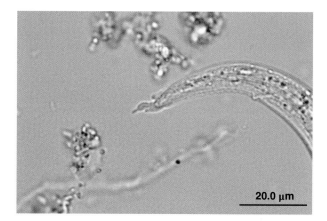

20.0 μm

Fig. 1.91 Detail of the tail of *Aelurostrongylus abstrusus* larva showing its characteristic subterminal spine that would be absent in other larvae found in feline feces. For further information on identification of lungworm larvae, see the section in this chapter "Identification of Nematode Larvae Recovered with Fecal Flotation or Baermann Procedures."

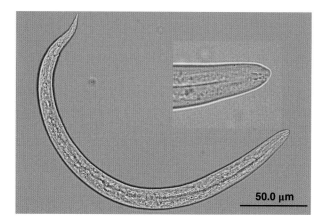

50.0 μm

Fig. 1.92 The tail of *Crenosoma* larvae has a slight deflection but lacks a definite kink or dorsal spine, allowing it to be differentiated from other lungworms. At the anterior end is a small cephalic button (inset). Larvae of *Crenosoma* can be differentiated from those of *Strongyloides* based on the morphology of the esophagus (Fig. 1.25).

Parasite: *Angiostrongylus vasorum* (Fig. 1.93)

Common name: French heartworm.

Taxonomy: Nematode (order Strongylida).

Geographic Distribution: Canada, Europe, South America, Africa. There is a single report of *A. vasorum* in a fox in the eastern United States based on histopathologic findings, but its endemicity has not been established.

Location in Host: Pulmonary arteries, right ventricle of dogs and foxes.

Life Cycle: First-stage larvae are passed in canine feces, and slugs, snails, and frogs act as intermediate hosts of the parasite. Frogs and birds also serve as paratenic hosts. Dogs and foxes are infected when they ingest intermediate hosts or paratenic hosts.

Laboratory Diagnosis: First-stage larvae in fresh feces are detected using the Baermann technique (most reliable) or fecal flotation. The larvae have a cephalic button on the anterior end, and there is a severe kink (S-shaped curve) in the tail, which has a dorsal spine.

Size: 340–399 × 13–17 µm

Clinical Importance: The parasite is a serious pathogen of dogs, causing potentially fatal cardiopulmonary disease. Ocular and central nervous system disease and bleeding disorders have also been reported.

Parasite: *Oslerus (= Filaroides) osleri* (Figs. 1.94 and 1.95)

Taxonomy: Nematode (order Strongylida). Two other closely related species (*Filaroides hirthi*, *F. milksi*) occur in the respiratory system of dogs but are rare and even more rarely cause disease.

Geographic Distribution: Worldwide.

Location in Host: Lumenal nodules in the tracheal bifurcation in dogs, coyotes, wolves, dingoes, and foxes.

Life Cycle: Infection follows ingestion of first-stage larvae from sputum or vomitus of an infected dog or other canid. This life cycle varies from that of other strongylid lungworms because the first larval stage is infective for the definitive host. Typically, the third larval stage is the infective form.

Laboratory Diagnosis: Diagnosis is best achieved by visual observation of the nodules on tracheal endoscopic examination. First-stage larvae may be detected in feces by $ZnSO_4$ centrifugal flotation or in transtracheal wash samples. The Baermann technique is *not* the method of choice because larvae passed in the feces are usually moribund or dead. The tail of the first-stage larva has an S-shaped sinus wave curve but lacks a dorsal spine. The first-stage larvae of *O. osleri* are indistinguishable from those of *F. hirthi*.

Size:	Larvae recovered from feces	232–266 µm
	Larvae recovered from trachea	325–378 µm

Clinical Importance: This is an uncommon infection in dogs in North America. Younger animals tend to be more severely affected than older ones. Respiratory distress, chronic cough, and weight loss can occur. Heavily infected animals may die.

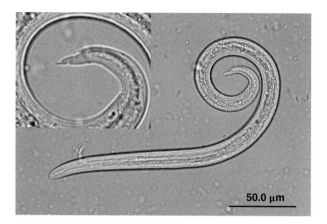

Fig. 1.93 *Angiostrongylus vasorum* first-stage larva. This species is uncommon in North America. Larvae can be differentiated from those of *Filaroides* and *Oslerus* in canine feces by the presence of the subterminal dorsal spine. The inset shows the S-shaped curve and the dorsal spine. The tail of *Aelurostrongylus abstrusus* (Fig. 1.91) is similar in appearance.

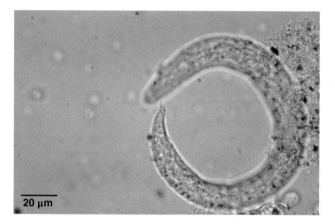

Fig. 1.94 First-stage *Oslerus* larva in dog feces. The larvae have a kinked tail, but the accessory spine seen in *Aelurostrongylus* and *Angiostrongylus* larvae is not present. Photo courtesy of Dr. Jeffrey F. Williams, Vanson HaloSource, Inc., Redmond, WA.

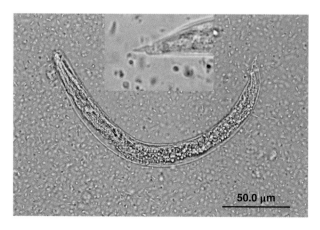

Fig. 1.95 First-stage larva of *Filaroides hirthi*, which is similar in appearance to *Oslerus osleri* and *Filaroides milksi*. The inset shows the tail with a kink, but not an accessory spine.

Parasite: ***Ollulanus tricuspis*** (Fig. 1.96)

Taxonomy: Nematode (order Strongylida).

Geographic Distribution: Europe, North America, parts of South America, Australia.

Location in Host: Adult worms are found in the stomach of cats and other felids.

Life Cycle: Adult female worms in the stomach produce third-stage larvae that primarily leave the host in vomitus. Infection of cats occurs through ingestion of these larvae in vomitus.

Laboratory Diagnosis: Infection is diagnosed by identification of larvae or the small adults in vomitus, using the Baermann test. Rarely, stages of the parasite may be seen in feces, but they are usually digested before reaching the environment.

Size:	Third-stage larvae	500 μm
	Adults	700–1000 μm

Clinical Importance: Infection can cause chronic gastritis and vomiting in cats. Colony and feral cats are most often infected.

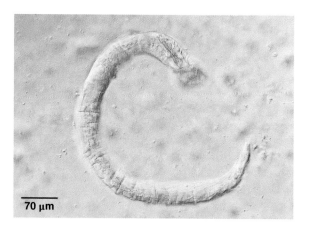

Fig. 1.96   Adult male *Ollulanus tricuspis* in a fecal sample. Larvae and adult worms are only rarely present in feces. Vomitus should be examined to diagnose infection. These worms can easily be differentiated from ascarids that may be vomited up by cats. The ascarid worms are several inches in length, while *Ollulanus* adults only reach a maximum length of 1 mm. Photo courtesy of Dr. Robert Ridley, College of Veterinary Medicine, Kansas State University, Manhattan, KS.

Parasite: ***Dipylidium caninum*** (Figs. 1.97–1.99, 1.105, 1.106)

Common name: Double-pored or cucumber seed or flea tapeworm.

Taxonomy: Cestode.

Geographic Distribution: Worldwide.

Location in Host: Small intestine of dogs and cats.

Life Cycle: Animals acquire infection through the ingestion of larval cysticercoids contained in fleas or, less frequently, in chewing lice (*Trichodectes*, *Felicola*). Arthropod intermediate hosts become infected by the ingestion of egg packets/segments.

Laboratory Diagnosis: Tapeworm segments in the perianal area or in feces are often observed by owners. Specific diagnosis is made by identification of egg packets recovered from segments. Occasionally, eggs and/or egg packets are detected on fecal flotation examinations, but flotation is very insensitive and most infections will be missed.

Size:	Egg packets	120–200 µm (contain an average of 25–30 eggs)
	Eggs	35–60 µm

Clinical Importance: Infections of this common tapeworm are generally subclinical; however, the passage of segments from the rectum may induce anal pruritus. *Dipylidium caninum* is zoonotic, with young children at greatest risk of acquiring infections from ingesting the infected flea or louse intermediate host.

DOGS AND CATS

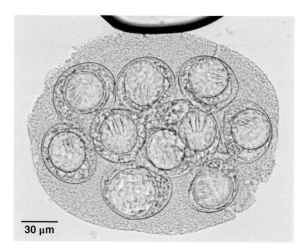

Fig. 1.97 *Dipylidium caninum* eggs, each containing a hexacanth embryo, occur in packets of about 25–30 eggs. The hooks are readily visible inside the eggs shown here. (Conboy, Gary. Cestodes of Dogs and Cats in North America. Veterinary Clinics of North America: Small Animal Practice. Elsevier, 2009.)

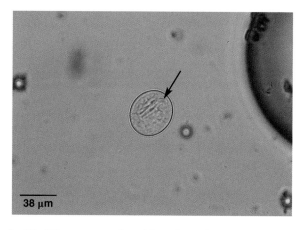

Fig. 1.98 Occasionally, *Dipylidium* eggs are released from the packets and may be detected individually on fecal flotation. Note the clear, thin shell wall of the egg and the refractile hooks (*arrow*) of the embryo.

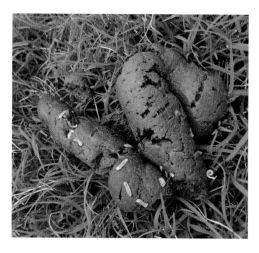

Fig. 1.99 *Dipylidium caninum* segments on the surface of a canine fecal sample. Photo courtesy of Dr. Kathryn Duncan, College of Veterinary Medicine, Oklahoma State University, Stillwater, OK.

Parasite: ***Taenia* spp.** (Figs. 1.100–1.103, 1.105, 1.106)

Taxonomy: Cestode. Numerous species infect small animals, including *T. taeniaeformis* in cats and *T. pisiformis*, *T.* (=*Multiceps*) *multiceps*, *T. hydatigena*, *T. ovis* in dogs.

Geographic Distribution: Worldwide.

Location in Host: Small intestine of dogs, cats, and various wild carnivores.

Life Cycle: Carnivores acquire infections through the ingestion of the immature meta-cestode stage (morphologic forms include cysticerci, coenuri, and strobilocerci) in the tissues of prey animals. Prey animals become infected with the metacestode through the ingestion of food contaminated with eggs passed in carnivore feces.

Laboratory Diagnosis: Eggs are detected when free in the feces by flotation techniques. Generally, however, eggs are passed from the host contained in tapeworm segments. Therefore, fecal flotation tends to be a poor indicator of infection status.

Size: 25–40 μm in diameter

Clinical Importance: Infections in the definitive host are generally subclinical; however, the passage of segments from the rectum may induce anal pruritus. *Taenia taeniaeformis* (small-rodent intermediate host) and *T. pisiformis* (rabbit intermediate host) are common species infecting pet cats and dogs, respectively. Metacestode infection in the intermediate hosts can cause disease (*T. multiceps*) or meat condemnation (*T. ovis*).

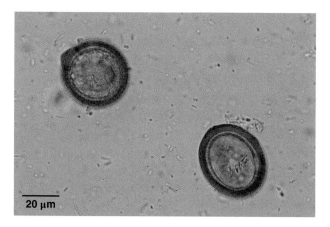

Fig. 1.100 *Taenia* eggs are brown with a thick shell wall (embryophore) and contain a hexacanth embryo (six hooks). Three-four refractile hooks are visible in the egg on the lower right of the photo. Note the radial striations in the wall of the egg.

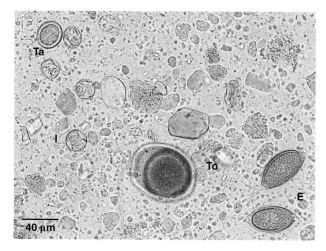

Fig. 1.101 Eggs of *Eucoleus* (E), *Toxocara* (To), and *Taenia* (Ta) and oocysts of *Cystoisospora* (I) in a feline fecal sample. Photo courtesy of Dr. Robert Ridley, College of Veterinary Medicine, Kansas State University, Manhattan, KS.

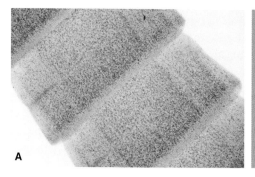

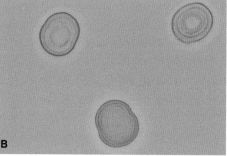

Fig. 1.102 Tapeworm segments from an animal (A) can usually be easily identified as such by squashing the segment between two slides and identifying the eggs. Sometimes, however, segments are passed that contain no eggs. These can still be identified as segments by observing the numerous small, round, transparent bodies, called "calcareous corpuscles," which produce the stippled effect (A) and are shown at higher magnification in (B). Photo (B) courtesy of Dr. Manigandan LeJeune, Animal Health Diagnostic Center, Cornell University, Ithaca, NY.

Parasite: ***Echinococcus*** spp. (Figs. 1.103, 1.105, 1.106)

Common name: Dwarf dog or fox tapeworm.

Taxonomy: Cestode. A number of species are found worldwide infecting domestic and wild canids and felids. *Echinococcus granulosus*, *E. canadensis* and *E. multilocularis* have the widest distribution and all infect dogs and wild canids. Cats can be infrequently infected with *E. multilocularis*.

Geographic Distribution: *Echinococcus granulosus* and *E. canadensis* are found worldwide; *E. multilocularis* occurs in the United States, Canada, and in parts of Europe and Asia.

Location in Host: Small intestine.

Life Cycle: Carnivores acquire infections through the ingestion of larvae (metacestodes) in the tissues of prey animals. Prey animals become infected with the metacestode through the ingestion of eggs passed in carnivore feces.

Laboratory Diagnosis: Like the eggs of *Taenia*, *Echinococcus* eggs have a thick shell wall with radial striations (embryophore). The six hooks of the hexacanth embryo allow it to be distinguished from pollen grains or other debris. The eggs of *Taenia* and *Echinococcus* are morphologically identical.

Size: 25–40 μm in diameter

Clinical Importance: Adult parasite infections in the definitive host are subclinical. *Echinococcus* spp. are important due to their zoonotic potential. Human infection with the metacestode stage can cause serious disease and death. Rarely, the metacestode stage can develop in dogs that ingest eggs. Resulting disease is similar to that seen in humans.

Parasite: ***Mesocestoides*** spp. (Figs. 1.104–1.106)

Taxonomy: Cestode. Species include *M. canislagopodis*, *M. lineatus*, *M. literatus*, *M. vogae*.

Geographic Distribution: Worldwide (except Australia).

Location in Host: Small intestine of dogs, cats, various wild mammals, and birds.

Life Cycle: The life cycle is not completely known. Dogs and cats acquire infections through ingestion of tetrathyridia contained in the tissues of various reptile, amphibian, bird, and mammal intermediate hosts. Eggs are passed in motile segments in the feces of infected dogs and cats. The first intermediate host and the form of the first larval stage of *Mesocestoides* are unknown.

Laboratory Diagnosis: Club-shaped segments are passed in the feces. Eggs are contained in a round parauterine organ at the broad end of the segment. Eggs are rarely found free in the feces of definitive hosts but would, presumably, be detected by fecal flotation.

Size: Eggs 30–40 μm in diameter

Clinical Importance: Infection of the definitive host with the adult tapeworm is usually subclinical. Fatal peritonitis due to large numbers of tetrathyridia or acephalic metacestodes has been reported in dogs acting as hosts to the larval stages.

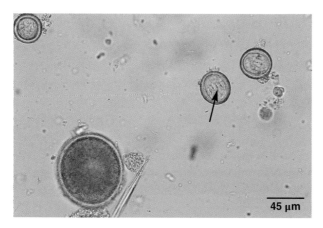

Fig. 1.103   Embryonic hooks are visible in the two *Taenia* or *Echinococcus* eggs in this photo (*arrow*). Hooks can be used to differentiate tapeworm eggs from similar artifacts like pollen grains. The eggs of *Taenia* and *Echinococcus* are morphologically identical. A *Toxocara* egg is also present.

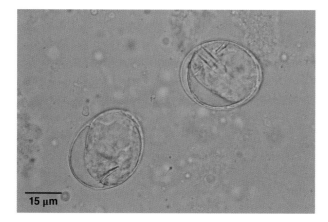

Fig. 1.104   *Mesocestoides* eggs have a thin, clear, smooth shell wall and contain a hexacanth embryo. The hooks of the embryo are readily visible.

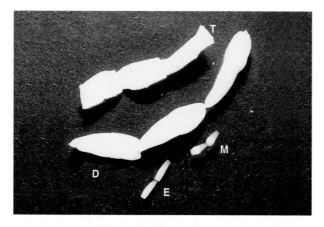

Fig. 1.105   Mature tapeworm segments passed in the feces may be observed by owners and presented for identification. The size and shape of these segments are quite characteristic: *Taenia* segments (T) are square to rectangular in shape, *Dipylidium* segments (D) are more barrel-shaped, and *Mesocestoides* has club-shaped segments (M). *Echinococcus* (E) segments are small and are often overlooked. Identification can be confirmed by examining eggs from the segments.

Parasite: ***Diphyllobothrium (=Dibothriocephalus) latum*** (Fig. 1.107)

Common name: Broad fish tapeworm.

Taxonomy: Cestode. Dogs and cats can also be infected with *D. dendriticum*.

Geographic Distribution: Northern Hemisphere and South America.

Location in Host: Small intestine of dogs, cats, pigs, humans, and various other fish-eating mammals.

Life Cycle: Eggs passed in the feces of the final host hatch coracidia, which are ingested by freshwater copepods (first intermediate hosts). Fish eat the copepods containing the next larval stage (procercoids), which develop into the plerocercoids (infective stage) in the fish. Predatory fish can acquire plerocercoids through ingestion of infected smaller fish. Mammalian definitive hosts acquire infections through the ingestion of plerocercoids contained in the tissues of fish.

Laboratory Diagnosis: The eggs can be detected in feces using a sedimentation technique. Lengths of reproductively spent segments are occasionally passed in the feces.

Size: Eggs 58–76 × 40–51 μm

Clinical Importance: Uncommon in pets in North America. Infections are generally subclinical in dogs and cats. Dogs and cats do not serve as direct sources of infection for humans. Human infection with this tapeworm may lead to the development of vitamin B_{12} deficiency.

Parasite: ***Spirometra*** **spp.** (Fig. 1.108)

Common name: Zipper tapeworm.

Taxonomy: Cestode.

Geographic Distribution: *Spirometra mansonoides* occurs in North and South America, and *S. erinaceieuropaei* occurs in Asia and Europe. Other species have been reported in Africa and Asia.

Location in Host: Small intestine of cats, dogs, and wild animals.

Life Cycle: Dogs and cats acquire infections by the ingestion of frogs, snakes, rodents, or birds containing plerocercoids (known as spargana). Eggs passed in the feces of dogs and cats hatch coracidia, which are eaten by freshwater copepods and develop into procercoids. The second intermediate hosts (frogs, snakes, etc.) acquire plerocercoids by feeding on the copepods.

Laboratory Diagnosis: The yellow-brown eggs can be detected in feces using a sedimentation technique but are also often recovered in flotation procedures. Lengths of reproductively spent segments are occasionally passed in the feces.

Size: Eggs 65–70 × 35–37 μm

Clinical Importance: Infections in the definitive hosts are usually subclinical, although vomiting has been reported. Cats can also serve as paratenic hosts, with plerocercoids surviving in various tissues (sparganosis) and causing clinical signs depending on location.

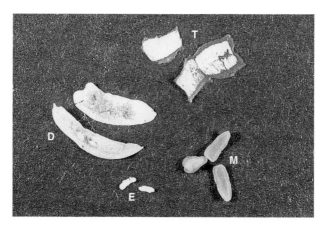

Fig. 1.106 Within hours of passing from the host, tapeworm segments lose their motility and dry up. Clients may find dried tapeworm segments in resting areas of dogs and cats. The dried segments still retain their characteristic shape. Shown in this photo are *Taenia* (T), *Echinococcus* (E), *Dipylidium* (D), and *Mesocestoides* (M) segments.

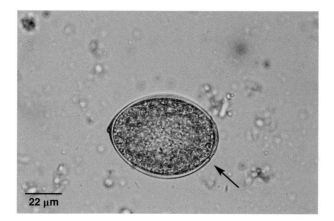

22 μm

Fig. 1.107 Unlike common tapeworms, *Diphyllobothrium* eggs lack hooks and resemble trematode eggs. They are light brown and operculate (*arrow*). They contain an undifferentiated embryo surrounded by yolk cells that completely fill the space within the eggshell. A pore in the shell wall at the pole opposite to the operculum is often visible due to the slight bit of protein protruding from it.

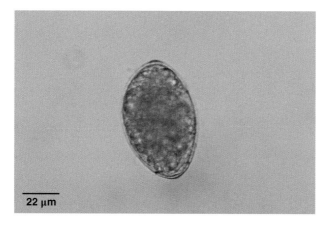

22 μm

Fig. 1.108 The operculate eggs of *Spirometra* also resemble trematode eggs. They contain an undifferentiated embryo and yolk cells completely fill the space within the eggshell. The eggs are asymmetrical about the long axis. The operculum in this egg is at the lower end.

Parasite: *Alaria* spp. (Figs. 1.109 and 1.110)

Taxonomy: Trematode.

Geographic Distribution: Worldwide.

Location in Host: Small intestine of dogs, cats, and various wild carnivores.

Life Cycle: Eggs are passed in the feces of the mammalian host. Following larval development in a snail intermediate host, a second intermediate host (frog) is infected. Infection of dogs and cats occurs by ingestion of frogs or various paratenic hosts harboring the larval stage (mesocercaria). Transmammary transmission has been reported in cats.

Laboratory Diagnosis: The most reliable method is detection of eggs by sedimentation examination of feces, although sometimes eggs may be detected on fecal flotation.

Size: 98–134 × 62–68 μm

Clinical Importance: Infections are generally nonpathogenic in dogs and cats. *Alaria* is a potentially serious zoonotic risk to humans through the ingestion of raw or improperly cooked frogs containing mesocercaria.

Parasite: *Paragonimus kellicotti* (Fig. 1.111)

Taxonomy: Trematode.

Geographic Distribution: North America. Other species of *Paragonimus* that infect domestic animals, humans, and wildlife occur in South and Central America, Africa, and Asia.

Location in Host: Lung parenchyma of cats, dogs, pigs, goats, minks, and various other wild mammals.

Life Cycle: Snails are infected by miracidia that emerge from eggs released in the feces of definitive hosts. Crayfish serve as the second intermediate host. Dogs and cats acquire infection by ingesting the metacercaria in the tissues of crayfish or paratenic hosts.

Laboratory Diagnosis: A sedimentation technique (recommended) or fecal flotation (less reliable) can be used to detect the yellow-brown, operculate eggs, which have a thickened ridge in the shell wall along the line of the operculum. Cysts may be evident on radiographs.

Size: 75–118 × 42–67 μm

Clinical Importance: Infection may be subclinical or cause eosinophilic bronchitis and granulomatous pneumonia, resulting in chronic cough and lethargy. In some cases pneumothorax may develop due to rupture of cysts. Infections can be fatal.

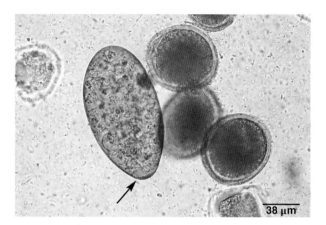

Fig. 1.109 *Alaria* eggs are large, operculate, yellow-brown in color and contain an undifferentiated embryo surrounded by yolk cells. The operculum in this egg is difficult to see but is marked by a slight discontinuity in the shell (*arrow*). *Toxocara* eggs are also present. Photo courtesy of Dr. Yoko Nagamori, College of Veterinary Medicine, Oklahoma State University, Stillwater, OK.

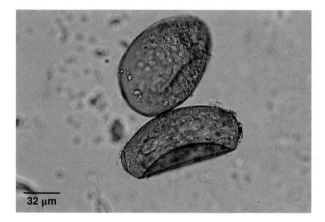

Fig. 1.110 Sometimes *Alaria* spp. eggs are detected using the centrifugal flotation technique; however, egg morphology may be altered: the eggs appear collapsed or folded due to the osmotic pressure associated with the high specific gravity of the flotation solution.

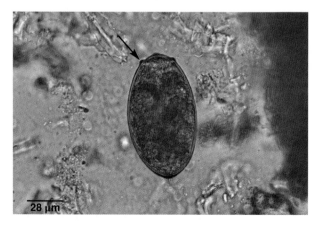

Fig. 1.111 *Paragonimus* eggs have an undifferentiated embryo when passed in the feces. The yellow-brown, operculate eggs can be identified by the characteristic thickened ridge in the shell wall along the line of the operculum (*arrow*). Collapsed eggs may be seen in flotation preparations.

Parasite: **Nanophyetus salmincola** (Fig. 1.112)

Common name: Salmon poisoning fluke.

Taxonomy: Trematode.

Geographic Distribution: Pacific Northwest region of North America.

Location in Host: Small intestine of dogs, cats, and various other piscivorous carnivores.

Life Cycle: Dogs and cats are infected by the ingestion of metacercariae in the tissues of salmonid fish (second intermediate hosts). Snails serve as the first intermediate host.

Laboratory Diagnosis: Eggs can be detected by sedimentation examination of feces.

Size: 72–97 × 35–55 μm

Clinical Importance: *Nanophyetus salmincola* serves as a vector for the causal agent of salmon poisoning disease (*Neorickettsia helminthoeca*) and Elokomin fluke fever (*Neorickettsia* sp.). Salmon poisoning disease is extremely pathogenic in dogs.

Parasite: **Heterobilharzia americana** (Figs. 1.113 and 1.114)

Taxonomy: Trematode.

Geographic Distribution: Southeast and south-central United States.

Location in Host: Mesenteric and hepatic portal veins of dogs and various wildlife species.

Life Cycle: Eggs released in the feces of dogs produce ciliated larvae (miracidia) that develop in a snail intermediate host. Cercariae that are released from the snail intermediate host infect dogs and wildlife through direct skin penetration.

Laboratory Diagnosis: Eggs can be detected by sedimentation examination of feces in saline (or 5% formol-saline). It is important to use saline in the procedure because eggs are stimulated to hatch when they contact water. The free-swimming miracidia can be observed by placing the sediment in water after performing the sedimentation procedure with saline.

Size: Eggs 74–113 × 60–80 μm

Clinical Importance: Infection with *H. americana* in dogs is uncommon in most areas, Infection can cause chronic diarrhea, anorexia, and emaciation. *Heterobilharzia* also has zoonotic importance as one of the causal agents of cercarial dermatitis (swimmer's itch) in humans.

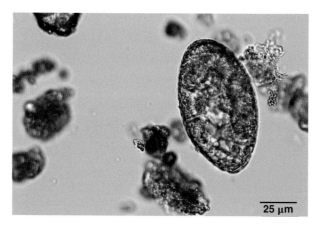

Fig. 1.112 The operculated eggs of *Nanophyetus* contain an undifferentiated embryo surrounded by yolk cells.

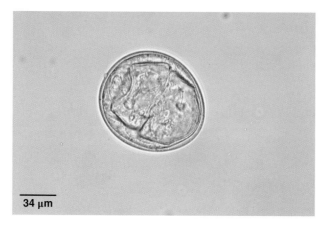

Fig. 1.113 The large, elliptical eggs of *Heterobilharzia americana* have a smooth, thin shell wall and contain a fully formed miracidium. The shell wall of the egg lacks an operculum. Photo courtesy of Dr. Bruce Hammerberg and Dr. James Flowers, College of Veterinary Medicine, North Carolina State University, Raleigh, NC.

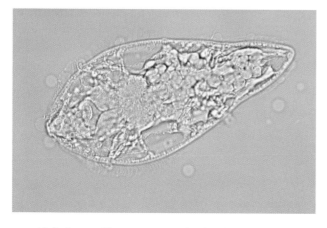

Fig. 1.114 On contact with freshwater, *H. americana* eggs hatch, releasing a ciliated miracidium stage. To prevent hatching of the eggs, a sedimentation procedure for diagnosis should be performed using saline instead of water. Photo courtesy of Dr. Bruce Hammerberg and Dr. James Flowers, College of Veterinary Medicine, North Carolina State University, Raleigh, NC.

Parasite: ***Platynosomum concinnum*** (also known as *P. fastosum, P. illiciens*) (Figs. 1.115, 1.116)

Common name: Lizard poisoning fluke.

Taxonomy: Trematode.

Geographic Distribution: Southeastern United States, South America, Caribbean, West Africa. Other flukes that may be found in the bile or pancreatic ducts in North America include *Eurytrema procyonis, Metorchis conjunctus* and *Parametorchis* spp.

Location in Host: Gall bladder and bile ducts of cats.

Life Cycle: Adult worms produce eggs that are passed in the feces of cats. The life cycle is complex, involving snail, crustacean, and amphibian or reptile intermediate hosts. Cats are infected following ingestion of lizards or amphibians containing larvae.

Laboratory Diagnosis: A sedimentation procedure is most effective for recovering the relatively small, operculate eggs of *Platynosomum*.

Size: 34–50 × 20–35 μm

Clinical Significance: Light infections are asymptomatic. Heavily infected cats may show signs of weight loss and hepatomegaly that can be severe and fatal.

Parasite: ***Cryptocotyle lingua*** (Fig. 1.117)

Taxonomy: Trematode.

Geographic Distribution: Northern temperate marine coastal regions of the world.

Location in Host: Intestine.

Life Cycle: Snails are infected by larval stages emerging from eggs released in the feces of infected definitive hosts. Fish serve as the second intermediate host. Dogs, cats, and birds become infected by ingesting metacercariae, visible as small black spots on the skin of fish.

Laboratory Diagnosis: A sedimentation technique (recommended) or fecal flotation (less reliable) can be used to detect these small, undifferentiated, yellow-brown, operculate eggs. The eggs are elliptical-shaped with one end narrower than the other. The operculum occurs at the narrower end and is difficult to see.

Size: 32–50 × 18–25 μm

Clinical Significance: Clinical disease due to infection with this intestinal fluke appears to be rare. Enteritis may occur in cases of heavy infections. Cats appear to be less susceptible to infection.

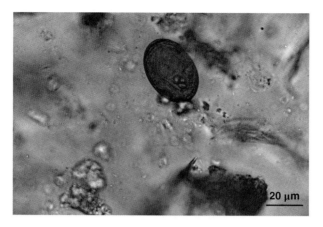

Fig. 1.115 The small brown eggs of *Platynosomum* have an operculum at one end, contain a fully formed miracidium, and may not be seen with routine flotation procedures. Photo courtesy of Dr. Heather Walden, College of Veterinary Medicine, University of Florida, Gainesville, FL.

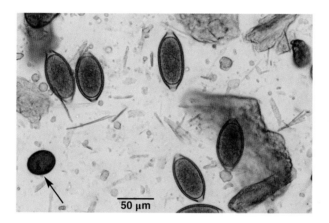

Fig. 1.116 *Platynosomum* (arrow) and *Trichuris* eggs in the feces of a cat. Both parasites are unlikely to be encountered in the United States outside the southeast. Photo courtesy of Dr. Jennifer Ketzis, School of Veterinary Medicine, Ross University, St. Kitts, W.I.

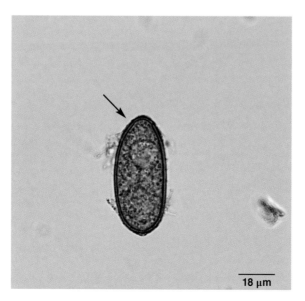

Fig. 1.117 *Cryptocotyle lingua* egg detected on fecal sedimentation of feces from a dog. The operculum of *Cryptocotyle* is difficult to see; it occurs on the narrower pole of the egg (*arrow*). The eggs are undifferentiated when passed in the feces.

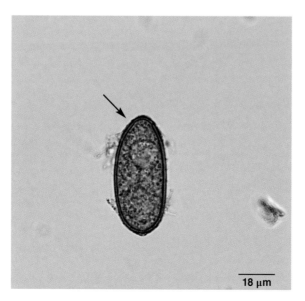

Parasite: *Metorchis* **spp.,** *Eurytrema* **spp.** (Fig. 1.118)

Taxonomy: Trematode.

Geographic Distribution: Europe, Asia, North America.

Location in Host: Bile ducts and gallbladder (*Metorchis*), pancreatic ducts (*Eurytrema*) of wild carnivores, rarely dogs and cats.

Life Cycle: Snails are infected by larval stages emerging from eggs in feces of definitive hosts that become infected following ingestion of a second intermediate host (fish in the case of *Metorchis* and probably an arthropod for *Eurytrema*).

Laboratory Diagnosis: A sedimentation technique would be most effective.

Size: *Metorchis* 24–30 × 13–16 µm, *Eurytrema* 45–53 × 29–36 µm

Clinical Significance: Infection in dogs and cats is rare, but may be associated with disease of infected organ.

Parasite: *Linguatula* **spp.** (Fig. 1.119)

Taxonomy: Pentastomid.

Geographic Distribution: Most infections from Africa and Asia.

Location in Host: Nasal passages, frontal sinuses of canids and, less often, felids.

Life Cycle: Eggs shed in nasal discharge or feces of infected hosts. Herbivores are intermediate hosts with larvae in tissues infecting the final host when ingested.

Laboratory Diagnosis: Centrifugal fecal flotation with solutions of ≥1.25 SG.

Size: 90–133 × 54–88 µm

Clinical Significance: In dogs infection may be asymptomatic or produce increased nasal discharge and sneezing. Humans can serve as intermediate hosts or, rarely, definitive hosts.

Parasite: *Macracanthorhynchus ingens* (Fig. 1.120)

Taxonomy: Acanthocephala.

Geographic Distribution: North America.

Location in Host: Intestine of raccoons, black bears, rarely dogs.

Life Cycle: Eggs shed in feces of infected hosts. Larvae infect definitive hosts when millipede intermediate hosts carrying larvae are ingested.

Laboratory Diagnosis: A sedimentation test would be most effective for detecting eggs.

Size: 90–110 × 50–65 µm

Clinical Significance: Dogs are rarely infected with this parasite.

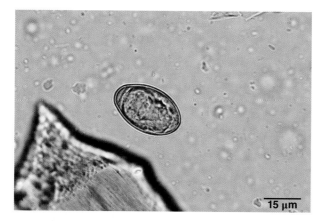

Fig. 1.118   *Metorchis* is another genus of flukes present in wild animals that may occasionally infect dogs and cats.

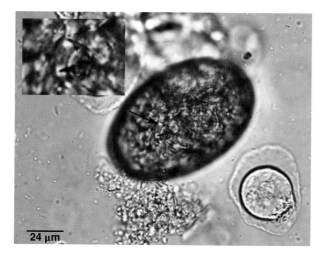

Fig. 1.119   Large eggs of *Linguatula* may be seen in dogs in North America with a history of travel to an endemic area. Careful examination at high power should reveal the presence of several hooks, in the parasite embryo (arrow and inset). Photo courtesy of Dr. Yoko Nagamori, College of Veterinary Medicine, Oklahoma State University, Stillwater, OK.

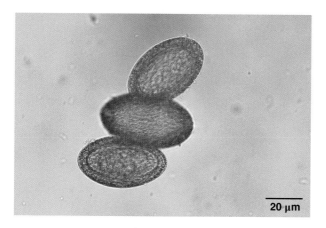

Fig. 1.120   *Macracanthorhynchus ingens* eggs. Acanthocephalan eggs contain a larva with spines, which may be seen inside eggs. Dogs are also rarely infected with another acanthocephalan parasite, *Oncicola canis*. Photo courtesy of Dr. Heather Walden, College of Veterinary Medicine, University of Florida, Gainesville, FL.

Ruminants and Camelids

Helminth Eggs, Larvae and Protozoan Cysts
found in freshly voided feces of
Cattle

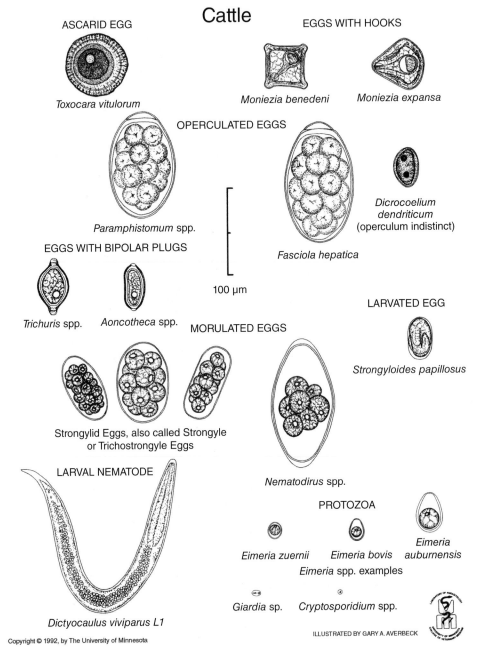

ASCARID EGG

Toxocara vitulorum

EGGS WITH HOOKS

Moniezia benedeni

Moniezia expansa

OPERCULATED EGGS

Paramphistomum spp.

Dicrocoelium dendriticum (operculum indistinct)

Fasciola hepatica

EGGS WITH BIPOLAR PLUGS

Trichuris spp.

Aoncotheca spp.

100 µm

LARVATED EGG

Strongyloides papillosus

MORULATED EGGS

Strongylid Eggs, also called Strongyle or Trichostrongyle Eggs

Nematodirus spp.

LARVAL NEMATODE

PROTOZOA

Eimeria zuernii

Eimeria bovis

Eimeria auburnensis

Eimeria spp. examples

Giardia sp.

Cryptosporidium spp.

Dictyocaulus viviparus L1

ILLUSTRATED BY GARY A. AVERBECK

Fig. 1.121   Parasites found in bovine feces. Figure courtesy of Dr. Bert Stromberg and Mr. Gary Averbeck, College of Veterinary Medicine, University of Minnesota, Minneapolis, MN.

Helminth Eggs, Larvae and Protozoan Cysts
found in freshly voided feces of
Sheep, Goats and Camelids

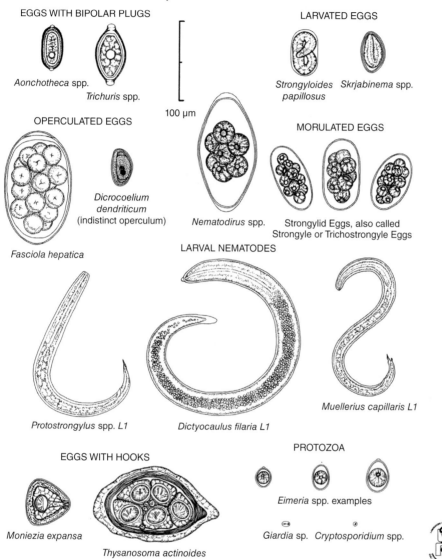

EGGS WITH BIPOLAR PLUGS

Aonchotheca spp.

Trichuris spp.

100 μm

LARVATED EGGS

Strongyloides   Skrjabinema spp.
papillosus

OPERCULATED EGGS

Dicrocoelium
dendriticum
(indistinct operculum)

Fasciola hepatica

MORULATED EGGS

Nematodirus spp.   Strongylid Eggs, also called
Strongyle or Trichostrongyle Eggs

LARVAL NEMATODES

Muellerius capillaris L1

Protostrongylus spp. L1   Dictyocaulus filaria L1

EGGS WITH HOOKS

Moniezia expansa

Thysanosoma actinoides

PROTOZOA

Eimeria spp. examples

Giardia sp. Cryptosporidium spp.

ILLUSTRATED BY GARY A. AVERBECK

RUMINANTS AND
CAMELIDS

Fig. 1.122   Parasites found in feces of sheep and goats. Figure courtesy of Dr. Bert Stromberg and Mr. Gary Averbeck, College of Veterinary Medicine, University of Minnesota, Minneapolis, MN.

Table 1.7. Representative treatments for selected parasites of ruminants and camelids

Parasite	Effective treatments	Dose, route, and regimen
Cryptosporidium parvum	[a]Halofuginone lactate	Administer according to label directions. Begin within 48 h of birth for prevention, within 24 h of diarrhea for treatment
Eimeria spp.	Amprolium Decoquinate Lasalocid Monensin Sulfamethiazine	Administer according to label directions for prevention or treatment. Use in small ruminants/camelids may require modification of dose
	[a]Toltrazuril	Administer according to label directions
Gastrointestinal nematodes of pastured and feedlot cattle (see label for specific indications)	Albendazole, [a]closantel, doramectin, eprinomectin, [a]febantel, fenbendazole, ivermectin, levamisole, morantel tartrate, moxidectin, [a]netobimin, oxfendazole	Administer according to label directions
Gastrointestinal nematodes of dairy cattle >20 months of age (see label for specific indications)	Eprinomectin (pour-on only), fenbendazole, morantel tartrate, moxidectin (pour-on only)	Administer according to label directions
Gastrointestinal nematodes of goats (see label for specific indications)	Albendazole, [a]closantel, [a]doramectin, fenbendazole, [a]ivermectin, [a]levamisole, morantel tartrate, [a]moxidectin	Administer according to label directions; elevated dose often required for goats
Gastrointestinal nematodes of sheep (see label for specific indications)	Albendazole, [a]closantel, [a]derquantel-abamectin, [a]doramectin, [a]febantel, [a]fenbendazole, ivermectin, levamisole, [a]mebendazole, [a]monepantel, moxidectin, [a]netobimin, [a]oxfendazole	Administer according to label directions
Dictyocaulus viviparus	Fenbendazole, eprinomectin, ivermectin, moxidectin	Administer according to label directions
Muellerius capillaris	[a]Fenbendazole, [a]ivermectin, [a]moxidectin	Effective when administered at label-approved or elevated dose
Toxocara vitulorum	[a]Doramectin (injectable), [a]fenbendazole, [a]ivermectin (injectable), [a]moxidectin (injectable)	Effective when administered at label-approved dose. Efficacy demonstrated for injectable but not pour-on macrocyclic lactones
Moniezia spp.	Albendazole	Administer according to label directions
Fasciola hepatica	Albendazole, clorsulon, [a]closantel	Administer according to label directions

[a] Not label-approved in the United States.
Additional information on parasite treatments can be found in Chapter 7.

RUMINANTS AND CAMELIDS

Protozoan Parasites

Parasite: **Eimeria spp.** (Figs. 1.46, 1.123–1.130, 1.133, 1.136, 1.145)

Common name: Coccidia.

Taxonomy: Protozoa (coccidia).

Geographic Distribution: Worldwide.

Location in Host: Many host-specific species of *Eimeria* infect the intestinal tract of domestic ruminants and camelids.

Life Cycle: Fecal oocysts sporulate in the environment and infect intestinal cells following ingestion. Asexual and sexual reproduction are followed by the production of oocysts that exit the host in manure. Sporulated oocysts can survive for long periods under favorable environmental conditions.

Laboratory Diagnosis: Oocysts are found by fecal flotation techniques. Species identification is difficult and may require microscopic exam of sporulated (infective) oocysts. Although the number of oocysts in feces has been used as an indicator of clinical disease, high numbers of oocysts can also be present in the absence of clinical signs.

Size: Approximately 12–45 µm in length (oocyst), depending on species

Clinical Importance: Most ruminants become infected with coccidia at an early age, and low-level infection persists through adulthood. While infection is often subclinical, coccidiosis is a common cause of diarrhea in young ruminants. Signs range from mild diarrhea to severe, bloody diarrhea.

Not all species of *Eimeria* are equally pathogenic. Of 12 species of common bovine *Eimeria*, clinical disease is usually associated with *E. bovis*, *E. zuernii*, or, less commonly, *E. alabamensis*. Similarly, *E. bakuensis*, *E. ahsata*, and *E. ovinoidalis* are pathogenic ovine *Eimeria* species. In goats, *E. airlongi*, *E. caprina*, *E. ninakohlyakimovae*, and *E. christenseni* have been associated with clinical disease. Fewer species of coccidia occur in camelids than in ruminants. They all have been reported to cause clinical disease, although in the United States, *E. macusaniensis* is considered most pathogenic.

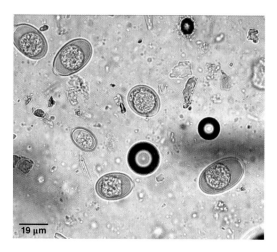

Fig. 1.123   Ruminants and camelids are infected with a variety of *Eimeria* spp. The oocysts of most of these species are colorless, have a thin wall, and are oval or round. When seen in fresh feces, oocysts contain a single cell.

Table 1.8. **Common *Eimeria* species of cattle**

Name	Average size (μm)	Range (μm)	Length:width (range)	Notes
Eimeria alabamensis	**19 × 13**	13–25 × 11–17	Not established	• No micropyle • **Pyriform** (sub-ellipsoidal or sub-cylindrical) • Colorless to greyish lavender • Wall – thin & delicate • Mildly pathogenic
Eimeria auburnensis	**38 × 23**	32–46 × 19–28	L:W **1.67** (1.32–2.08)	• Flat micropyle • **Elongate ovoid** (sub-ellipsoidal to notably tapered) • Oocyst wall typically smooth rarely rough (mammillations) • Yellowish brown • Mildly pathogenic
Eimeria bovis	**28 × 20**	23–34 × 17–23	L:W **1.37** (1.1–1.8)	• Flat micropyle • **Stoutly egg-shaped/ovoid** (tapered towards micropylar/blunted narrow end) • Yellowish • Most pathogenic
Eimeria brasiliensis	**38 × 27**	31–49 × 21–33	Not established	• Micropyle • Polar cap (may be collapsed) • **Ovoidal** • Colorless to yellowish or pinkish • Occasionally plaques on wall • Nonpathogenic
Eimeria bukidnonensis	**47.4 × 33**	43–51 × 30–35	L:W **1.4** (1.3–1.8)	• Micropyle • **Piriform** • **Brown radially striated/speckled wall** • Mildly pathogenic
Eimeria canadensis	**33 × 23**	28–38 × 20–29	L:W **1.39** (1.2–1.6)	• Micropyle • **Ellipsoidal** but varies from cylindrical to stoutly ellipsoidal • Colorless to pale yellow • Nonpathogenic • Oocyst wall 1 μm in middle, thins as it tapers
Eimeria cylindrica	**23 × 14**	16–30 × 12–17	L:W **1.67** (1.3–2.0)	• No micropyle • **Cylindrical** (vary from ellipsoidal to narrow cylinder) • Colorless • Mildly pathogenic
Eimeria ellipsoidalis	**17 × 13**	12–27 × 10–18	L:W **1.30** (1.0–1.6)	• No micropyle • Predominantly **ellipsoidal** (also spherical to subspherical) • Colorless • Mildly pathogenic
Eimeria pellita	**40 × 28**	36–41 × 26–30	Not established	• Flat micropyle • **Ovoid** • Brown • Thick **velvety** walls • Nonpathogenic
Eimeria subspherica	**11 × 10**	9–14 × 8–13	Not established	• No micropyle • **Subspherical** but vary from spherical to bluntly ellipsoidal • Thin oocyst wall • Colorless • More **fragile appearance** compared to *E. ellipsoidalis* or *E. zuernii* • Nonpathogenic
Eimeria wyomingensis	**39.9 × 28.3**	36–44 × 26–30	Not established	• Micropyle • **Ovoid** • Yellowish-brown • Nonpathogenic
Eimeria zuernii	**17.8 × 15.6**	15–22 × 13–18	L:W **1.14** (1.0–1.4)	• No micropyle • **Spherical to bluntly ellipsoidal** • Colorless • Most pathogenic

Information compiled by Dr. Manigandan Lejeune, Animal Health Diagnostic Center, Cornell University, Ithaca, NY. *Source*: Bowman, D.D. Georgis' Parasitology for Veterinarians 11th edition. 2021. Elsevier.

RUMINANTS AND CAMELIDS

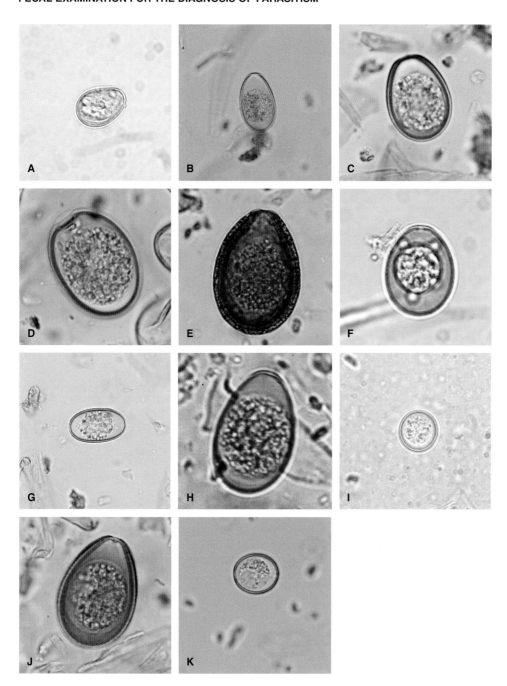

Fig. 1.124   Bovine *Eimeria* oocysts (relative sizes not accurate; see Table 1.8): (A) *E. alabamensis*, (B) *E. auburnensis*, (C) *E. bovis*, (D) *E. brasiliensis*, (E) *E. bukidnonensis*, (F) *E. canadensis*, (G) *E. cylindrica/ellipsoidalis*, (H) *E. pellita*, (I) *E. subspherica*, (J) *E. wyomingensis*, (K) *E. zuernii*. (A, F, H, I) Courtesy of Dr. Aaron Lucas, Virginia-Maryland College of Veterinary Medicine, Virginia Tech, Blacksburg, VA. Other photos courtesy of Dr. Manigandan Lejeune, Animal Health Diagnostic Center, Cornell University, Ithaca, NY.

Table 1.9. Common *Eimeria* species of sheep

Name	Goat equivalent	Average Size (µm)	Range (µm)	Length:width (range)	Notes
Eimeria ahsata	N/A	33–40 × 20–26	29–48 × 17–30	L:W **1.52** (1.1–1.8)	• Micropyle • Polar cap - dome shaped • **Ellipsoidal** to ovoid • Faint pink • Very pathogenic
Eimeria bakuensis	*Eimeria arlongi*	27–31 × 20–21	23–36 × 16–24	L:W **1.41** (1.3–1.6)	• Micropyle • Polar cap (dome- to mound-shaped) • **Ovoid to ellipsoid** (generally straight sides), Yellow-brown • Pathogenic
Eimeria crandallis	*Eimeria hirci*	22–23 × 18–19	17–28 × 14–22	L:W **1.11** (1.0–1.35)	• Micropyle • Polar cap • **Spherical to broadly ellipsoidal** • Colorless • May cause diarrhea
Eimeria faurei	*Eimeria aspheronica*	29–32 × 21–23	24–37 × 18–28	Not established	• Micropyle: 'Cup-shaped' inward projection • **Ovoid (egg-shaped)** • Light colored • Oocyst wall with faint external coat • Mildly pathogenic
Eimeria granulosa	*Eimeria jolchejevi*	29–32 × 21–24	22–37 × 17–26	Not established	• Micropyle • Polar cap prominent (easily dislodged) • Oocyst wall lightly colored with thick inner layer • **Broad shouldered urn like/piriform/bluntly ellipsoidal** • Nonpathogenic
Eimeria intricata	*Eimeria korcharli*	46–51 × 32–39	39–59 × 27–47	L:W **1.47** (1.3–1.8)	• Micropyle • Polar cap • **Ellipsoid** • Oocyst wall 3 layered-**Opaque**, rough, brown, **striated** • Mildly pathogenic
Eimeria ovinoidalis	*Eimeria ninakohlyakimovae*	23 × 18	16–28 × 14–23	L:W **1.27** (1.1–1.5)	• Micropyle barely seen • **Ovoid to ellipsoidal** • Colorless • Very pathogenic
Eimeria pallida	*Eimeria pallida*	14–15 × 10–11	12–20 × 8–15	L:W **1.43** (12–1.7)	• Micropyle not seen • **Ellipsoidal** • Oocyst wall thin, Colorless, two layered with a single dark refraction line on inner edge • Nonpathogenic • Narrower than *Eimeria parva*
Eimeria parva	*Eimeria alijevi*	15-18 × 13.5-15	12–23 × 10–19	L:W **1.18** (1.0–1.5)	• Micropyle not seen • **Roundish** • Oocyst wall pale yellow, two layered with two dark refraction lines on each side of inner layer • Mildly pathogenic
Eimeria punctata	*Eimeria punctata*	21–26 × 18–19	18–28 × 16–21	L:W **1.20** (1.1–1.3)	• Micropyle • Polar cap • **Ellipsoidal/Subspherical to ovoid** • Cone-shaped pits on wall/pitted like a thimble • Non pathogenic

Information compiled by Dr. Maniganden Lejeune, Animal Health Diagnostic Center, Cornell University, Ithaca NY. *Source*: Bowman, D.D. *Georgis' Parasitology for Veterinarians* 11th edition. 2021. Elsevier.

Table 1.10. Common *Eimeria* species of goats

Name	Sheep equivalent	Average Size (μm)	Range (μm)	Length: width (range)	Notes
Eimeria arloingi	*Eimeria bakuensis*	**28 × 21**	22–35 × 16–26	**L:W 1.3–1.6** (1.1–2.1)	• Micropyle • Polar cap • **Elongate ellipsoidal** • 2 layers (outer colorless, inner brownish yellow) • Pathogenic
Eimeria aspheronica	*Eimeria faurei*	**29–33 × 22–24**	24–37 × 18–26	**L:W 1.2–1.4** (1.1–1.6)	• Micropyle: 'Cup-shaped' inward projection • **Ovoid (egg-shaped)** • Oocyst wall colorless • A small knob associated with micropyle on inside of oocyst • Mildly pathogenic
Eimeria caprina	N/A	**32 × 23**	27–40 × 19–26	**L:W 1.4** (1.2–2.1)	• Micropyle • **Ellipsoid to oval** • 2 layers (outer brownish yellow, inner colorless) • Nonpathogenic
Eimeria caprovina	N/A	**30 × 24**	26–36 × 21–28	**L:W 1.3** (1.1–1.5)	• Micropyle • **Ellipsoidal/ovoid/subspherical** • 2 layers (outer colorless, inner brownish yellow)
Eimeria christenseni	N/A	**38–41 × 25–28**	31–46 × 22–31	**L:W 1.5–1.6** (1.2–1.8)	• Micropyle • **Ovoid** • 2 layered (outer colorless to pale yellow, Inner brownish yellow & wrinkled at micropyle end • Pathogenic
Eimeria korcharli	*Eimeria intricata*	**45 × 37**	41–50 × 34–37	Not established	• Micropyle • Polar cap • **Ellipsoid** • Oocyst wall 3 layered-**Opaque**, rough, brown, **striated** • Mildly pathogenic
Eimeria hirci	*Eimeria crandallis*	**21–23 × 16–19**	18–29 × 14–21	**L:W 1.2–1.3** (1.1–1.7)	• Micropyle • Polar cap • **Spherical to broadly ellipsoidal** • 2 layers (outer colorless, inner brownish yellow) • May cause diarrhea
Eimeria jolchejevi	*Eimeria granulosa*	**31–33 × 20–23**	26–37 × 18–26	**L:W 1.4–1.5** (1.2–1.7)	• Micropyle • Polar cap prominent (easily dislodged) • **Broad shouldered urn like**/ piriform/bluntly ellipsoidal • Oocyst wall lightly colored with thick brownish yellow inner layer • Nonpathogenic
Eimeria ninakohlyakimovae	*Eimeria ovinoidalis*	**24–25 × 18–21**	20–28 × 4–24	**L:W 1.2–1.3** (1.0–1.5)	• Micropyle barely seen • **Ovoid to ellipsoidal** • Colorless • Very pathogenic
Eimeria pallida	*Eimeria pallida*	**16 × 12**	13–18 × 10–14	**L:W 1.3** (1.2–1.6)	• Micropyle not seen • **Ellipsoidal** • Oocyst wall thin, Colorless, two layered with a single dark refraction line on inner edge • Nonpathogenic • Narrower than *Eimeria alijevi*
Eimeria alijevi	*Eimeria parva*	**17–20 × 14–19**	15–23 × 12–22	**L:W 1.1–1.2** (1.1–2.1)	• Micropyle not seen • **Roundish** • Oocyst wall pale yellow, two layered with two dark refraction lines on each side of inner layer • Mildly pathogenic • Less common in goats
Eimeria punctata	*Eimeria punctata*	**26 × 20**	21–31 × 15–23	**L:W 1.3** (1.2–1.7)	• Micropyle • Polar cap • **Ellipsoidal/Subspherical to ovoid**, greenish yellow • Cone-shaped pits on wall/pitted like a thimble • Non pathogenic

Information compiled by Dr. Maniganden Lejeune, Animal Health Diagnostic Center, Cornell University, Ithaca NY. *Source:* Bowman, D.D. *Georgis' Parasitology for Veterinarians* 11th edition. 2021. Elsevier.

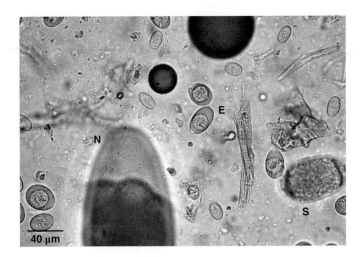

Fig. 1.125   Small ruminants are infected with a variety of coccidia species, although few are highly pathogenic. Sheep and goats are infected by different *Eimeria* spp. (E), although oocysts from the two host species are often indistinguishable. Slightly out of focus in this photo are an egg of *Nematodirus* (N) and a typical strongylid egg (S).

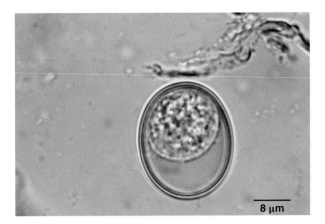

Fig. 1.126   The oocyst shown here is *E. ninakohlyakimovae* from a goat. A similar oocyst is produced by *E. ovoinodalis* in sheep. Both species can be pathogenic in their respective hosts. Photo courtesy of Dr. Manigandan Lejeune, Animal Health Diagnostic Center, Cornell University, Ithaca, NY.

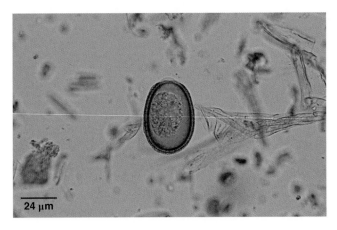

Fig. 1.127   Many, but not all, *Eimeria* species have a cap that covers the micropyle, which can be seen at the upper end of this oocyst. The micropyle cap (or polar cap), if present, is helpful in identifying the genus in dogs that have eaten feces of other animal species. The photo shows the oocyst of *Eimeria intricata*, a parasite of sheep. The oocyst is brown and larger than other ovine *Eimeria*.

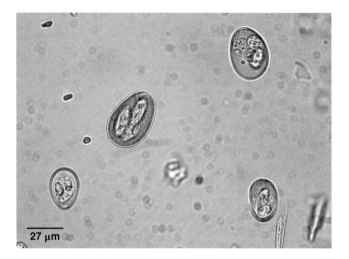

Fig. 1.128   In this bovine fecal sample, several fully sporulated *Eimeria* oocysts can be seen. In some cases, examination of the sporulated oocyst is required for confirmation of identification of the *Eimeria* species. In many clinical cases, specific identification is not performed. Photo courtesy of Dr. Aaron Lucas, Virginia-Maryland College of Veterinary Medicine, Virginia Tech, Blacksburg, VA.

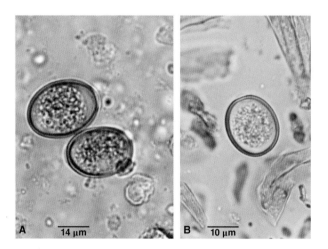

Fig. 1.129   *Eimeria llamae* (A) and the smaller *E. punonensis* (B) are coccidia of New World camelids. Photos courtesy of Dr. Manigandan Lejeune, Animal Health Diagnostic Center, Cornell University, Ithaca, NY.

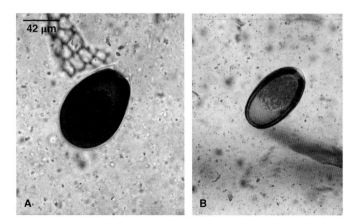

Fig. 1.130   New World camelids are also infected with two species of *Eimeria* that produce large brown oocysts, which can be confused: *E. macusaniensis* (A) and *E. ivitaensis* (B). The oocysts of *E. macusaniensis* are pear-shaped, while those of *E. ivitaensis* are more elongated and elliptical in shape.

Parasite: *Cryptosporidium* spp. (Figs. 1.131 and 1.132)

Taxonomy: Protozoa (coccidia). Ruminants are infected with several *Cryptosporidium* species, including *C. parvum, C. andersoni, C. bovis, C. ubiquitum,* and *C. xiaoi.*

Geographic Distribution: Worldwide.

Location in Host: *Cryptosporidium parvum* is an intestinal parasite of ruminants, camelids, and other mammals. Other species parasitize the small intestine or stomach (abomasum).

Life Cycle: Ruminants are infected by ingestion of oocysts. Oocysts are infective as soon as they are passed in manure and are very resistant to environmental conditions.

Laboratory Diagnosis: The small oocysts of *Cryptosporidium* spp. can be detected with centrifugal flotation exam using Sheather's sugar solution. Fecal smears can also be stained with acid-fast stains or examined by immunodiagnostic techniques. Species identification requires molecular analysis.

Size: 4–8 μm in diameter depending on species

Clinical Importance: Infections may be subclinical or cause diarrhea of varying severity, especially in young animals. *Cryptosporidium parvum* is a widely reported zoonotic species. Other *Cryptosporidium* species may also be zoonotic.

Parasite: *Giardia duodenalis*, also identified as *G. lamblia, G. intestinalis, G. bovis,* etc. (Figs. 1.53–1.59, 1.133)

Taxonomy: Protozoa (flagellate). The taxonomy of *Giardia* species is currently undergoing revision. Isolates of the parasite are currently assigned to assemblages based on genetic analysis. Isolates of hoofed stock typically belong to Assemblage E.

Geographic Distribution: Worldwide.

Location in Host: Small intestine of ruminants and camelids.

Life Cycle: *Giardia* cysts passed in the feces infect other animals when ingested in the environment. Following excystation, trophozoites inhabit the small intestine.

Laboratory Diagnosis: Cysts of *Giardia* can be found in fecal samples using centrifugal flotation procedures (33% $ZnSO_4$ flotation solution preferred). Trichrome-stained fecal smears and immunodiagnostic tests can also be used.

Size: Cysts   9–13 × 7–9 μm
           Trophozoites   12–17 × 7–10 μm

Clinical Importance: Many animals are infected, particularly when young. Clinical disease is uncommon, but there are some reports of parasite impact on growth in young animals.

RUMINANTS AND CAMELIDS

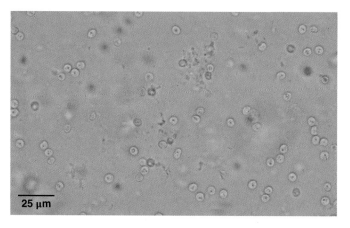

Fig. 1.131 The small oocysts of *Cryptosporidium* are best seen using the high-dry objective (40×) on the microscope. They are highly refractile and often appear to have a single black dot in the center.

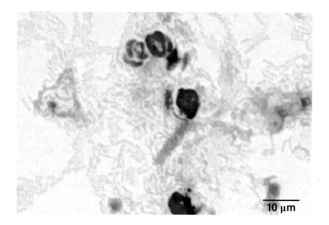

Fig. 1.132 *Cryptosporidium* oocysts can also be detected in acid fast-stained fecal smears. Photo source: CDC/ Public Health Image Library (https://phil.cdc.gov/Details.aspx?pid=7829).

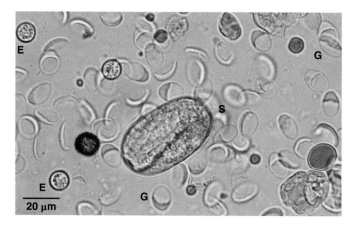

Fig. 1.133 This calf fecal sample contains a larvated *Strongyloides* egg (S) as well as numerous collapsed *Giardia* cysts (G). Several small *Eimeria* oocysts (E) are also present. Most coccidia oocysts are larger than *Giardia* cysts.

Parasite: ***Buxtonella sulcata*** (Fig. 1.134).

Taxonomy: Protozoa (ciliate).

Geographic Distribution: Worldwide.

Location in Host: Cecum of ruminants.

Life Cycle: The life cycle has not been fully described. Trophozoites are present in the cecum and cysts pass out of the host in the manure.

Laboratory Diagnosis: Cysts may be seen in manure samples examined by sedimentation test procedures and rarely by fecal flotation procedures.

  Size: Cyst 40–60 μm

Clinical Significance: No clinical significance has been reported.

Helminth Parasites

Parasite: **Strongylid Parasites of Ruminants and Camelids** (Figs. 1.16, 1.128, 1.135–1.140, 1.145)

  Common name: Various, including brown stomach worm, barber pole worm, hookworm, nodular worm, strongyles, trichostrongyles.

Taxonomy: Nematodes (order Strongylida). Numerous genera belong to this group, including *Ostertagia*, *Haemonchus*, *Cooperia*, *Trichostrongylus*, *Teladorsagia*, *Mecistocirrus*, *Oesophagostomum*, *Bunostomum*, *Chabertia*, *Camelostrongylus*, and *Lamanema*.

Geographic Distribution: Worldwide.

Location in Host: Gastrointestinal tract of ruminant and camelid hosts. The genera infecting these hosts are largely the same, although species may vary.

Life Cycle: Adult worms in the gastrointestinal tract produce eggs that develop in manure in the environment. Infective larvae are released onto pasture, where they are ingested by grazing hosts.

Laboratory Diagnosis: Eggs are detected by routine or quantitative fecal flotation procedures and are similar in appearance. For diagnosis of genera, culture of feces and identification of infective third-stage larvae may be performed. Quantitative egg counts are useful in designing and evaluating parasite control programs. Molecular testing to identify parasite genus is also available.

  Size: Approximately 65–100 × 34–50 μm, depending on species

Clinical Importance: Virtually all grazing animals are infected with strongylid parasites, and many infections are asymptomatic. Young, nonimmune animals are most susceptible to subclinical and clinical disease, which may include diarrhea, anemia, hypoproteinemia, reduced growth, and death in severe cases. The species of greatest importance vary with host and region.

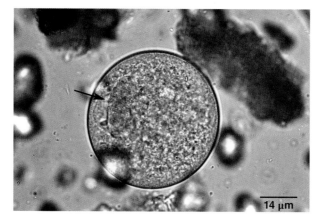

Fig. 1.134 Cyst of *Buxtonella sulcata*. These cysts may be seen in bovine fecal samples examined by sedimentation test and infrequently in bovine fecal flotation test preparations. The bean-shaped macronucleus characteristic of ciliates can be seen (arrow). Photo courtesy of Dr. Yoko Nagamori, College of Veterinary Medicine, Oklahoma State University, Stillwater, OK.

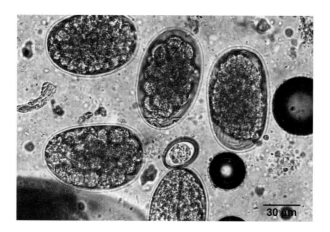

Fig. 1.135 The strongylid (also referred to as strongyle or trichostrongyle) egg is the helminth egg seen most often in ruminant and camelid feces. In fresh feces, eggs are thin shelled and oval in shape and contain a grapelike cluster of cells (morula). Development to the first larval stage occurs in the egg. Identification of eggs to a specific genus or species is not generally considered reliable because of substantial overlap in the sizes and shapes of eggs from different strongylid species.

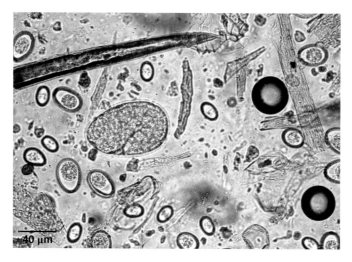

Fig. 1.136 Once strongylid eggs are exposed to oxygen and adequate temperature, development to the first larval stage begins. In warm conditions, partially (as seen in this photo) or fully formed larvae may be seen when samples are collected from the ground. In older samples, the eggs will hatch releasing the larvae, which cannot be easily identified. *Eimeria* oocysts are also present in this sample, representing several species, based on morphologic differences.

Parasite: **Nematodirus spp.** (Figs. 1.128, 1.137, 1.138)

  Common name: Thread-necked worm.

Taxonomy: Nematode (order Strongylida).

Geographic Distribution: Worldwide.

Location in Host: Several species are found in the small intestine of ruminants and camelids.

Life Cycle: Unlike most other strongylids, larvae develop to the infective stage within the egg. Ruminants are infected when they ingest the hatched infective larvae.

Laboratory Diagnosis: Large eggs present in routine or quantitative fecal flotation exams.

  Size: 152–260 × 67–120 µm, depending on species (a similar egg is produced by *Marshallagia marshalli*, a parasite of sheep in the western United States)

Clinical Importance: Most species of *Nematodirus* do not usually cause clinical disease. *Nematodirus battus*, however, is an important cause of lamb diarrhea in some parts of the world. *Nematodirus* infections may cause disease in young camelids.

Parasite: **Strongyloides papillosus** (Figs. 1.133, 1.139)

Taxonomy: Nematode (order Rhabditida).

Geographic Distribution: Worldwide.

Location in Host: Small intestine of ruminants and camelids.

Life Cycle: Eggs shed in the feces hatch, releasing first-stage larvae. After a period of free-living development in the environment, infective third-stage larvae are produced that infect the host by ingestion or penetration of the skin. Transmammary infection also occurs.

Laboratory Diagnosis: Eggs are detected by routine flotation techniques. They are smaller than strongylid eggs and contain a larva when passed in the feces.

  Size: 40–60 × 32–40 µm

Clinical Importance: Infection usually has no clinical significance, although very heavy infection may produce severe diarrhea in young animals.

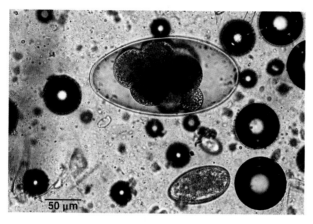

Fig. 1.137   Egg of *Nematodirus* sp. This is one of the few strongylid eggs of ruminants that can be easily identified specifically because of its large size and two to eight distinctive, large cells inside the freshly passed egg. The eggs of *Marshallagia* spp. are similar in size to those of *Nematodirus*. *Marshallagia* spp. are found worldwide, but this genus is less common than *Nematodirus*. A much smaller typical strongylid egg is also present in the photo.

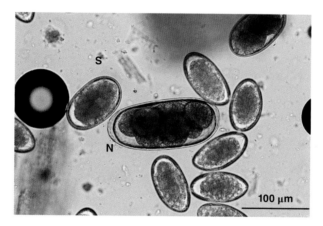

Fig. 1.138   Ovine fecal sample containing strongylid eggs (S), and a *Nematodirus battus* egg (N), which is usually browner in color than the eggs of other *Nematodirus* species.

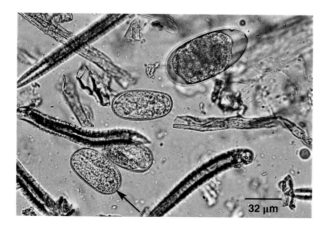

Fig. 1.139   *Strongyloides* eggs may be confused with strongylid eggs. The two egg types can be easily distinguished because *Strongyloides* eggs are smaller and contain a fully formed larva when passed in the feces (arrow). Eggs are primarily seen in samples from immature animals. Photo courtesy of Dr. Yoko Nagamori, College of Veterinary Medicine, Oklahoma State University, Stillwater, OK.

Parasite: **Trichuris spp.** (Figs. 1.140–1.142)

Common name: Whipworm.

Taxonomy: Nematode (order Enoplida). Several species (*T. ovis*, *T. discolor*, etc.) occur in ruminants.

Geographic Distribution: Worldwide.

Location in Host: Cecum and colon of ruminants and camelids.

Life Cycle: Eggs produced by adults in the large intestine are passed in the feces. After a minimum of 3 weeks in the environment, eggs reach the infective stage and can infect a host when ingested.

Laboratory Diagnosis: Identification of brown, bipolar-plugged eggs in fecal flotation preparations.

Size: 70–80 × 30–42 µm

Clinical Importance: Eggs of *Trichuris* are often found in ruminant fecal samples. Clinical disease (diarrhea) is rare and associated with heavy infection.

Parasite: **Aonchotheca (= Capillaria) spp.** (Figs. 1.141–1.143)

Taxonomy: Nematode (order Enoplida). These parasites (*A. bovis* in cattle, *A. longipes* in sheep) were formerly included in the genus *Capillaria*. Camelids are also infected with *Aonchotheca* and at least one other capillarid species.

Geographic Distribution: Worldwide.

Location in Host: Small intestine of ruminants and camelids.

Life Cycle: Parasite eggs are shed from the host in manure. Infection follows ingestion of infective eggs in the environment.

Laboratory Diagnosis: Eggs with bipolar plugs are detected by fecal flotation procedures. Although they are similar to *Trichuris* (whipworm) eggs, *Aonchotheca* spp. eggs are smaller.

Size: 45–50 × 22–25 µm

Clinical Importance: *Aonchotheca* infection in ruminants is considered clinically insignificant.

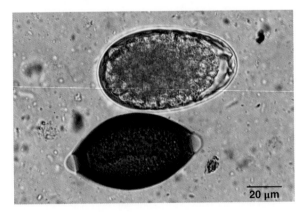

Fig. 1.140   *Trichuris* eggs are common in ruminant feces. They have a thick, brown shell and polar plug at each end. In this photo from an ovine fecal sample a *Trichuris* egg and a strongylid egg are present.

RUMINANTS AND CAMELIDS

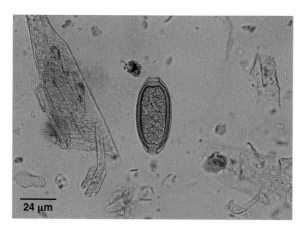

Fig. 1.141   This bipolar *Aonchotheca* (*Capillaria*) egg can be confused with *Trichuris* eggs but is smaller and less brown.

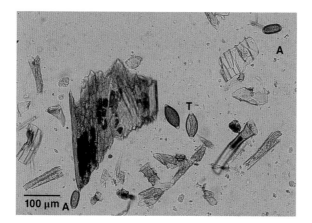

Fig. 1.142   Ruminant fecal sample containing both *Trichuris* (T) and *Aonchotheca* (A) eggs.

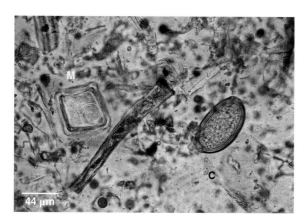

Fig. 1.143   Camelids can be infected with *Aonchotheca* sp. but are also parasitized by another capillarid, which produces a distinctively larger egg with asymmetric bipolar plugs. Neither species appears to have clinical significance. A large capillarid egg (C) is shown with a *Moniezia* egg (M).

Parasite: ***Toxocara (Neoascaris) vitulorum*** (Fig. 1.144)

Common name: Roundworm.

Taxonomy: Nematode (order Ascaridida).

Geographic Distribution: Worldwide, but rare in cattle in North America.

Location in Host: Small intestine of cattle and bison.

Life Cycle: Cattle are infected following the ingestion of larvated eggs in the environment. Larvae migrate into tissues and form a somatic reservoir that is activated in pregnancy. Egg-producing adult infections occur primarily in calves as a result of transmammary transmission.

Laboratory Diagnosis: Detection of typical ascarid-type eggs with flotation procedures.

Size: 75–95 × 60–75 µm

Clinical Importance: Infection with adult worms occurs in calves less than 6 months of age. Small to moderate infection may be tolerated without signs of disease, but diarrhea, weight loss, and death can occur in heavy infection.

Parasite: ***Skrjabinema* spp.** (Fig. 1.145)

Common name: Pinworm.

Taxonomy: Nematode (order Oxyurida).

Geographic Distribution: Worldwide.

Location in Host: Cecum of sheep, goats, some wild ruminant species, and some camelids.

Life Cycle: Female worms deposit eggs on the perianal skin. Eggs fall off the host, become dispersed in the environment, and are eaten by other animals.

Laboratory Diagnosis: Eggs are rarely seen in routine fecal exams as they are not deposited in feces.

Size: 47–63 × 27–36 µm

Clinical Importance: Clinically insignificant.

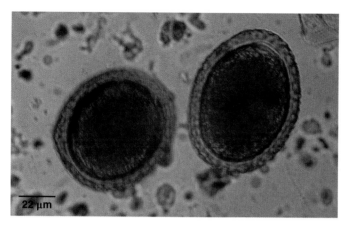

Fig. 1.144 *Toxocara vitulorum* eggs have the thick shell typical of ascarids. *Toxocara* is rarely seen in cattle in North America. Photo courtesy of Dr. Gil Myers, Myers Parasitological Service, Magnolia, TN and Dr. Eugene Lyons, Department of Veterinary Science, University of Kentucky, Lexington, KY.

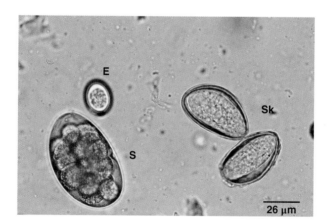

Fig. 1.145 *Skrjabinema* (Sk), the ruminant pinworm. Pinworm eggs often appear flattened on one side. These eggs are rarely found in fecal exams because they are not passed in the feces. A strongylid egg (S) and *Eimeria* (E) oocyst are also present. Photo courtesy of Dr. Yoko Nagamori, College of Veterinary Medicine, Oklahoma State University, Stillwater, OK.

Parasite: ***Muellerius capillaris, Protostrongylus* spp.** (Figs. 1.146–1.150)

Taxonomy: Nematodes (order Strongylida).

Geographic Distribution: Worldwide.

Location in Host: Lung parenchyma of sheep, goats, and some deer.

Life Cycle: Infection of small ruminants follows ingestion of infected snail or slug inter-mediate hosts while grazing. Snails are infected when they eat first-stage larvae in the feces.

Laboratory Diagnosis: The Baermann test is used for detection of first-stage larvae. *Muellerius* has a kinked tail with an accessory spine, in contrast to the plain tail of *Protostrongylus*.

Size:	*Muellerius*	300–320 µm
	Protostrongylus	340–400 µm

Clinical Importance: Most cases are asymptomatic. Heavy infections may cause clinical disease, especially in goats infected with *Muellerius*.

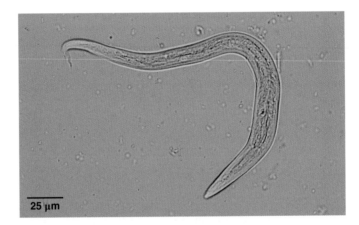

Fig. 1.146   Iodine-stained *Muellerius* larva.

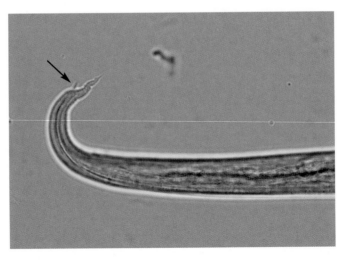

Fig. 1.147   *Muellerius* larvae can be easily identified by the presence of a kinked tail and accessory spine (*arrow*) at the end of the tail.

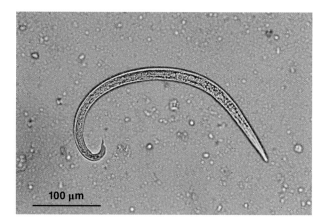

Fig. 1.148 *Parelaphostrongylus*, a parasite of white-tailed deer, produces first-stage larvae that look very similar to those of *Muellerius*. Infection of small ruminants and camelids with larvae of this parasite may produce neurologic disease, but the parasite does not reach the adult stage in domestic animals and the larvae are present only in feces of white-tailed deer.

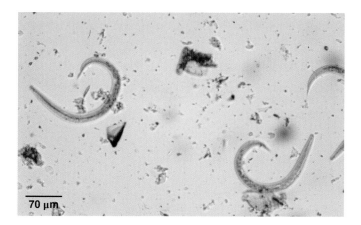

RUMINANTS AND CAMELIDS

Fig. 1.149 *Protostrongylus* larvae have a plain tail without the kink and accessory spine seen in *Muellerius* larvae. Photo courtesy of Dr. Alvin Gajadhar, Centre for Animal Parasitology, CFIA, Saskatoon, Saskatchewan, Canada.

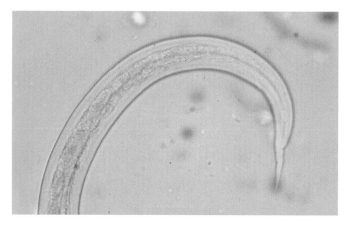

Fig. 1.150 Higher magnification view of the simple tail of a *Protostrongylus* first-stage larva in feces. Photo courtesy of Dr. Alvin Gajadhar, Centre for Animal Parasitology, CFIA, Saskatoon, Saskatchewan, Canada.

Parasite: **Dictyocaulus spp.** (Figs. 1.151 and 1.152)

Common name: Lungworm.

Taxonomy: Nematode (order Strongylida). Species include *D. viviparus* (cattle, camelids), *D. filaria* (sheep, goat, camelids), *D. cameli* (camel).

Geographic Distribution: Worldwide.

Location in Host: Trachea, bronchi, and bronchioles.

Life Cycle: First-stage larvae are passed in the feces of the host. Infective third-stage larvae develop on pasture and are ingested during grazing. Larvae migrate from the intestine to the respiratory tract and become mature.

Laboratory Diagnosis: The Baermann test is used to detect first-stage larvae in fresh feces. Some larvated eggs may also be present in fresh feces.

Size:	*D. viviparus*	300–360 μm
	D. filaria	550–580 μm

Clinical Importance: Heavy infections may cause severe respiratory signs, especially in cattle. Disease is usually seen in young animals before immunity develops.

Parasite: **Moniezia spp.** (Figs. 1.143, 1.153, 1.154)

Common name: Tapeworm.

Taxonomy: Cestode. Species include *M. benedeni* and *M. expansa*.

Geographic Distribution: Worldwide.

Location in Host: Small intestine of ruminants and camelids.

Life Cycle: Tapeworm eggs are shed in segments from the host. Ruminants are infected following ingestion of the intermediate host (free-living pasture mites) containing the tapeworm larvae.

Laboratory Diagnosis: Eggs may be found in fecal flotation tests, but infection is usually recognized when owners see tapeworm segments on the animal or in the environment.

Size: 65–75 μm in diameter

Clinical Importance: In general, little clinical importance, although there are anecdotal reports that heavy infection may cause reduced growth in young animals.

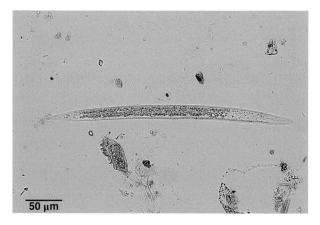

Fig. 1.151 *Dictyocaulus viviparus* first-stage larva. Intestinal cells contain characteristic dark food granules. *Dictyocaulus filaria* larvae have a small knob at the anterior end that is not present in *D. viviparus* larvae. Photo courtesy of Dr. Manigandan Lejeune, Animal Health Diagnostic Center, Cornell University, Ithaca, NY.

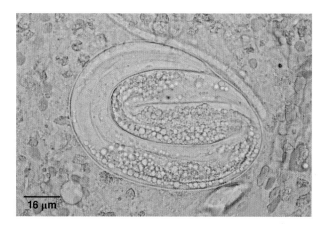

Fig. 1.152 Although *Dictyocaulus* larvae are most often seen in fecal samples, unhatched eggs may also be found in feces and samples collected from the trachea. The dark food granules are evident even in this unhatched *Dictyocaulus* larva. Photo courtesy of Dr. Jeffrey F. Williams, Vanson HaloSource, Inc., Redmond, WA.

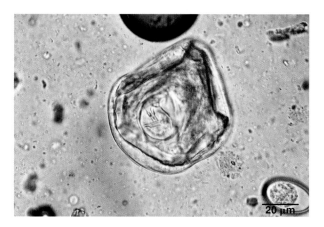

Fig. 1.153 Eggs of *Moniezia* are often square or triangular, unlike the more common round or oval shape of other parasite eggs. The presence of the embryo with its six hooks clearly identifies these structures as tapeworm eggs. In this egg, four hooks are visible.

Parasite: ***Thysanosoma, Stilesia*** (Fig. 1.155)

Taxonomy: Cestodes.

Geographic Distribution: *Stilesia* is found in Europe, Africa, and Asia, while *Thysanosoma* is confined to North and South America. In the United States, its distribution appears to be limited to the western states.

Location in Host: Bile ducts of ruminants, especially sheep, and camelids.

Life Cycle: Although these tapeworms have not been extensively studied, it is thought that their intermediate hosts may be oribatid mites and psocid insects. Like *Moniezia*, the definitive host is infected following ingestion of the intermediate host.

Laboratory Diagnosis: Tapeworm segments are passed in the feces and eggs may be found in fecal flotation tests.

   Size: Approximately 30 × 20 μm

Clinical Importance: These tapeworms have no economic importance unless they are present in large enough numbers to cause liver condemnation.

Parasite: ***Fasciola hepatica*** (Figs. 1.156–1.158)

   Common name: Liver fluke.

Taxonomy: Trematode.

Geographic Distribution: Worldwide. A similar species, *F. gigantica*, is also found in Africa, Asia, and Hawaii.

Location in Host: Adults in the bile ducts of cattle, sheep, goats, camelids, and a variety of other animals, including dogs, horses, and humans.

Life Cycle: Miracidia hatch from the eggs and invade an appropriate snail host. Cercariae emerging from the snail encyst on vegetation and are ingested by host animals. Larvae leave the gastrointestinal tract and migrate through the liver to reach the bile ducts.

Laboratory Diagnosis: Large brown eggs are detected using a sedimentation procedure. Eggs may be difficult to detect and not indicative of the level of infection in a herd. A commercially available apparatus, the Flukefinder, simplifies the sedimentation procedure (see the section "Fecal Sedimentation").

   Size: 130–150 × 63–90 μm

Clinical Importance: *Fasciola* infections in ruminants may cause significant production losses. Sheep are particularly susceptible, and heavy infection may be fatal. Chronically infected animals can develop anemia and unthriftiness. A similar parasite, *Fascioloides magna*, is the liver fluke of white tailed deer. Migration of *F. magna* larvae in other ruminants, especially small ruminants, may cause hepatic disease.

RUMINANTS AND CAMELIDS

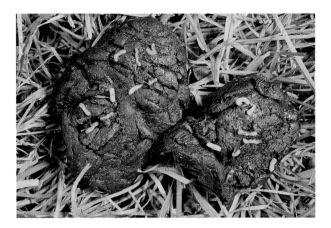

Fig. 1.154   Owners may be alarmed by the presence of *Moniezia* segments in the feces of their animals, although tapeworms have little clinical significance. Tapeworm segments are seen most often in the manure of young animals. Photo courtesy of Dr. Jeffrey F. Williams, Vanson HaloSource, Inc., Redmond, WA.

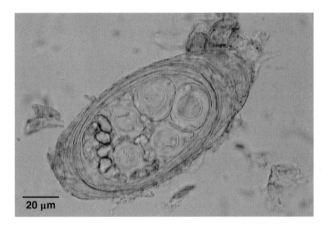

Fig. 1.155   Packet of *Thysanosoma* eggs from a sheep. The eggs lack the pyriform apparatus seen in *Moniezia* eggs. Hooks can be seen in some of the eggs. The entire packet of eggs is 124 × 62 μm. Photo courtesy of Dr. Ellis C. Greiner, College of Veterinary Medicine, University of Florida, Gainesville, FL.

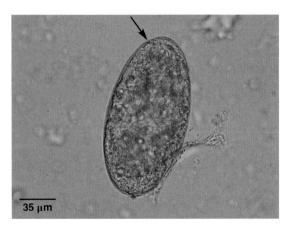

Fig. 1.156   *Fasciola hepatica* egg. These large eggs have an operculum (*arrow*) and look similar to eggs of rumen flukes, although *Paramphistomum* eggs are slightly larger (about 160 μm) and less brown in color.

Parasite: ***Paramphistomum* spp.** (Figs. 1.157 and 1.158)

Common name: Rumen fluke.

Taxonomy: Trematode. Other genera belonging to this family include *Cotylophoron* and *Calicophoron*.

Geographic Distribution: Worldwide.

Location in Host: Adult flukes in the rumen of cattle, sheep, other ruminants, and camelids.

Life Cycle: Eggs passed in the feces of the host animal hatch in water, liberating miracidia, which infect snails. Following development in the snail, cercariae are released, which encyst on vegetation. Definitive hosts are infected by ingesting fluke metacercariae while grazing.

Laboratory Diagnosis: Eggs of paramphistomes are similar to those of *Fasciola*. They are best recovered using a sedimentation procedure, but examination of fecal material will not detect immature flukes, which are the most pathogenic stage of infection.

Size: Approximately 114–175 × 65–100 μm, depending on species

Clinical Importance: Clinical disease is rare in North America. In other parts of the world, larval paramphistomes in the duodenum and upper ileum are reported to cause enteritis leading to diarrhea, emaciation, and death in severe cases.

Parasite: ***Dicrocoelium dendriticum*** (Fig. 1.159)

Taxonomy: Trematode.

Geographic Distribution: Europe, Asia, sporadic occurrence in North America.

Location in Host: Bile ducts of domestic and wild ruminants, pigs, dogs, horses, rabbits.

Life Cycle: Larvae in eggs are ingested by snails. Ants act as the second intermediate host, and the final host is infected while grazing. Larval flukes enter bile ducts directly and do not migrate through the liver.

Laboratory Diagnosis: A sedimentation test will detect the small, brown, operculate eggs in the feces.

Size: 38–45 × 22–30 μm

Clinical Importance: In heavy infections, extensive cirrhosis of the liver can develop, leading to anemia and weight loss.

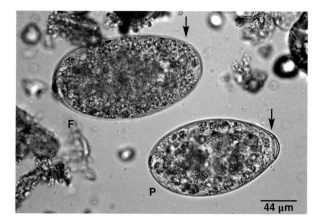

Fig. 1.157 *Fasciola hepatica* (F) and *Paramphistomum* (P) eggs. The two eggs are very similar but the browner color of *Fasciola* is easily seen in this photo. The operculum of each egg is indicated by an arrow. Photo courtesy of Dr. Yoko Nagamori, College of Veterinary Medicine, Oklahoma State University, Stillwater, OK.

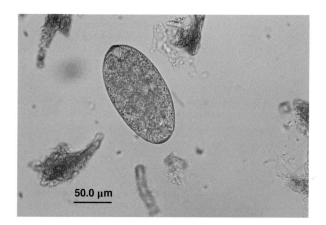

Fig. 1.158 Egg of *Fascioloides magna*, the liver fluke of white-tailed deer. These eggs are similar in size and appearance to those of *F. hepatica*. Because patent infections do not develop in domestic livestock, eggs will not be present in their feces.

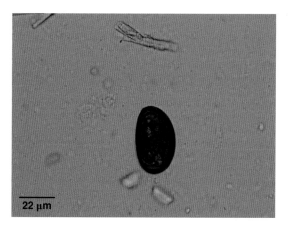

Fig. 1.159 *Dicrocoelium dendriticum* eggs contain a fully formed miracidium, tend to be flattened on one side, and are smaller than eggs of *Fasciola* and the paramphistome flukes.

RUMINANTS AND CAMELIDS

Parasite: *Eurytrema* **spp. including** *E. coelomaticum, E. pancreaticum* (Fig. 1.160)

Taxonomy: Trematode.

Geographic Distribution: Asia, parts of South America.

Location in Host: Adult flukes are found in the pancreatic ducts of small ruminants, cattle, camels, pigs, and occasionally humans. Flukes are also occasionally found in the bile ducts and small intestine.

Life Cycle: The eggs produced by adult flukes leave the host in manure. Snails are the first intermediate host. A grasshopper or cricket second intermediate host transmits the infection when ingested by the final host.

Laboratory Diagnosis: A sedimentation test will detect the small, brown eggs in the feces.

   Size: 44–48 × 23–36 μm

Clinical Importance: Many infections are subclinical. Heavy worm burdens can cause fibrosis of the ducts and pancreatic atrophy, resulting in weight loss and poor condition.

Parasite: *Schistosoma* **spp.** (Fig. 1.161)

Taxonomy: Trematode. Several species infect ruminants, camels, horses, and pigs, including *S. bovis*, *S. mattheei*, and *S. japonicum*.

Geographic Distribution: Africa, Asia.

Location in Host: Most important species are found in the portal mesenteric veins of the host.

Life Cycle: Eggs in host feces hatch in water, releasing the miracidia, which enter the snail intermediate host. Cercariae produced by multiplication within the snail are released and penetrate the skin of the definitive host. There is no second intermediate host in the life cycle.

Laboratory Diagnosis: A saline sedimentation procedure is used to detect eggs in manure. Fecal examination is most useful in early infection because egg production declines as infection progresses. Eggs do not have an operculum and most are spindle-shaped. In some species, a spine is present on one end of the egg.

   Size: 130–280 × 38–85 μm, depending on species

Clinical Importance: Disease results from the host reaction to the presence of parasite eggs in tissue. Clinical signs may occur in heavy infections, including diarrhea, anemia, and wasting.

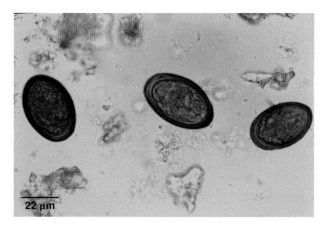

Fig. 1.160 The eggs of *Eurytrema* are similar in appearance to those of *Dicrocoelium*. Photo courtesy of Dr. Alvin Gajadhar, Centre for Animal Parasitology, CFIA, Saskatoon, Saskatchewan, Canada.

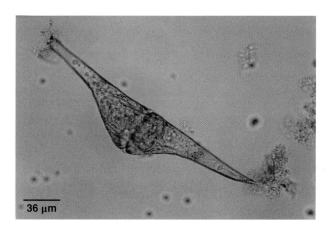

Fig. 1.161 Ruminant schistosomes typically produce a spindle-shaped egg. This egg of *Schistosoma spindale*, an Asian species, has a spine at one end. Photo courtesy of Dr. Alvin Gajadhar, Centre for Animal Parasitology, CFIA, Saskatoon, Saskatchewan, Canada.

Horses

In comparison to dogs, cats, and ruminants, the diversity of parasite eggs and cysts frequently encountered in equine feces is much reduced. The most common finding in equine samples is the strongylid egg. Horses are infected with many strongylid species, although individual species cannot be determined by morphologic characteristics of eggs alone. The parasites shown in this section can also infect other equid species. Parasites illustrated in other sections may not be extensively covered here and references are given to figures elsewhere in the book.

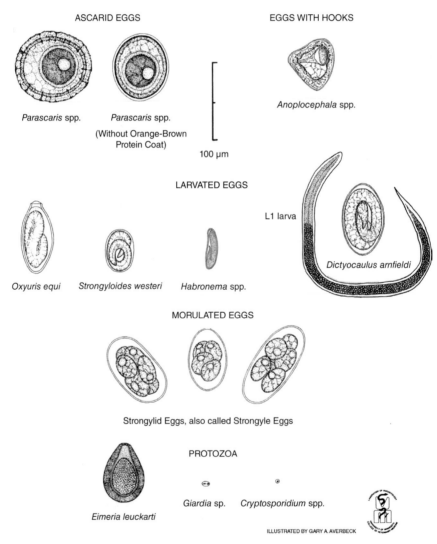

Fig. 1.162   Parasites found in fecal samples of horses. Figure courtesy of Dr. Bert Stromberg and Mr. Gary Averbeck, College of Veterinary Medicine, University of Minnesota, Minneapolis, MN.

Table 1.11. **Representative treatments for selected parasites of horses**

Parasite	Effective treatments	Dose, route, and regimen
Eimeria leuckarti *Giardia* sp. *Cryptosporidium* spp.	None indicated	NA, rarely associated with clinical disease
Strongylus spp. (large strongyles)	Fenbendazole, ivermectin, moxidectin, oxibendazole, pyrantel pamoate, pyrantel tartrate	Administer according to label directions
Cyathostomins (small strongyles)	[a]Fenbendazole, ivermectin, moxidectin, [a]oxibendazole, [a]pyrantel pamoate, [a]pyrantel tartrate	Administer according to label directions
Parascaris equorum	Fenbendazole, [a]ivermectin, [a]moxidectin, oxibendazole, [a]pyrantel pamoate, pyrantel tartrate	Administer according to label directions
Oxyuris equi	Fenbendazole, [b]ivermectin, [b]moxidectin, oxibendazole, pyrantel pamoate, pyrantel tartrate	Administer according to label directions
Trichostrongylus axei	Ivermectin, moxidectin	Administer according to label directions
Strongyloides westeri	Ivermectin, oxibendazole	Administer according to label directions
Habronema muscae *Habronema microstoma* *Draschia megastoma*	Ivermectin, [c]moxidectin	Administer according to label directions
Dictyocaulus arnfieldi	Ivermectin	Administer according to label directions
Anoplocephala perfoliata	Praziquantel	Administer according to label directions; equine formulations available in combination with macrocyclic lactones
	Pyrantel pamoate	Administer according to label directions for tapeworm treatment

[a] Resistance or
[b] suboptimal efficacy to this treatment has been reported.
[c] Not label-approved against *H. microstoma* or *D. megastoma*.
NA: not applicable.
Additional information on parasite treatments can be found in Chapter 7.

HORSES

Protozoan Parasites

Parasite: ***Eimeria leuckarti*** (Fig. 1.163)

Taxonomy: Protozoa (coccidia).

Geographic Distribution: Worldwide.

Location in Host: Small intestine of horses and donkeys.

Life Cycle: Oocysts leave the host in the manure. Sporulation occurs in the environment, and new hosts are infected by ingestion of infective oocysts.

Laboratory Diagnosis: Infection is diagnosed by finding the large, deep-brown oocysts in the feces. A sedimentation procedure has been recommended, but oocysts can also be seen with flotation procedures.

Size: 80–88 × 55–59 µm

Clinical Importance: Infection appears to have little clinical significance in horses, although rare cases of diarrhea have been reported. Infections are seen only in young animals.

Parasite: ***Giardia duodenalis*, *Cryptosporidium* spp.** (Figs. 1.164 and 1.165)

Taxonomy: Protozoa (*Giardia*, flagellate; *Cryptosporidium*, coccidia).

Geographic Location: Worldwide.

Location in Host: Small intestine.

Laboratory Diagnosis: As in other hosts, *Giardia* cysts are most easily detected with 33% $ZnSO_4$ centrifugal flotation, and *Cryptosporidium* oocysts with Sheather's sugar centrifugal flotation. Both organisms can also be found in fecal smears with appropriate stains and by non-host-specific immunodiagnostic or molecular tests.

Clinical Importance: Both infections occur most frequently in young animals but are rarely associated with clinical disease.

HORSES

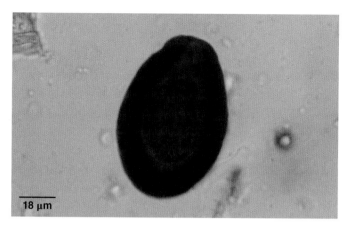

Fig. 1.163   The large size and deep-brown color of the oocysts of *E. leuckarti* make them very distinctive. They are seen in feces of young horses.

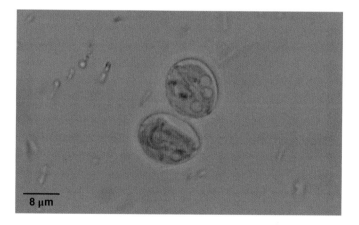

Fig. 1.164   Fecal flotation test containing iodine-stained *Giardia* cysts.

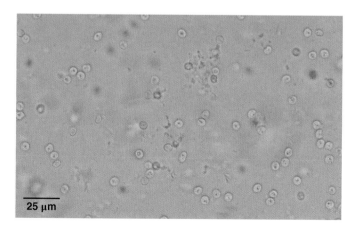

Fig. 1.165   *Cryptosporidium* oocysts in a sugar flotation preparation.

HORSES

Helminth Parasites

Parasite: **Equine Strongylid Parasites** (Figs. 1.166–1.168, 1.171, 1.179)

Common name: Various, including bloodworm, small and large strongyle.

Taxonomy: Nematode (order Strongylida). Numerous genera belong to this group, including the large strongyles (e.g., *Strongylus vulgaris*), the small strongyles (cyathostomins), and *Trichostrongylus axei*.

Geographic Distribution: Worldwide.

Location in Host: Cecum and colon (with the exception of *T. axei*, a parasite of the stomach).

Life Cycle: Eggs released by adult worms in the large bowel develop in feces in the environment. Infective larvae on pasture are ingested by grazing horses. Large and small strongyles undergo a period of development in the intestinal wall (small strongyles) or in extra-intestinal tissue (large strongyles) before maturing in the bowel lumen.

Laboratory Diagnosis: Eggs are detected on routine fecal flotation. Eggs are similar in appearance and are not routinely identified specifically. Quantitative egg counts are used in targeted selective treatment programs and testing for drug efficacy.

Size: Variable, with considerable overlap among species; eggs approximately 60–120 × 35–60 μm

Clinical Importance: Virtually all grazing horses are infected with strongylid parasites. Many low to moderate infections are subclinical, although they may cause reduced weight gain and performance. Young, nonimmune animals are most susceptible to clinical disease, which may include diarrhea, colic, and hypoproteinemia.

HORSES

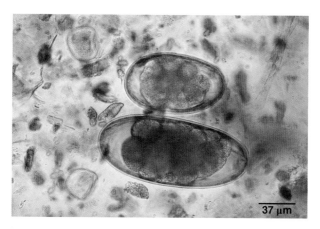

Fig. 1.166 Equine strongylid (strongyle) eggs in fresh fecal samples are typical of the order, with a thin shell surrounding a central group of cells (morula). In warm weather, larvae may form within 1–2 days. The two eggs shown here demonstrate the range of sizes in this group of worms, but in most cases there is too much overlap to identify parasite species. Photo courtesy of Dr. Manigandan Lejeune, Animal Health Diagnostic Center, Cornell University, Ithaca, NY.

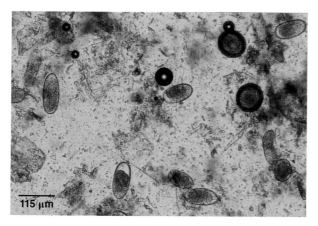

Fig. 1.167 Several equine strongylid eggs are present in this fecal sample. Two *Parascaris* (roundworm) eggs are also present.

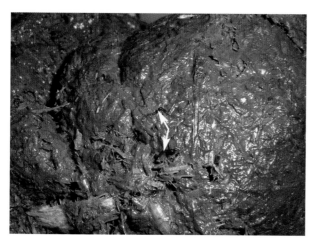

Fig. 1.168 Equine small strongyle larvae (*arrows*) in manure. These small (less than 2 cm) red larvae may be present in large numbers in manure of horses with acute larval cyathostominosis.

HORSES

Parasite: ***Parascaris* spp.** (Figs. 1.167, 1.169–1.171)

Common name: Roundworm.

Taxonomy: Nematode (order Ascaridida). This parasite genus was previously generally identified as *P. equorum*, but investigators have recently found that *P. univalens* is a common species.

Geographic Distribution: Worldwide.

Location in Host: Small intestine of horses and other equids.

Life Cycle: Infective larvae develop in eggs passed in the feces of horses. Infection occurs by ingestion of larvated eggs. Larvae migrate through the liver and lungs of the host before returning to the small intestine to mature.

Laboratory Diagnosis: Flotation procedures will detect the typical thick-shelled ascarid eggs.

Size: 90–100 µm in diameter

Following treatment with some anthelmintics, adult ascarids may be passed in manure. These worms will be much larger than any other equine helminths, with females reaching 50 cm in length.

Clinical Importance: Adult worms are common in young horses, infrequent in adults. Heavy infections can cause respiratory signs (from migrating larvae), ill-thrift, colic, diarrhea, and intestinal obstruction that may be fatal.

HORSES

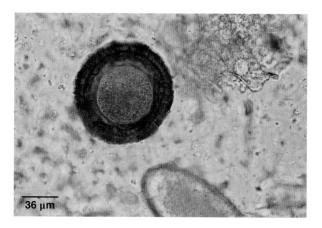

Fig. 1.169   *Parascaris* eggs are typical, thick-shelled ascarid eggs containing a single cell when passed in the feces. Figure 1.167 shows *Parascaris* eggs at a lower magnification.

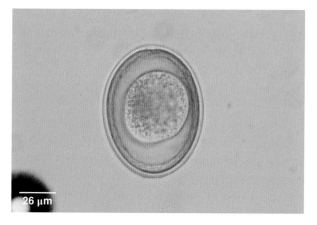

Fig. 1.170   *Parascaris* eggs may lose the rough, proteinaceous coat on the eggshell, but they can still be identified as ascarid eggs by the thick shell and single cell inside the freshly passed egg.

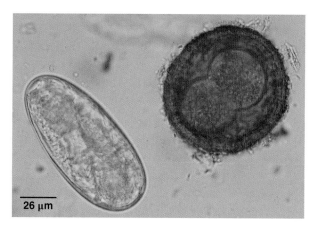

Fig. 1.171   Larvated strongylid egg and *Parascaris* egg that has undergone the first cell division. The fecal sample containing these eggs was fresh when collected but was not examined for some time, allowing development to occur.

Parasite: ***Strongyloides westeri*** (Fig. 1.172)

Common name: Threadworm.

Taxonomy: Nematode (order Rhabditida).

Geographic Distribution: Worldwide.

Location in Host: Small intestine.

Life Cycle: Patent infections develop primarily by transmammary infection of foals. Larvated eggs passed in the feces of foals lead to the development of infective larvae that can penetrate the skin or be ingested. In adult horses, larvae migrate to tissues and form a somatic larval reservoir.

Laboratory Diagnosis: Small, larvated eggs are detected by flotation procedures.

Size: 40–52 × 32–40 μm

Clinical Importance: Clinical disease occurs only in foals. Heavy burdens can produce severe diarrhea and dehydration. Respiratory signs may develop associated with larval migration.

Parasite: ***Oxyuris equi*** (Figs. 1.173 and 1.174)

Common name: Pinworm.

Taxonomy: Nematode (order Oxyurida). *Probstmayria vivipara* is a less common pinworm of horses.

Geographic Distribution: Worldwide.

Location in Host: Large intestine of horses and other equids.

Life Cycle: Horses ingest infective eggs. Adult female worms migrate to the perianal region and lay clusters of sticky eggs. These eventually are rubbed off the horse and contaminate the environment.

Laboratory Diagnosis: Because eggs are attached to hairs in the perianal region, they are not often seen in flotation tests. A more successful procedure for recovering eggs is the "Scotch tape test." A piece of clear adhesive tape is touched to the skin in the perianal area and then taped onto a microscope slide and examined. Pinworm eggs can easily be seen through the tape.

Size: 85–95 × 40–45 μm

Clinical Importance: Egg-laying activities of the female worms produce intense pruritus. Horses bite at and rub the perineal region, leading to a "rat-tailed" appearance and possible secondary trauma.

HORSES

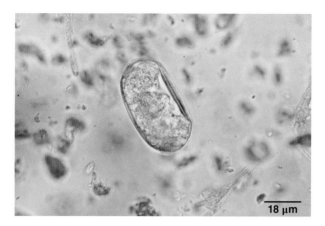

18 µm

Fig. 1.172   Egg of *Strongyloides westeri*, the horse threadworm. These eggs are usually seen only in the feces of young horses. *Strongyloides* eggs are already larvated when passed in the feces, and they are smaller than strongylid eggs. Figure 1.139 shows both *Strongyloides* and strongylid eggs of ruminants, which have a similar size relationship to the species found in horses. Photo courtesy of Dr. Manigandan Lejeune, Animal Health Diagnostic Center, Cornell University, Ithaca, NY.

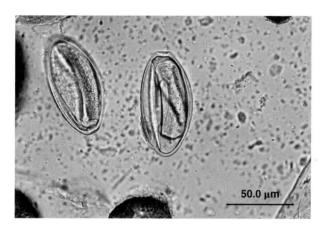

50.0 µm

Fig. 1.173   *Oxyuris* eggs are asymmetrical with a single polar plug. Eggs embryonate rapidly and may be seen with a larva inside.

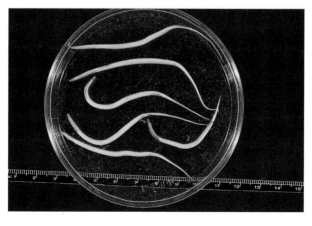

Fig. 1.174   Adult pinworms are occasionally seen in the feces of horses. Adult female *Oxyuris* can reach a maximum size of 10 cm and can be recognized by their thin, pointed tails. Male worms are much smaller. Photo courtesy of Dr. Jeffrey F. Williams, Vanson HaloSource, Inc., Redmond, WA.

HORSES

Parasite: ***Habronema microstoma, H. muscae, Draschia megastoma*** (Fig. 1.175)

Taxonomy: Nematodes (order Spirurida).

Geographic Distribution: Worldwide.

Location in Host: Stomach of horses and donkeys.

Life Cycle: Adult worms are found in the stomach; *D. megastoma* in tumor-like masses near the margo plicatus. Larvated eggs are passed in the feces and are ingested by fly larvae intermediate hosts. Infective worm larvae deposited by adult flies around the lips of horses make their way into the mouth and to the stomach.

Laboratory Diagnosis: The larvated eggs passed in the feces are too dense to float in most flotation solutions. A sedimentation procedure is recommended for detection.

    Size: 40–80 × 10–20 μm

Clinical Importance: Gastritis resulting in poor growth may develop. If flies deposit third-stage larvae on a wound, a condition known as "summer sore" can occur, in which larvae survive and prevent wound healing.

Parasite: ***Dictyocaulus arnfieldi*** (Figs. 1.152, 1.176 and 1.177)

        Common name: Lungworm.

Taxonomy: Nematode (order Strongylida).

Geographic Distribution: Worldwide.

Location in Host: Bronchi and bronchioles of horses and donkeys.

Life Cycle: Adult worms in the respiratory tract produce larvated eggs that hatch before or soon after leaving the host. Eggs and/or larvae are coughed up, swallowed, and passed in the feces. Larvae develop to the infective third stage in the environment and are ingested by grazing horses.

Laboratory Diagnosis: Larvated eggs may be detected in feces with flotation tests. However, eggs hatch rapidly or even before leaving the host, so the Baermann test for the first-stage larvae is the preferred technique for diagnosis. While lungworms readily mature in donkeys, they may not mature in horses, making diagnosis more difficult.

    Size: Eggs   74–96 × 46–58 μm
               Larvae   420–480 μm

Clinical Importance: Bronchitis and pneumonia may develop. Infections appear to be tolerated better by donkeys than by horses.

HORSES

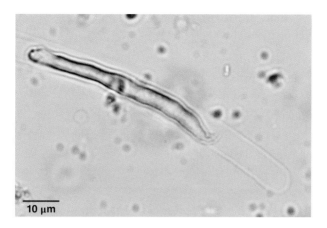

Fig. 1.175 Larvated egg of *Habronema* sp. The larva is surrounded by a thin shell. *Draschia* sp. eggs are similar. Photo courtesy of Dr. Manigandan Lejeune, Animal Health Diagnostic Center, Cornell University, Ithaca, NY.

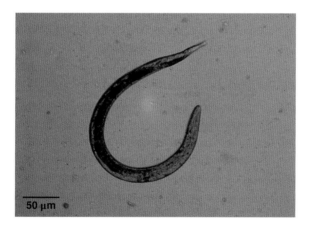

Fig. 1.176 The only parasitic nematode larvae that would be expected in the fresh feces of horses are those of *Dictyocaulus*. See also Figure 1.152 for *Dictyocaulus* eggs that may be seen in tracheal fluid samples. Photo courtesy of Dr. Craig Reinemeyer, East Tennessee Clinical Research, Knoxville, TN.

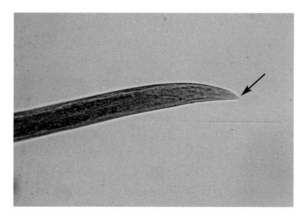

Fig. 1.177 Larvae of *Dictyocaulus arnfieldi*, the equid lungworm, have a small terminal projection at the posterior end (*arrow*) that can be seen with higher magnification.

HORSES

Parasite: *Anoplocephala perfoliata, A. magna,* **and** *Paranoplocephala mamillana* (Figs. 1.178 and 1.179)

Common name: Tapeworm.

Taxonomy: Cestodes.

Geographic Distribution: Worldwide.

Location in Host: Small intestine of horses and donkeys.

Life Cycle: Eggs passed in the feces are ingested by free-living pasture mites. Horses are infected during grazing when they ingest mites containing tapeworm cysticercoid larvae.

Laboratory Diagnosis: Flotation procedures for detection of eggs in fecal samples are used, but false-negative results are common. A test for detection of antibodies to *Anoplocephala* infection is available.

Size:	*A. perfoliata*	65–80 µm in diameter
	Other species	50–60 µm

Clinical Importance: Most tapeworm infections are asymptomatic. Disease has been associated with *A. perfoliata*. These parasites cluster at the ileo–cecal junction, where heavy infection can cause ulceration leading to perforation or intussusception.

Horses may also be infected with some of the trematode (fluke) parasites that affect ruminants. For information on these parasites, see Figures 1.156 and 1.161.

HORSES

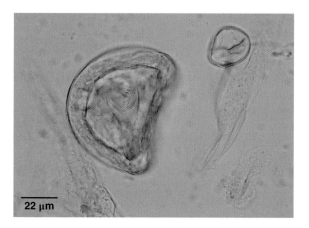

Fig. 1.178 The egg of the equine tapeworm *Anoplocephala* is similar in appearance to that of the ruminant tapeworm *Moniezia*. The eggs of both genera are often irregularly shaped. A pyriform apparatus surrounds the embryo, which has six hooks (hexacanth).

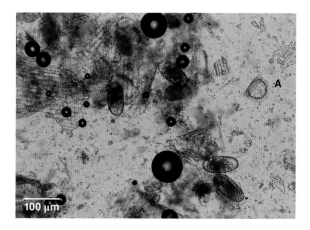

Fig. 1.179 *Anoplocephala* egg (A) and several equine strongylid eggs.

HORSES

Swine

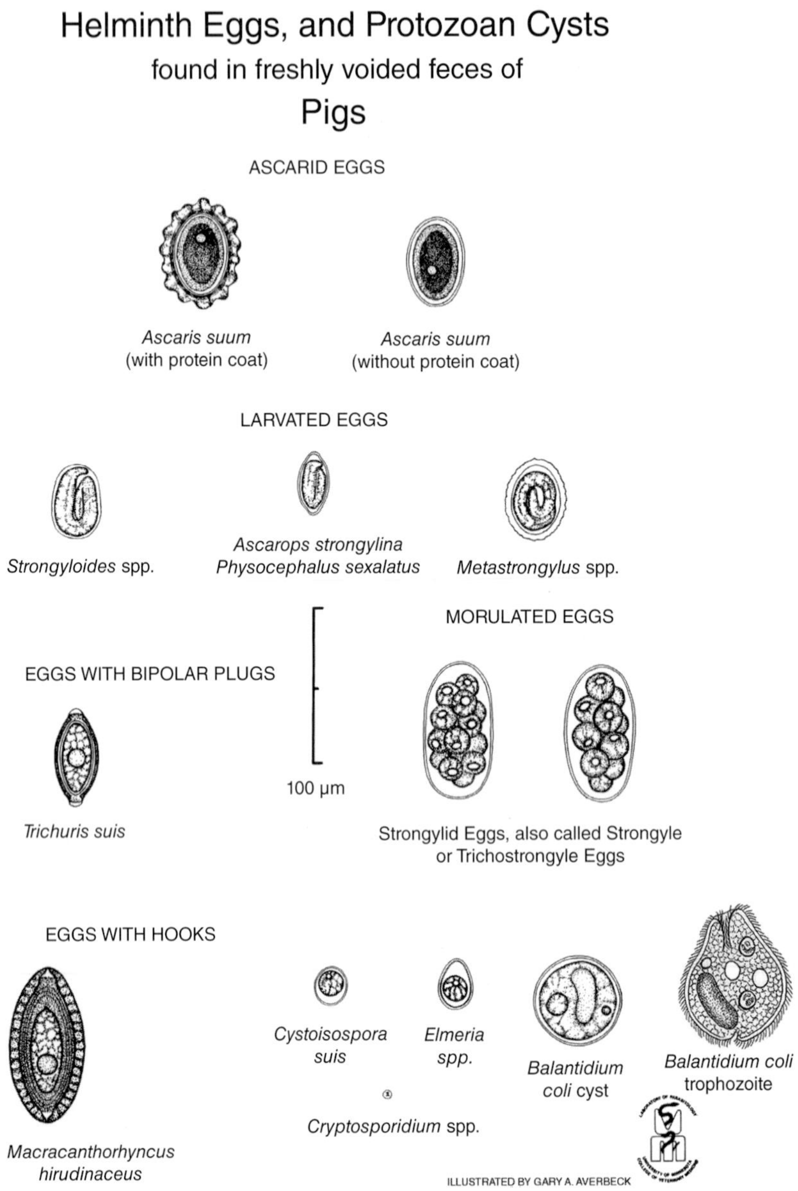

Helminth Eggs, and Protozoan Cysts
found in freshly voided feces of
Pigs

ASCARID EGGS

Ascaris suum
(with protein coat)

Ascaris suum
(without protein coat)

LARVATED EGGS

Strongyloides spp.

Ascarops strongylina
Physocephalus sexalatus

Metastrongylus spp.

MORULATED EGGS

EGGS WITH BIPOLAR PLUGS

100 µm

Trichuris suis

Strongylid Eggs, also called Strongyle
or Trichostrongyle Eggs

EGGS WITH HOOKS

                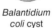   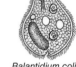

Cystoisospora
suis

Elmeria
spp.

Balantidium
coli cyst

Balantidium coli
trophozoite

Cryptosporidium spp.

Macracanthorhyncus
hirudinaceus

ILLUSTRATED BY GARY A. AVERBECK

Fig. 1.180   Parasites found in fecal samples of pigs. Figure courtesy of Dr. Bert Stromberg and Mr. Gary Averbeck, College of Veterinary Medicine, University of Minnesota, Minneapolis, MN.

Table 1.12. **Representative treatments for selected parasites of swine**

Parasite	Effective treatments	Dose, route, and regimen
Cystoisospora suis	[a]Toltrazuril	20 mg/kg PO, once
Ascaris suum	Dichlorvos, doramectin, fenbendazole, [b]hygromcyin B, ivermectin, levamisole, piperazine, pyrantel tartrate	Administer according to label directions
Trichuris suis	Dichlorvos, fenbendazole, [b]hygromcyin B	Administer according to label directions
Oesophagostomum spp.	Dichlorvos, doramectin, fenbendazole, [b]hygromcyin B, ivermectin, levamisole, pyrantel tartrate	Administer according to label directions
Metastrongylus spp.	Doramectin, fenbendazole, ivermectin, levamisole	Administer according to label directions
Strongyloides ransomi	Doramectin, ivermectin, levamisole	Administer according to label directions
Stephanurus dentatus	Doramectin, fenbendazole, ivermectin, levamisole	Administer according to label directions
Hyostrongylus rubidus	Doramectin, fenbendazole, ivermectin	Administer according to label directions
Macracanthorhynchus hirudinaceus	[c]Ivermectin	Administer according to label directions

[a] Not label-approved for use in pigs in the United States.
[b] Label-approved as an aid in the control of infection.
[c] Reported effective when administered according to label directions.
Additional information on parasite treatments can be found in Chapter 7.

PIGS

Protozoan Parasites

Parasite: **Cystoisospora (Isospora) suis** (Fig. 1.181)

Common name: Coccidia.

Taxonomy: Protozoa (coccidia).

Geographic Distribution: Worldwide.

Location in Host: Small intestine.

Life Cycle: Oocysts are shed in the feces and can sporulate rapidly in warm weather. Transmission occurs in the neonatal period with sows serving as a source of oocysts. Neonates are infected when they ingest sporulated (infective) oocysts.

Laboratory Diagnosis: *Cystoisopora* oocysts are detected in feces with flotation procedures. However, oocysts are shed at such a low rate in asymptomatic carriers that detection is very difficult. In clinically affected neonatal pigs, disease usually develops before oocysts are shed, and intestinal mucosal impression smears at necropsy are more effective for diagnosis.

Size: Oocysts are nearly spherical and approximately 18 × 20 μm

Clinical Importance: *Cystoisospora suis* can produce neonatal diarrhea in pigs (5–10 days of age) that may be severe and cause death.

Parasite: **Eimeria spp.** (Figs. 1.182 and 1.183)

Common name: Coccidia.

Taxonomy: Protozoa (coccidia). Eight species of porcine *Eimeria* have been described, including *E. scabra*, *E. deblieki*, *E. porci*, and *E. spinosa*.

Geographic Distribution: Worldwide.

Location in Host: Intestinal tract; location depends on species and stage of development.

Life Cycle: Oocysts are shed in the feces and sporulate rapidly in warm weather. Pigs are infected when they ingest sporulated (infective) oocysts.

Laboratory Diagnosis: *Eimeria* oocysts are detected in feces with flotation procedures.

Size: Oocysts vary with species, with a range of 11–35 × 9–20 μm

Clinical Importance: *Eimeria* spp. infections are common in swine but rarely produce clinical disease.

Swine may also be infected with *Cryptosporidium parvum* and *Giardia duodenalis*. These two protozoan parasites appear to have little clinical significance but may have zoonotic importance. For further information, see sections related to these parasites in the small animal and ruminant sections.

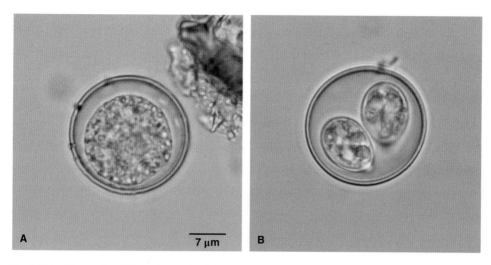

Fig. 1.181 Unsporulated (A) and sporulated (B) oocyst of *Cystoisospora suis*. Photos courtesy of Dr. Manigandan Lejeune, Animal Health Diagnostic Center, Cornell University, Ithaca, NY.

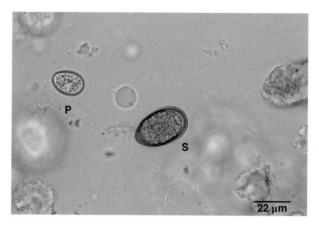

Fig. 1.182 Oocysts of *E. porci* (P) and *E. scabra* (S), two of the eight *Eimeria* species described from pigs. Photo courtesy of Dr. Manigandan Lejeune, Animal Health Diagnostic Center, Cornell University, Ithaca, NY.

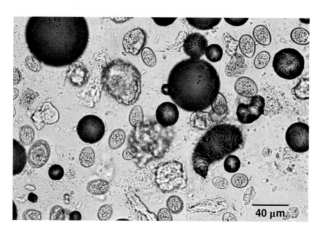

Fig. 1.183 Numerous *Eimeria* oocyts in a porcine fecal sample. Although common in pigs, *Eimeria* spp. infections have little clinical importance. Photo courtesy of Dr. Yoko Nagamori, College of Veterinary Medicine, Oklahoma State University, Stillwater, OK.

PIGS

Parasite: ***Balantidium (=Neobalantidium) coli*** (Figs. 1.184–1.186)

Taxonomy: Protozoa (ciliate).

Geographic Distribution: Worldwide.

Location in Host: Large intestine of swine; may also occasionally infect humans and other primates, camels, dogs, and other animals.

Life Cycle: Infection follows ingestion of cysts shed into the environment from infected swine. The only other stage of the life cycle is the motile trophozoite in the intestinal tract.

Laboratory Diagnosis: Motile trophozoites can be seen in direct fecal smears. Flotation tests are more sensitive for detecting cysts. The kidney-bean-shaped macronucleus is a distinctive feature.

Size:	Trophozoites	50–150 × 40–65 μm
	Cysts	40–60 μm

Clinical Importance: *Balantidium* infection is generally asymptomatic in swine, although bloody diarrhea may occur in some hosts.

PIGS

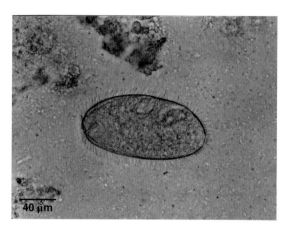

Fig. 1.184 *Balantidium coli* trophozoite in a direct saline smear. The cilia covering trophozoites can be seen as a halo surrounding the organism. Trophozoites are usually destroyed by fecal flotation procedures. Photo courtesy of Dr. Alvin Gajadhar, Centre for Animal Parasitology, CFIA, Saskatoon, Saskatchewan, Canada.

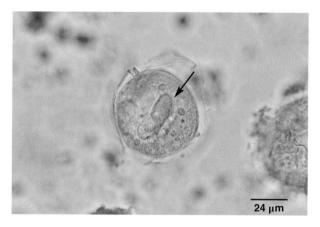

Fig. 1.185 The kidney-bean-shaped macronucleus, characteristic of ciliates, is present in this unstained *Balantidium* cyst in a porcine fecal sample (arrow). The macronucleus is usually easily seen in stained specimens. Photo courtesy of Dr. Manigandan Lejeune, Animal Health Diagnostic Center, Cornell University, Ithaca, NY.

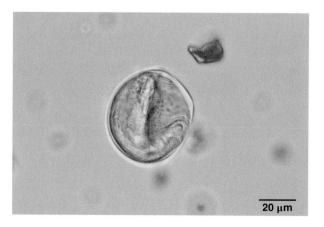

Fig. 1.186 Hyperosmotic flotation solutions can cause distortion of *Balantidium coli* cysts. This cyst, found in a ZnSO$_4$ centrifugal fecal flotation preparation, is partially collapsed. Photo courtesy of Dr. Manigandan Lejeune, Animal Health Diagnostic Center, Cornell University, Ithaca, NY.

PIGS

Helminth Parasites

Parasite: *Ascaris suum* (Fig. 1.187)

Common name: Roundworm.

Taxonomy: Nematode (order Ascaridida).

Geographic Distribution: Worldwide.

Location in Host: Small intestine.

Life Cycle: Pigs are infected when they ingest infective eggs in the environment. Following migration through the liver and lungs, adults develop in the small intestine. Like other ascarids, *A. suum* has very resistant eggs that can survive for years in the environment.

Laboratory Diagnosis: Eggs can be detected in feces with routine flotation procedures.

Size: 50–70 × 40–60 μm

Clinical Importance: *Ascaris suum* is a common and important parasite of swine, even in confinement systems. Larval migration through liver and lung may cause liver condemnation and predispose pigs to bacterial or viral pneumonia. Adult worms in the small intestine may cause reduced growth. Larvae can also migrate and cause disease in other animals and humans.

Parasite: **Hyostrongylus rubidus, Oesophagostomum spp.** (Figs. 1.188, 1.191)

Common name: Red stomach worm (*Hyostrongylus*), nodular worm (*Oesophagostomum*).

Taxonomy: Nematodes (order Strongylida).

Geographic Distribution: Worldwide.

Location in Host: Stomach (*Hyostrongylus*) and large intestine (*Oesophagostomum*) of wild and domestic swine.

Life Cycle: These parasites have a direct life cycle; eggs are shed in the feces and hatch in the environment. Swine are infected following ingestion of third-stage larvae.

Laboratory Diagnosis: Typical strongylid eggs are detected in fecal samples by flotation techniques. Eggs of *Hyostrongylus* and *Oesophagostomum* cannot be distinguished from each other or from less common strongylid parasites of swine, including *Trichostrongylus axei* and *Globocephalus*.

Size: 69–85 × 39–45 μm

Clinical Importance: These parasites are common in pastured swine. *Hyostrongylus* may cause ulcerative gastritis, resulting in anemia and reduced production. Host response to *Oesophagostomum* larvae in the wall of the intestinal tract leads to the development of nodules that, in heavy infections, can lead to enteritis and reduced production.

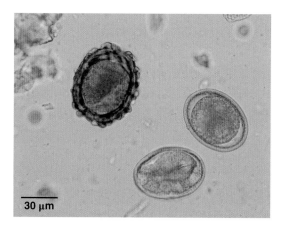

Fig. 1.187   Like other ascarid eggs, those of *Ascaris suum* contain a single cell surrounded by a thick shell when first passed in the feces. In some cases, the rough, brown outer layer of the shell may be absent, as seen in two of the eggs in this figure. *Ascaris suum* eggs are very similar in appearance to those of the human ascarid, *A. lumbricoides*.

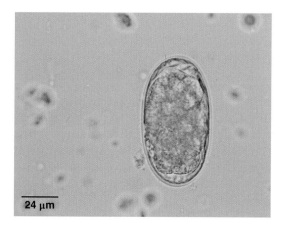

Fig. 1.188   *Hyostrongylus* and *Oesophagostomum* are the most common and important strongylid parasites of swine and produce indistinguishable eggs typical of this group of nematodes. Fecal culture and identification of third-stage larvae are necessary to identify parasite genus.

Parasite: ***Trichuris suis*** (Fig. 1.189)

  Common name: Whipworm.

Taxonomy: Nematode (order Enoplida).

Geographic Distribution: Worldwide.

Location in Host: Large intestine of wild and domestic pigs.

Life Cycle: *Trichuris* spp. have a direct life cycle. Pigs are infected following ingestion of infective eggs in the environment. Eggs leave the host in manure and are able to survive for long periods in the environment.

Laboratory Diagnosis: Eggs can be detected in routine fecal flotation tests.

  Size: 50–60 × 21–25 µm

Clinical Importance: This common helminth infection of swine may cause diarrhea and dehydration. Severe infections can produce bloody diarrhea.

Parasite: ***Strongyloides ransomi*** (Figs. 1.190 and 1.191)

  Common name: Threadworm.

Taxonomy: Nematode (order Rhabditida).

Geographic Distribution: Worldwide.

Location in Host: Small intestine.

Life Cycle: Larvated eggs are passed in the feces and hatch in the environment. After a free-living period in the environment, third-stage larvae are produced that infect pigs through either ingestion or skin penetration. Sows carrying larvae in the tissues transmit the parasite through the milk to their litters.

Laboratory Diagnosis: Eggs are detected in fecal samples using flotation techniques. The thin-shelled egg contains a larva in fresh fecal samples.

  Size: 45–55 × 26–35 µm

Clinical Importance: *Strongyloides* causes diarrhea in pigs as young as 10 days of age. Severe infections may be fatal.

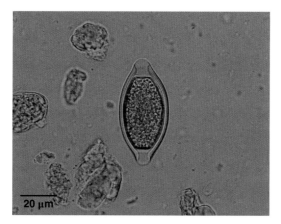

Fig. 1.189   Like other members of the genus, eggs of *Trichuris suis*, the swine whipworm, are football-shaped with a polar plug at each end.

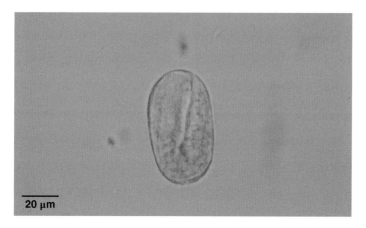

Fig. 1.190   Larvated *Strongyloides* eggs are usually present only in the feces of young pigs. Photo courtesy of Merial.

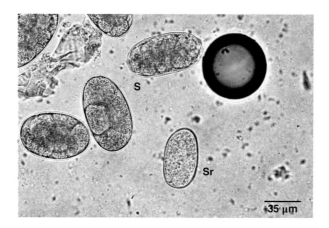

Fig. 1.191   The small *Strongyloides ransomi* egg (Sr) pictured here could be confused with strongylid eggs, but strongylid eggs (S) are larger and do not contain a larva in fresh fecal samples. The strongylid eggs in this photo are from *Oesophagostomum dentatum*. Photo courtesy of Dr. Yoko Nagamori, College of Veterinary Medicine, Oklahoma State University, Stillwater, OK.

Parasite: ***Metastrongylus* spp.** (Fig. 1.192)

　　Common name: Lungworm.

Taxonomy: Nematode (order Strongylida). Several species similar in life cycle and pathogenicity have been described.

Geographic Distribution: Worldwide.

Location in Host: Bronchi and bronchioles of domestic and wild pigs.

Life Cycle: Eggs containing a larva are passed in the feces of pigs. When earthworm intermediate hosts ingest the eggs, they hatch and develop to infective larvae. Swine are infected by ingestion of earthworms containing third-stage larvae.

Laboratory Diagnosis: Larvated eggs are detected in feces by flotation procedures.

　　Size: 51–63 × 33–42 µm

Clinical Importance: These parasites are uncommon in intensively raised swine. Heavy infections, especially in young pigs, can cause clinical respiratory disease.

Parasite: ***Physocephalus sexalatus, Ascarops strongylina*** (Figs. 1.193 and 1.194)

Taxonomy: Nematode (order Spirurida).

Geographic Distribution: Worldwide.

Location in Host: Stomach of domestic and wild pigs.

Life Cycle: Eggs containing larvae are passed in the feces, where they are ingested by beetle intermediate hosts. Pigs are infected following ingestion of larvae in the intermediate host.

Laboratory Diagnosis: A sedimentation procedure is recommended for detecting spirurid parasite eggs. The ellipsoidal eggs of both species are indistinguishable and are larvated when passed in the feces.

　　Size: 39–45 × 17–26 µm

Clinical Importance: Spirurid parasites are uncommon in intensively raised swine. Most infections are asymptomatic, but heavy infections may produce gastritis, leading to weight loss or failure to gain.

PIGS

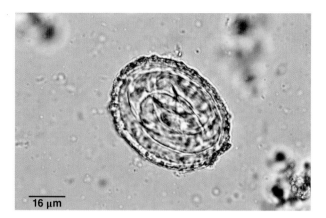

Fig. 1.192   In fresh fecal samples, *Metastrongylus* eggs contain a larva and have a thick shell with a rough surface. Photo courtesy of Dr. Yoko Nagamori, College of Veterinary Medicine, Oklahoma State University, Stillwater, OK.

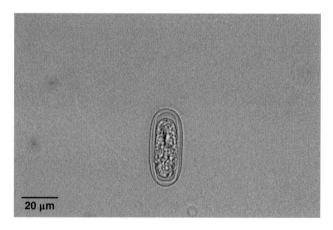

Fig. 1.193   Egg of *Physocephalus*. Photo courtesy of Merial.

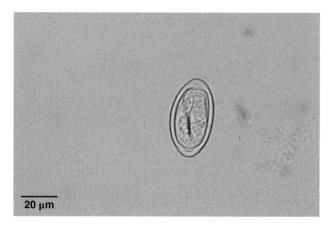

Fig. 1.194   *Ascarops* egg. Spirurid eggs are unlikely to be seen if standard flotation procedures are used. Their larvated eggs have a thick shell (easily appreciated in the *Physocephalus* egg), unlike the thin-shelled eggs of *Strongyloides* or *Metastrongylus*. Photo courtesy of Merial.

PIGS

Parasite: *Fasciola* **spp.,** *Eurytrema pancreaticum, Dicrocoelium dentriticum, Schistosoma* **spp.** (Figs. 1.156, 1.159, 1.160, 1.195)

Although swine are not considered to be the primary host for most trematodes, pigs may be infected with trematode parasites (*Fasciola* spp., *E. pancreaticum, D. dentriticum, Schistosoma* spp.) that also infect ruminants. Trematode infections of domestic swine would only be seen in pastured pigs because the complicated life cycle of flukes prevents transmission in confinement operations.

Parasite: *Macracanthorhynchus hirudinaceus* (Fig. 1.196)

Common name: Thorny-headed worm.

Taxonomy: Acanthocephalan.

Geographic Distribution: Worldwide.

Location in Host: Small intestine.

Life Cycle: Parasite eggs are passed in manure and ingested by beetle intermediate hosts. Swine are infected when they ingest infective larvae (cystacanths) in beetles.

Laboratory Diagnosis: Eggs are not consistently recovered by flotation procedures. A sedimentation procedure should also be performed.

Size: Variable, 67–110 × 40–65 μm

Clinical Importance: Acanthocephalan parasites have a proboscis covered with hooks. Attachment of the proboscis causes damage to the intestinal wall. Clinical signs range from none to diarrhea and weight loss. *Macracanthorhynchus* is unlikely to be present in total-confinement systems.

PIGS

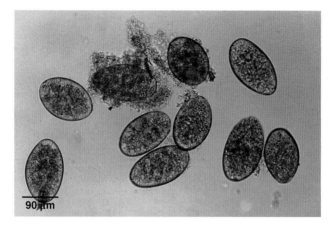

Fig. 1.195 *Fasciola* eggs. Trematode infections are rarely encountered in swine in North America, but are more common in other parts of the world where pigs range freely and infections also occur in other domestic animals. Photo courtesy of Dr. Alvin Gajadhar, Centre for Animal Parasitology, CFIA, Saskatoon, Saskatchewan, Canada.

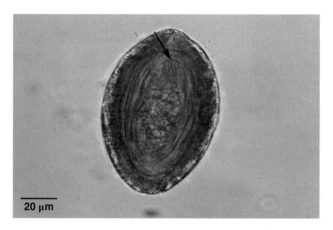

Fig. 1.196 *Macracanthorhynchus hirudinaceus* egg. The embryo (acanthor) is surrounded by several membranes and contains hooks at one end that are often visible (*arrow*). Common tapeworm eggs also contain hooks, but thorny-headed worm eggs have a more complex membranous structure and an elongated embryo. Photo courtesy of Dr. Alvin Gajadhar, Centre for Animal Parasitology, CFIA, Saskatoon, Saskatchewan, Canada.

PIGS

Birds

Protozoan Parasites

Parasite: ***Eimeria* spp., *Isospora* spp.** (Figs. 1.197–1.201, 1.211)

Common name: Coccidia.

Taxonomy: Protozoa (coccidia). *Eimeria* spp. are common in poultry and other Galliformes and Columbriformes. *Isospora* spp. are more common in Passeriformes, Psittaciformes, and Piciformes. Species of coccidia are host specific. *Caryospora*, *Sarcocystis*, and *Atoxoplasma* are other coccidia genera that infect some birds.

Geographic Distribution: Worldwide.

Location in Host: Primarily in the gastrointestinal tract.

Life Cycle: These parasites have a typical coccidia life cycle. Birds ingest infective oocysts from the environment. Sexual and asexual multiplication most often occurs within cells of the intestinal tract (some species are found in other organs). Development culminates in the production of oocysts, which are passed in the feces.

Laboratory Diagnosis: *Eimeria* oocysts are detected with routine flotation procedures. Sporulation of oocysts may be required for species identification.

Size: Approximately 10–45 μm in length (oocysts), depending on species

Clinical Importance: Coccidia are common parasites of domestic and wild birds. Many infections are asymptomatic, but under some circumstances coccidia may cause severe diarrhea and death. *Eimeria* spp. are among the most important pathogens in modern poultry confinement operations.

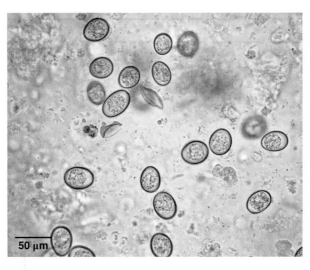

Fig. 1.197 *Eimeria* spp. oocysts from a chicken. *Eimeria* species are common parasites of wild and domestic birds. Individual birds may be infected with multiple coccidia species.

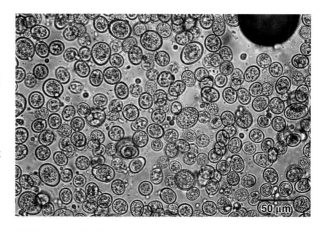

Fig. 1.198 After reaching the environment, *Eimeria* oocysts sporulate; the length of time required for this process is determined by temperature but may take only a few days. Birds may be simultaneously infected with multiple *Eimeria* species. This chicken sample shows oocysts of different sizes representing several different species. Photo courtesy of Dr. Yoko Nagamori, College of Veterinary Medicine, Oklahoma State University, Stillwater, OK.

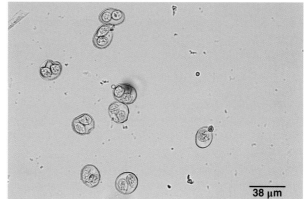

Fig. 1.199 *Isospora* spp. can also be found in birds, as seen in this fecal sample from a zebra finch. Sporulated *Isospora* spp. oocysts contain two sporocysts. Photo courtesy of Dr. Manigandan Lejeune, Animal Health Diagnostic Center, Cornell University, Ithaca, NY.

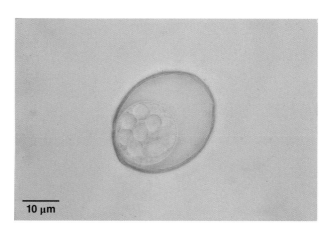

Fig. 1.200 *Caryospora* oocyst. The sporulated oocyst of this genus contains a single sporocyst with eight sporozoites. Photo courtesy of Dr. David Baker, School of Veterinary Medicine, Louisiana State University, Baton Rouge, LA.

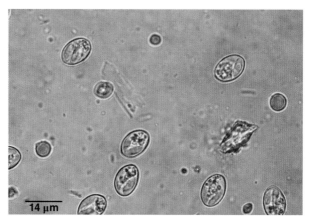

Fig. 1.201 *Sarcocystis* is another coccidia genus that may be found in the feces of carnivorous birds that act as the definitive host of the parasite. Oocysts sporulate in the host, and small sporocysts are passed in the feces. Photo courtesy of Dr. Yoko Nagamori, College of Veterinary Medicine, Oklahoma State University, Stillwater, OK.

Parasite: ***Cryptosporidium* spp.** (Fig. 1.202)

Taxonomy: Protozoa (coccidia). Avian species of this genus include *C. baileyi* and *C. meleagridis*. The latter species has been found to be infective for humans and some other mammals, as well as birds.

Geographic Distribution: Worldwide.

Location in Host: Gastrointestinal, respiratory, and/or urinary tracts depending on host.

Life Cycle: Infection of the bird host follows ingestion of the infective oocyst. Development and reproduction occur in the epithelial cells of the gastrointestinal and respiratory tract primarily. In some bird species, the urinary tract is affected.

Laboratory Diagnosis: Oocysts can be detected with the Sheather's sugar flotation procedure. Acid-fast or other staining procedures of fecal smears can also be used, as well as fecal immunodiagnostic tests.

   Size: 4–6 μm in diameter

Clinical Importance: Depending on the body systems affected, birds may show diarrhea, coughing, sneezing, and dyspnea or renal disease. Severe infection may cause death. *Cryptosporidium meleagridis* can infect humans.

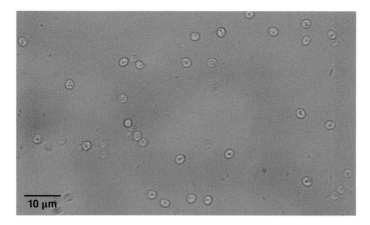

Fig. 1.202 *Cryptosporidium* spp. oocysts in birds are similar in appearance to those of mammalian species. Slides should be examined using the 40× lens of the microscope.

Parasite: **Gastrointestinal Flagellates** (Figs. 1.203 and 1.204; see also Figs. 1.53–1.59 for illustrations of *Giardia*)

Taxonomy: Protozoa (flagellates). Several genera are found in the avian digestive tract, including *Trichomonas*, *Cochlosoma*, *Histomonas*, *Giardia*, *Spironucleus* (= *Hexamita*), and *Chilomastix*.

Geographic Distribution: Worldwide.

Location in Host: *Trichomonas gallinae* is found in the upper digestive system; *Histomonas* in the cecum and liver; and *Cochlosoma*, *Giardia*, and *Spironucleus* in the intestines.

Life Cycle: Most avian flagellates have only a trophozoite stage. They are transmitted from bird to bird by direct contact and contaminated food or water. Feeding of young birds by adults can also transmit *T. gallinae*, while *Histomonas* can be carried in the eggs of the cecal roundworm, *Heterakis*. *Giardia* trophozoites encyst in the intestinal tract. Cysts passed in the feces are ingested by birds. *Chilomastix* also forms cysts.

Laboratory Diagnosis: *Trichomonas* trophozoites have anterior flagella and an undulating membrane. They can usually be detected in smears made from exudates or lesions in the oral cavity, esophagus, and crop. *Giardia* cysts can be recovered by $ZnSO_4$ centrifugal flotation. *Chilomastix* cysts are rarely found in feces. *Giardia*, *Spironucleus*, and *Cochlosoma* trophozoites may be seen in very fresh fecal smears. *Spironucleus* has no sucking disk, unlike *Giardia* and *Cochlosoma*. *Histomonas* is unlikely to be detected in fecal smears.

Size:		
	Trichomonas	8–14 μm in length, depending on species
	Giardia trophozoites	10–20 × 5–15 μm
	Giardia cysts	10–14 × 8–10 μm
	Cochlosoma	6–10 × 4–6.5 μm
	Spironucleus	5–12 × 2–7 μm
	Chilomastix	6–24 × 3–10 μm

Clinical Importance: Pigeons and raptors are particularly susceptible to trichomoniasis of the upper digestive tract. Affected birds may show depression and weakness with characteristic plaques and accumulation of cheesy material in the mouth, esophagus, and crop. Severe infections may be fatal. Although many *Giardia* infections are asymptomatic, the parasite can cause diarrhea, depression, and debilitation, particularly in young psittacines. Feather picking associated with infection has also been described. *Histomonas* is the cause of blackhead in turkeys. Other flagellates may also produce diarrhea, but many infections are asymptomatic. None of these avian flagellates has zoonotic importance.

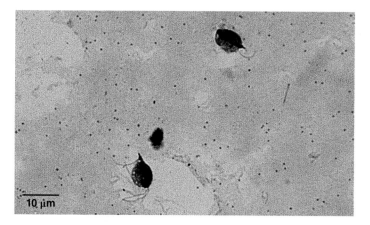

Fig. 1.203   *Trichomonas* spp. in birds have an undulating membrane and several anterior flagella. They can be seen in smears made from lesions in the upper gastrointestinal tract. The presence of caseous lesions in the esophagus and crop is also helpful in diagnosis.

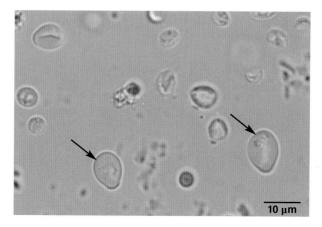

Fig. 1.204   *Chilomastix* is a genus of intestinal flagellate found in birds, pigs, and primates. Infections are usually considered of no pathogenic importance, but the lemon-shaped parasite cysts (arrow) may be seen in fecal samples. Photo courtesy of Dr. Manigandan Lejeune, Animal Health Diagnostic Center, Cornell University, Ithaca, NY.

Helminth Parasites

Parasite: *Capillaria* spp., *Eucoleus* spp. (Figs. 1.205–1.207, 1.213)

Taxonomy: Nematode (order Enoplida). A variety of species can be found in domestic and wild birds.

Geographic Distribution: Worldwide.

Location in Host: Various locations in the gastrointestinal tract, depending on species.

Life Cycle: Eggs are passed in the feces of the host and become infective in the environment. Some species, such as *C. obsignata*, have a direct life cycle, while others have been shown to use an earthworm intermediate host.

Laboratory Diagnosis: Bipolar-plugged eggs can be detected in the feces with flotation techniques.

Size: Approximately 45–70 μm in length, depending on species

Clinical Importance: Capillarid parasites can cause severe inflammation wherever species occur in the digestive tract, including the esophagus, crop, and intestines. Heavy infections may be fatal.

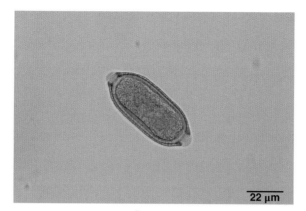

Fig. 1.205   Eggs of *Capillaria* spp. are very common in the feces of domestic and wild birds. The bipolar-plugged eggs have a thick shell and are typically yellowish. This *Capillaria* egg was present in a fecal sample from a superb starling. *Capillaria* spp. are uncommon in poultry maintained in total-confinement systems. Photo courtesy of Dr. Manigandan Lejeune, Animal Health Diagnostic Center, Cornell University, Ithaca, NY.

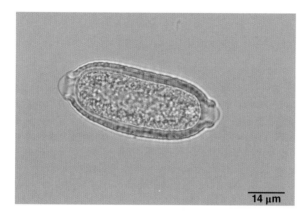

Fig. 1.206   Egg of *Eucoleus dispar* from a sharp-shinned hawk. Photo courtesy of Dr. Manigandan Lejeune, Animal Health Diagnostic Center, Cornell University, Ithaca, NY.

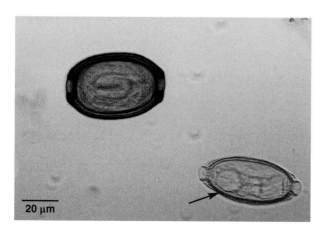

Fig. 1.207   *Capillaria* sp. egg in an owl (*arrow*). The larger, browner egg belongs to *Trichosomoides* sp., a parasite of the bladder of rats. Because parasite eggs of prey are sometimes found in predator feces, it is important to appreciate the normal array of parasites found in a host so spurious parasites can be correctly identified. Photo courtesy of Dr. Stephen Smith, Virginia-Maryland College of Veterinary Medicine, Virginia Tech, Blacksburg, VA.

Parasite: **Avian Ascarids** (Figs. 1. 208–1.210)

Common name: Roundworm, cecal worm (*Heterakis*).

Taxonomy: Nematodes (order Ascaridida). *Ascaridia* spp. and *Heterakis* spp. are common in poultry and many wild bird hosts. *Subulura* spp. occur less commonly in poultry and various other species of birds. *Porroceacum* spp. and *Contracecum* spp. are also found in a variety of bird hosts.

Geographic Distribution: Worldwide.

Location in Host: Intestinal tract; *Heterakis* spp. and *Subulura* spp. parasitize the ceca of birds.

Life Cycle: Eggs are passed in the feces of the bird host and develop to the infective stage in the environment. Birds become infected when they ingest infective eggs. Earthworms may act as transport hosts.

Laboratory Diagnosis: Thick-shelled eggs are detected with flotation procedures. Eggs of *Ascaridia* and *Heterakis* are similar in size and morphology and may be difficult to differentiate. Eggs of *Subulura* are larvated.

Size:	*Ascaridia*	77–94 × 43–55 μm
	Heterakis	66–79 × 41–48 μm
	Subulura	51–86 × 45–76 μm

Clinical Importance: Larvae of *Ascaridia* appear to be the most pathogenic stage and may cause enteritis in the prepatent period. Heavy burdens of adult worms can cause enteritis and intestinal obstruction. *Heterakis* is primarily important in poultry as a vector of *Histomonas meleagridis* (blackhead), which can be a serious disease of turkeys. The protozoan is carried from bird to bird in the eggs and larvae of *Heterakis*. Fatal infections of *Heterakis isolonche* due to nodular typhlitis have been reported in pheasants.

BIRDS, RODENTS, RABBITS, REPTILES

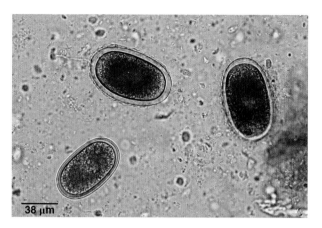

Fig. 1.208   A smooth, thick shell is seen in both *Ascaridia* spp. and *Heterakis* spp. eggs. This sample from a chicken shows two larger *Ascaridia* eggs and a single smaller *Heterakis* egg. The eggs of these two genera may be difficult to distinguish. Photo courtesy of Dr. Yoko Nagamori, College of Veterinary Medicine, Oklahoma State University, Stillwater, OK.

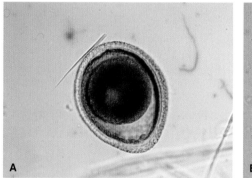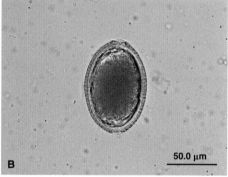

Fig. 1.209   Another ascarid genus found in ducks and wild birds is *Porrocecum*, which has eggs with a rough shell similar in appearance to that of many mammalian ascarid species. Some *Porrocecum* eggs have polar plugs. (A) was found in feces from a Harris hawk, and (B) was from a great horned owl.

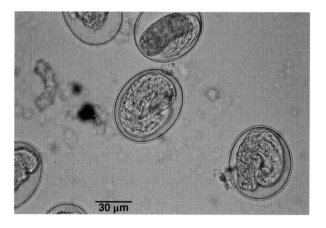

Fig. 1.210   *Subulura brumpti* eggs in the feces of a chicken. Unlike most ascarids, the relatively thick-walled eggs of subulurids are larvated when passed in the feces, but species identification may be difficult. Photo courtesy of Dr. Erin Burton, University of Minnesota College of Veterinary Medicine, St. Paul, MN.

Parasite: ***Trichostrongylus tenuis, Amidostomum* spp., and Other Avian Strongylids** (Fig. 1.211)

Taxonomy: Nematodes (order Strongylida). *Trichostrongylus tenuis* and *Amidostomum* spp. occur in domestic and game birds.

Geographic Distribution: Worldwide.

Location in Host: Cecum and intestines of game birds, poultry, and wild birds.

Life Cycle: Eggs are passed from the host in the feces. First-stage larvae hatch from the eggs, develop to the infective stage in the environment, and develop to the adult stage when ingested by the avian host.

Laboratory Diagnosis: Typical thin-shelled strongylid eggs can be detected with flotation procedures.

Size:	Varies with species	
	T. tenuis	65–75 × 35–42 μm
	Amidostomum anseri	85–110 × 50–82 μm

Clinical Importance: Heavy infections of *T. tenuis* can produce severe enteritis with resulting hemorrhagic diarrhea, weight loss, and death.

Parasite: ***Syngamus* spp.** (Figs. 1.212 and 1.213)

Common name: Gapeworm.

Taxonomy: Nematode (order Strongylida).

Geographic Distribution: Worldwide.

Location in Host: Trachea and bronchi of numerous domestic and wild birds. Species of a similar genus, *Cyathostoma*, are found in some aquatic birds and birds of prey.

Life Cycle: Eggs are produced by females in the trachea and are coughed up, swallowed, and passed out of the host in the feces. Infective larvae may be eaten directly from the environment by the avian host, or they may be ingested by an earthworm or molluscan transport host that is eaten, in turn, by a bird.

Laboratory Diagnosis: Ellipsoidal, bipolar eggs are seen in the feces with flotation procedures.

Size: 80–110 × 40–50 μm

Clinical Importance: Young birds are most severely affected. Large numbers of parasites and exudate obstruct the airways and can suffocate the host. The parasite's common name originates from the gaping and gasping of infected birds as they attempt to breathe. *Syngamus* is uncommon in total-confinement poultry systems.

BIRDS, RODENTS, RABBITS, REPTILES

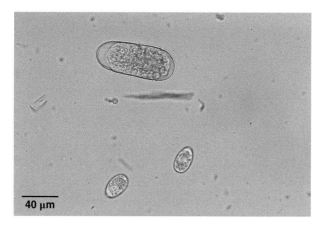

Fig. 1.211 Strongylid egg and coccidia oocysts in an avian fecal sample.

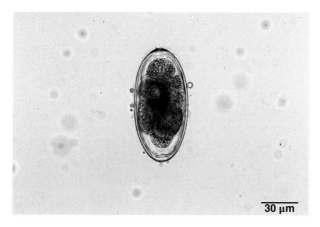

Fig. 1.212 *Syngamus* sp. egg from a crow. This is a common parasite of wild birds and poultry kept outside. Unlike most strongylid eggs, *Syngamus* eggs have bipolar plugs.

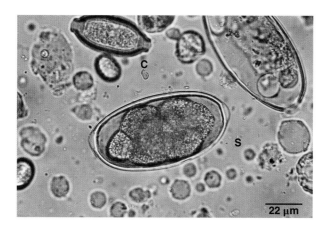

Fig. 1.213 Like *Syngamus*, eggs of *Capillaria* and *Eucoleus* spp. have bipolar plugs. However, the eggs of *Syngamus* are larger and contain several well-defined cells (morula) when passed in the feces. In this specimen from a pheasant, an egg of both *Syngamus* (S) and *Capillaria* (C) is present. Photo courtesy of Dr. Manigandan Lejeune, Animal Health Diagnostic Center, Cornell University, Ithaca, NY.

Parasite: *Dispharynx, Echinuria, Tetrameres, Cheilospirura (Acuaria), Serratospiculum,* and Others (Figs. 1.214–1.216)

Taxonomy: Nematodes (order Spirurida).

Geographic Distribution: Worldwide.

Location in Host: Species are found throughout the digestive tract. *Serratospiculum* parasitizes the respiratory tract of some wild birds.

Life Cycle: Adults (except *Serratospiculum*) are located in the digestive tract. Eggs are passed in the feces and are ingested by various arthropod intermediate hosts. Birds are infected by ingesting an intermediate host carrying infective larvae.

Laboratory Diagnosis: Flotation and sedimentation techniques can be used to detect the relatively small, larvated eggs in feces.

     Size: Approximately 30–55 × 20–35 μm, depending on species

Clinical Importance: Most infections with this group of parasites are not highly pathogenic. However, *Tetrameres* and *Dispharynx* in large numbers in the proventriculus may cause weight loss and reduced production. In poultry, members of this group of parasites are rare in total-confinement management systems.

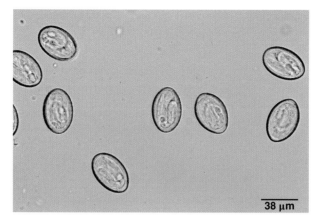

Fig. 1.214   Spirurid egg in the feces of a double-crested cormorant. Larvae are visible within the eggs.

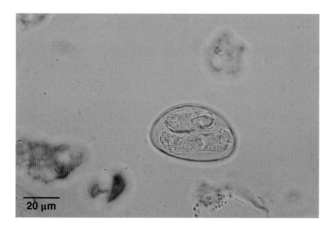

Fig. 1.215   Spirurid egg in the feces of a red-tailed hawk. The larva within the egg is clearly visible. Photo courtesy of Dr. Stephen Smith, Virginia-Maryland College of Veterinary Medicine, Virginia Tech, Blacksburg, VA.

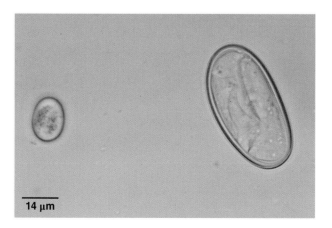

Fig. 1.216   *Tetrameres* egg in the feces of a homing pigeon. Like other spirurid eggs, this *Tetrameres* egg is larvated when passed in the feces, but further specific identification is difficult. Also pictured is a coccidia oocyst. Photo courtesy of Dr. Robert Ridley, College of Veterinary Medicine, Kansas State University, Manhattan, KS.

BIRDS, RODENTS, RABBITS, REPTILES

Parasite: *Echinostoma* spp., *Echinoparyphium*, *Prosthogonimus* spp., and Others (Figs. 1.217 and 1.218)

Common name: Fluke.

Taxonomy: Trematode.

Geographic Distribution: Worldwide.

Location in Host: Domestic and wild birds are parasitized by many fluke species. Adults can be found in various body systems, including the intestines and respiratory and reproductive tracts.

Life Cycle: Adult worms produce eggs that leave the host principally via the digestive tract. The first intermediate host is a mollusk, and a variety of animals act as second intermediate host depending on the fluke species (with the exception of schistosomes, which do not require a second intermediate host).

Laboratory Diagnosis: Fluke eggs in feces are best detected with a sedimentation technique because of their higher density. Fluke eggs are typically operculated and brown.

Size: Highly variable with species, approximately 20–100 μm in length

Clinical Importance: Many fluke infections are of low pathogenicity. Some genera of importance in domestic poultry are *Echinostoma* and *Echinoparyphium*, which may cause enteritis, and *Prosthogonimus*, a parasite of the oviduct, which can cause abnormal egg production and peritonitis. Because of their complex life cycles, flukes will be seen only in birds with access to intermediate hosts and will not occur in poultry confinement operations.

BIRDS, RODENTS, RABBITS, REPTILES

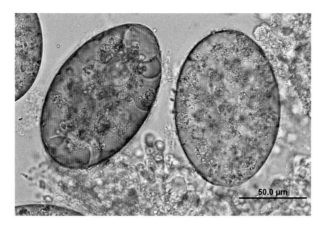

Fig. 1.217   Fluke eggs in avian feces. The operculum is not readily visible in these trematode eggs.

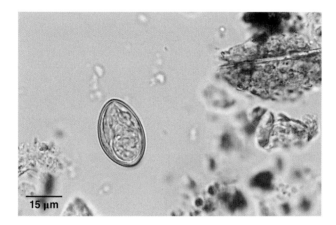

Fig. 1.218   The developing miracidium can be seen inside this avian trematode egg found in feces from a bird of prey.

Parasite: ***Davainea* spp., *Choanotaenia* spp., *Raillietina* spp., *Hymenolepis* spp., and Others** (Figs. 1.219, 1.220)

Common name: Tapeworm.

Taxonomy: Cestode.

Geographic Distribution: Worldwide.

Location in Host: Small intestine of a wide variety of domestic and wild birds.

Life Cycle: Eggs are passed in the feces. Insects are the most common intermediate hosts, but other invertebrates may also be used by some species (e.g., the intermediate host of *Davainea* is a mollusk).

Laboratory Diagnosis: Although proglottids are intermittently passed in the feces, detection of eggs by fecal exam is unreliable, and diagnosis is usually made at necropsy.

Size: Varies with species; individual eggs of many species are approximately 50–80 μm; some species have large egg packets

Clinical Importance: Many tapeworm infections are asymptomatic. However, some are serious pathogens; for example, *Davainea proglottina* and *Raillietina echinobothrida* can cause severe enteritis and death in domestic poultry. Tapeworms are common in unconfined poultry with access to the intermediate hosts.

BIRDS, RODENTS, RABBITS, REPTILES

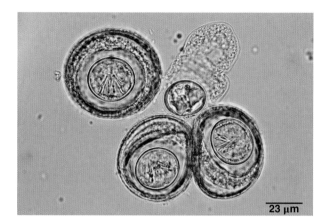

Fig. 1.219   *Raillietina* sp. eggs from a chicken. The embryonic hooks are clearly visible, and this character-istic is very helpful in recognizing tapeworm eggs. Photo courtesy of Dr. Manigandan Lejeune, Animal Health Diagnostic Center, Cornell University, Ithaca, NY.

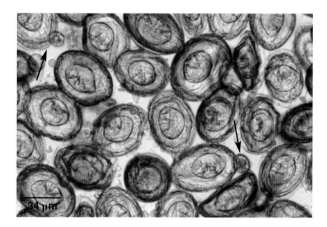

Fig. 1.220   Tapeworm eggs from a magpie. Scattered among the cestode eggs are occasional coccidia oocysts (*arrows*). Photo courtesy of Dr. Alvin Gajadhar, Centre for Animal Parasitology, CFIA, Saskatoon, Saskatchewan, Canada.

Parasite: ***Polymorphus* spp., *Filicollis* spp., and Others** (Figs. 1.221 and 1.222)

Common name: Thorny-headed worm.

Taxonomy: Acanthocephalan.

Geographic Distribution: Worldwide.

Location in Host: Digestive system.

Life Cycle: Eggs are passed in the feces of the host. Infective larvae develop in arthropod intermediate hosts and infect birds when they are ingested.

Laboratory Diagnosis: Eggs are not consistently recovered by flotation procedures. A sedimentation procedure should also be performed.

Size: Approximately 50–100 µm in length, depending on species

Clinical Importance: Thorny-headed worms are primarily parasites of free-ranging and wild birds because of their complex life cycles. Heavy infections may cause diarrhea and debilitation.

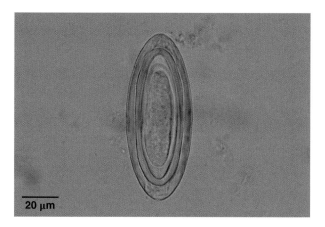

Fig. 1.221   Egg of a thorny-headed worm (*Centrorhynchus*) from the feces of a barred owl. Acanthocephalan eggs have several internal layers surrounding the larva (acanthor). Photo courtesy of Dr. Ellis C. Greiner, College of Veterinary Medicine, University of Florida, Gainesville, FL.

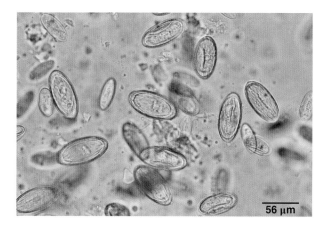

Fig. 1.222   Acanthocephalan (*Plagiorhynchus* sp.) eggs in the feces of an eastern blue bird. Photo courtesy of Dr. Manigandan Lejeune, Animal Health Diagnostic Center, Cornell University, Ithaca, NY.

BIRDS, RODENTS, RABBITS, REPTILES

Rodents and Rabbits

Protozoan Parasites

Parasite: *Eimeria* **spp.** (Figs. 1.223–1.225)

　　　　　Common name: Coccidia.

Taxonomy: Protozoa (coccidia).

Geographic Distribution: Worldwide.

Location in Host: A variety of species parasitize the intestinal tract of rodents and rabbits. *Eimeria stiedae* is found in the bile ducts of rabbits.

Life Cycle: Oocysts passed in the feces can sporulate quickly and infect the host when ingested. Asexual and sexual reproduction occurs in cells of the gastrointestinal tract.

Laboratory Diagnosis: Oocysts can be detected in feces by centrifugal or simple flotation techniques. Oocysts are elliptical to spherical-shaped.

　　Size: Approximately 10–45 × 10–30 μm, depending on species

Clinical Importance: Some species are nonpathogenic. Pathogenic intestinal coccidia can cause anorexia, weight loss, profuse diarrhea, and death. *Eimeria stiedae* infection of the rabbit liver can cause anorexia, diarrhea, distended abdomen, and death.

　　Rodents may also be infected with species of *Giardia* and *Cryptosporidium* (see Figs. 1.50 and 1.53–1.59).

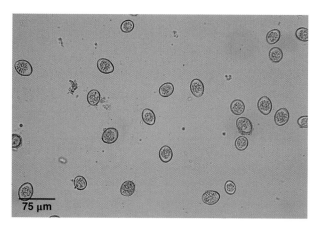

Fig. 1.223 *Eimeria* oocysts have smooth, clear cyst walls and contain a single round cell when freshly passed. The oocysts in this figure are *Eimeria nieschulzi*, a parasite of rats. Photo courtesy of Dr. George Conder, Pfizer Veterinary Medicine Pharmaceuticals Clinical Development, Pfizer, Inc., Kalamazoo, MI.

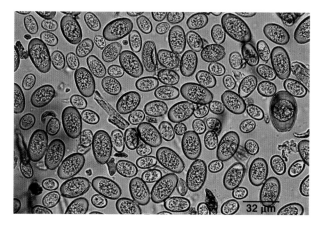

Fig. 1.224 Rodent and rabbit hosts may be infected with multiple species of coccidia. Oocysts of more than one species of rabbit *Eimeria* were detected in this sample. Photo courtesy of Dr. Yoko Nagamori, College of Veterinary Medicine, Oklahoma State University, Stillwater, OK.

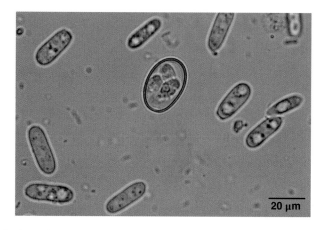

Fig. 1.225 Once in the environment, oocysts undergo sporulation to the infective stage. Sporulated oocysts of *Eimeria* contain four sporocysts, each containing two sporozoites (individual organisms). The sporocysts can clearly be seen inside this rabbit *Eimeria* sp. oocyst. Surrounding the oocyst are several elongated nonpathogenic yeast organisms that are very common in rabbit feces.

Helminth Parasites

Parasite: ***Syphacia obvelata*** (Fig. 1.226)

>   Common name: Pinworm.

Taxonomy: Nematode (order Oxyurida).

Geographic Distribution: Worldwide.

Location in Host: Large intestine of mice and gerbils.

Life Cycle: Eggs passed in the feces quickly become infective. Rodents develop infection following ingestion of larvated eggs.

Laboratory Diagnosis: When present in the feces, eggs can be detected by routine flotation techniques. Eggs are normally found on the skin in the perineal region of infected animals.

>   Size: 100–142 × 30–40 μm

Clinical Importance: Infections are typically subclinical.

Parasite: ***Aspiculuris tetraptera*** (Fig. 1.227)

>   Common name: Pinworm.

Taxonomy: Nematode (order Oxyurida).

Geographic Distribution: Worldwide.

Location in Host: Large intestine of mice.

Life Cycle: The life cycle is similar to that of *Syphacia oblevata*. Adult pinworms develop following ingestion of infective eggs.

Laboratory Diagnosis: Eggs can be detected in feces by centrifugal or simple flotation techniques. The eggs are ellipsoidal with a distinctive double shell wall and contain an undifferentiated embryo in fresh feces.

>   Size: 70–98 × 29–50 μm

Clinical Importance: Infections are usually subclinical.

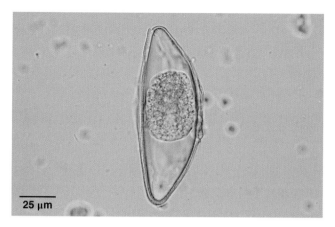

Fig. 1.226   *Syphacia* egg in feces from a gerbil. Eggs of *Syphacia* have a smooth, clear shell wall; are flat on one side; and contain an undifferentiated morula in fresh fecal samples.

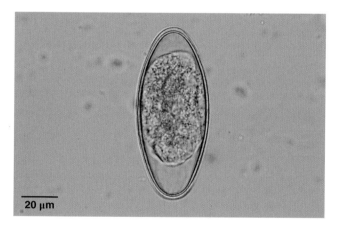

Fig. 1.227   *Aspiculuris* eggs have narrowed poles and a smooth, clear, double shell wall. Pinworms are common in rodents.

Parasite: ***Passalurus ambiguus*** (Fig. 1.228)

Common name: Pinworm.

Taxonomy: Nematode (order Oxyurida).

Geographic Distribution: Worldwide.

Location in Host: Cecum of rabbits.

Life Cycle: Eggs are passed in the feces of infected rabbits. The eggs become infective within a short period and infect the next host when ingested.

Laboratory Diagnosis: Eggs can be detected in feces by flotation techniques. The eggs have a smooth, clear shell wall that is flat on one side.

Size: 95–103 × 43 μm

Clinical Importance: Infections are usually subclinical.

Parasite: ***Paraspidodera uncinata, Heterakis spumosa*** (Fig. 1.229)

Taxonomy: Nematodes (order Ascaridida).

Geographic Distribution: Worldwide.

Location in Host: Cecum of guinea pigs (*Paraspidodera*) and rats (*Heterakis*).

Life Cycle: Eggs passed in the feces develop to the infective stage and infect the host when they are ingested.

Laboratory Diagnosis: Fecal flotation procedures can be used to recover these thick-shelled eggs.

Size: *Heterakis*   55–60 × 40–55 μm

           Paraspidodera   43 × 31 μm

Clinical Importance: Infection is usually subclinical. These parasites are seen primarily in wild rats and guinea pigs raised on dirt.

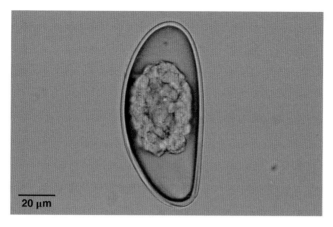

Fig. 1.228   *Passalurus ambiguus* eggs have an operculum-like structure at one end (not clearly visible in this example), and the eggs contain an undifferentiated morula in fresh fecal samples.

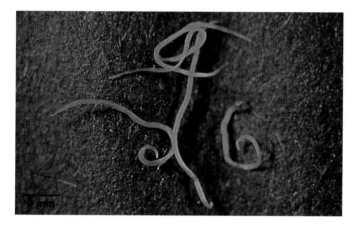

Fig. 1.229   Specimens of *Paraspidodera uncinata*, the cecal worm of guinea pigs. The eggs produced by this cecal nematode of rodents are similar to those of the avian cecal worm, *Heterakis* (Fig. 1.194). Photo courtesy of Dr. David Baker, School of Veterinary Medicine, Louisiana State University, Baton Rouge, LA.

BIRDS, RODENTS, RABBITS, REPTILES

Parasite: ***Heligmosomoides polygyrus, Nippostrongylus braziliensis, Obeliscoides cuniculi, Graphidium strigosum*** (Fig. 1.230)

Taxonomy: Nematodes (order Strongylida).

Geographic Distribution: Worldwide.

Location in Host: Stomach (*Obeliscoides, Graphidium*) of rabbits; small intestine of rats (*Nippostrongylus*) and mice (*Heligmosomoides*).

Life Cycle: Eggs passed in the feces develop into first-stage larvae, which hatch and continue development in the environment. In most cases, the definitive host is infected by ingesting third-stage larvae, but larvae of *Nippostrongylus braziliensis* usually penetrate the skin of the final host.

Laboratory Diagnosis: Fecal flotation procedures will recover the typical strongylid eggs produced by these parasites.

   Size: 52–106 × 28–58 µm (eggs), depending on species

Clinical Importance: Parasites belonging to this group of nematodes are unlikely to occur in caged rabbits and rodents but are common in wild animals. Infection is usually subclinical.

Parasite: ***Hymenolepis* spp.** (Figs. 1.231 and 1.232)

   Common name: Dwarf tapeworm of humans (*Hymenolepis nana*).

Taxonomy: Cestode. The most common species in domestic rodents is *Hymenolepis* (= *Vampirolepis*) *nana*. Other species infecting rodents are *H. diminuta* and *H. microstoma*.

Geographic Distribution: Worldwide.

Location in Host: Small intestine of rodents (mouse, rat, hamster). Humans and other primates also serve as hosts for *H. nana*.

Life Cycle: Eggs passed in the feces of definitive hosts are ingested by beetle intermediate hosts. Rodents and humans are infected following ingestion of the intermediate host containing cysticercoids. Infection with adult *H. nana* can also follow ingestion of the egg.

Laboratory Diagnosis: Eggs with six embryonic hooks are detected by either centrifugal or simple fecal flotation examination.

   Size: *H. nana*   40–45 × 34–37 µm

              H. diminuta   60–88 × 52–81 µm

Clinical Importance: Infections are usually subclinical. Heavy infections, particularly in young animals, can result in poor growth and rarely intestinal impaction and death.

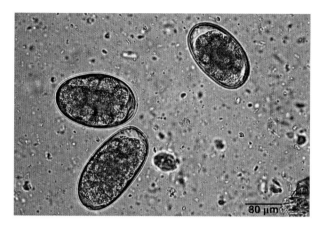

Fig. 1.230   Strongylid eggs in the feces of rabbits and rodents are similar to those produced by species in other common domestic hosts. These eggs were observed in the feces of a rabbit. Photo courtesy of Dr. Yoko Nagamori, College of Veterinary Medicine, Oklahoma State University, Stillwater, OK.

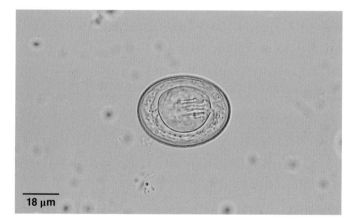

Fig. 1.231   *Hymenolepis nana* infects rodents and primates. Eggs are elliptical in shape with a smooth, clear shell wall and contain an embryo with six hooks. There are two knoblike protrusions at each end of the embryo. Like eggs of other common tapeworms, hooks are visible within the embryo.

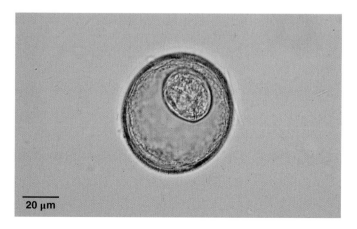

Fig. 1.232   Other species of *Hymenolepis* found in rodents have larger, rounder eggs than *H. nana*. Hymenolepid eggs are seen occasionally in fecal samples of dogs and cats that have recently eaten rodents.

Parasite: *Cittotaenia* spp. (Fig. 1.233)

　　　　Common name: Rabbit tapeworm.

Taxonomy: Cestode.

Geographic Distribution: Worldwide.

Location in Host: Small intestine of rabbits and hares.

Life Cycle: Eggs are ingested by free-living oribatid mites and develop into the cysticercoid larval stage. Rabbits are infected when they ingest the infected mites.

Laboratory Diagnosis: Fecal flotation procedures will recover *Cittotaenia* eggs.

　　Size: 64 μm in diameter

Clinical Importance: Heavy infections may cause weight loss.

Reptiles

Parasite: *Entamoeba, Cryptosporidium, Eimeria, Isospora, Caryospora,* other protozoa (Figs. 1.234–1.238)

Taxonomy: Protozoa.

Geographic Distribution: Worldwide.

Location in Host: Gastrointestinal tract.

Life Cycle: Reptiles are infected by ingestion of cysts or oocysts that are passed in host feces.

Laboratory Diagnosis: *Eimeria, Caryospora,* and *Cryptosporidium* oocysts and *Nyctotherus* cysts can be detected by fecal flotation techniques (the centrifugal flotation procedure with Sheather's sugar solution is recommended for *Cryptosporidium*). Wet mounts of feces or colonic washings can be examined for *Entamoeba* trophozoites and cysts and *Nyctotherus* trophozoites. Fecal smears may also be stained with Wright's stain or Giemsa stain.

Clinical Importance: *Cryptosporidium serpentis* may cause chronic hypertrophic gastritis in snakes, associated with weight loss and regurgitation. *Entamoeba invadens* can cause bloody diarrhea and hepatitis in snakes and some tortoise and lizard hosts. Weight loss and enteritis may accompany infection with *Eimeria* (all reptiles) and *Caryospora* (primarily snakes). *Nyctotherus* and several other intestinal protozoan organisms are considered commensal in most hosts but may become pathogenic if the host is immunosuppressed.

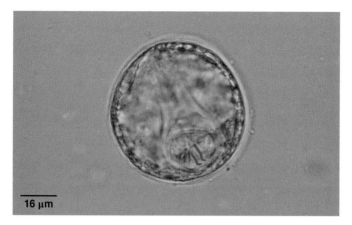

16 μm

Fig. 1.233   *Cittotaenia* eggs are quite similar in appearance to *Hymenolepis* eggs. The hooks in the tapeworm embryo are usually easily seen.

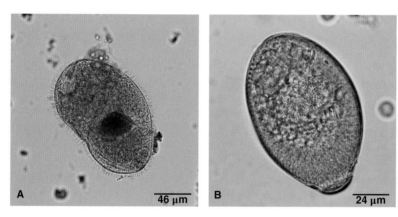

A   46 μm   B   24 μm

Fig. 1.234   Trophozoite (A) and cyst (B) of the commensal ciliate *Nyctotherus* in feces from an iguana. The trophozoites can be seen in fecal smears; cysts can be recovered with flotation procedures. Photos courtesy of Dr. Manigandan Lejeune, Animal Health Diagnostic Center, Cornell University, Ithaca, NY.

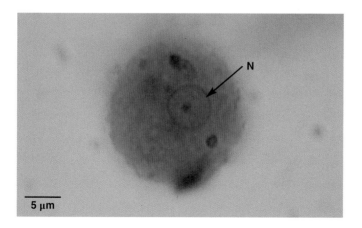

N

5 μm

Fig. 1.235   *Entamoeba invadens* trophozoite in a stained fecal smear from a Burmese python. A single nucleus (N) is seen in the trophozoite, and they are approximately 16 μm in size. Trophozoite movement can be seen in a wet mount of fresh feces. Photo courtesy of Dr. Ellis C. Greiner, College of Veterinary Medicine, University of Florida, Gainesville, FL.

BIRDS, RODENTS,
RABBITS, REPTILES

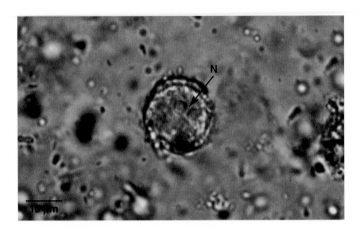

Fig. 1.236   Cyst of *Entamoeba invadens* in an iodine-stained smear of reptile feces. Two of the four nuclei (N) present in the cyst can be seen (*arrow*). Cysts are 11–20 μm. Photo courtesy of Dr. Thomas Nolan, School of Veterinary Medicine, University of Pennsylvania, Philadelphia, PA.

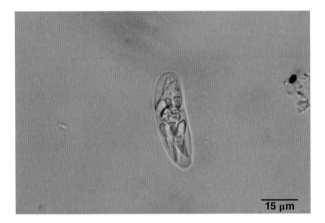

Fig. 1.237   Sporulated *Caryospora* oocyst in the feces of a loggerhead turtle. Oocysts of prey coccidia species may be found in the feces of carnivorous reptiles. Photo courtesy of Dr. Heather Walden, College of Veterinary Medicine, University of Florida, Gainesville, FL.

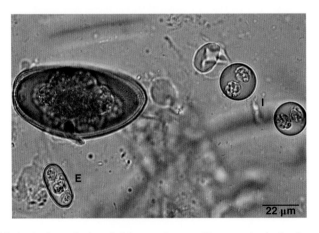

Fig. 1.238   Coccidia in the feces of a bearded dragon. *Isospora* (I) oocysts in the 2-cell stage and a sporulated *Eimeria*-like (E) oocyst are present. A large oxyurid egg is also present. Photo courtesy of Dr. Yoko Nagamori, College of Veterinary Medicine, Oklahoma State University, Stillwater, OK.

Parasite: **Reptile Helminths** (Figs. 1.238–1.254)

Taxonomy: Nematodes, cestodes (tapeworms), trematodes (flukes), acanthocephalans (thorny-headed worms), and pentastomid parasites.

Geographic Distribution: Worldwide.

Location in Host: Helminth parasites can be found in a variety of body systems, although those detected by fecal exam are primarily gastrointestinal or respiratory system parasites.

Life Cycle: Life cycle varies widely depending on the species. Some nematodes have a direct life cycle. Other nematodes and the remaining helminth groups all require at least one intermediate host.

Laboratory Diagnosis: Eggs are detected in feces by flotation or sedimentation procedures.

Clinical Importance: As in other hosts, low levels of helminth infection are usually well tolerated by reptiles. Heavy infections may result in clinical disease, especially in young or immunosuppressed animals. The complex life cycles of most flukes, tapeworms, and thorny-headed worms make these parasites uncommon in reptiles bred in captivity.

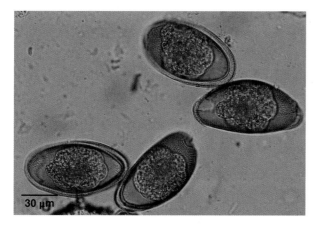

Fig. 1.239   Oxyurid (pinworm) eggs are frequently encountered in reptile feces. These eggs are usually elongated and may appear flat on one side. The eggs shown here are from a bearded dragon.

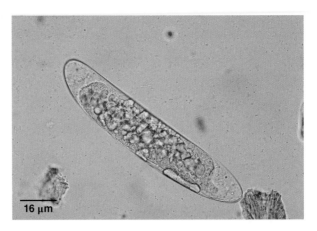

Fig. 1.240   Pinworm egg from a turtle.

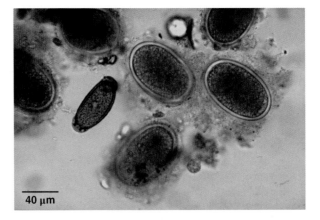

Fig. 1.241   Reptiles may be infected with the same groups of helminth parasites that infect other vertebrates. The photo shows examples of reptile capillarid and ascarid eggs.

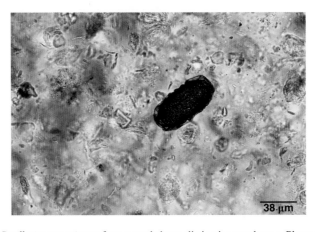

Fig. 1.242   This *Capillaria serpentia* egg from a turtle has a distinctive rough coat. Photo courtesy of Dr. Manigandan Lejeune, Animal Health Diagnostic Center, Cornell University, Ithaca, NY.

BIRDS, RODENTS, RABBITS, REPTILES

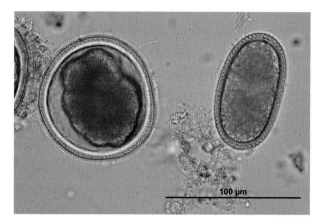

Fig. 1.243 Eggs of the ascarids *Hexametra* and *Spinicauda* in the feces of a chameleon.

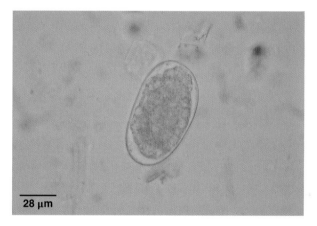

Fig. 1.244 *Kalicephalus* sp. egg from a python. This is one of the genera of strongylid nematodes parasitizing reptiles. Eggs of this nematode group are thin shelled. In fresh feces, reptile strongylid eggs may be larvated or contain a morula (cluster of cells), like the one shown here. Photo courtesy of Dr. Ellis C. Greiner, College of Veterinary Medicine, University of Florida, Gainesville, FL.

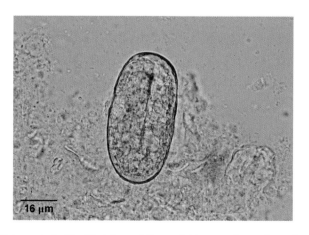

Fig. 1.245 Rhabditid nematodes like *Rhabdias* and *Strongyloides* occur in reptiles and amphibians. This egg was present in the feces of a rat snake. The larvated eggs are smaller than strongylid eggs.

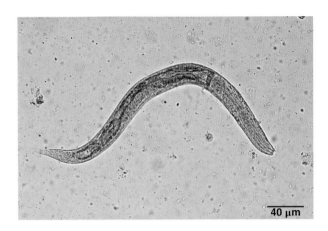

Fig. 1.246   *Rhabdias* is a common lungworm of frogs. First-stage larvae are passed in the feces.

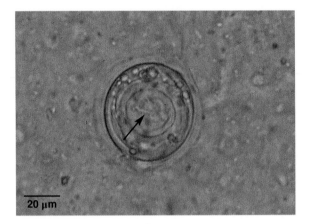

Fig. 1.247   Tapeworm egg from a water moccasin. This egg is surrounded by a gelatinous layer with one hook of the hexacanth embryo visible (*arrow*).

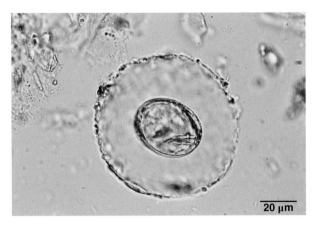

Fig. 1.248   Tapeworm egg from an anole. This egg is also surrounded by a clear gelatinous layer.

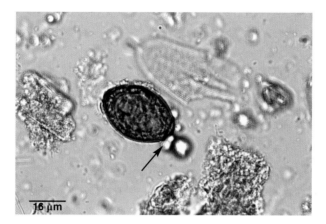

Fig. 1.249 Fluke (trematode) infections are common in wild reptiles, especially those associated with water. The operculum is clearly visible (*arrow*) in this fluke egg from an anole.

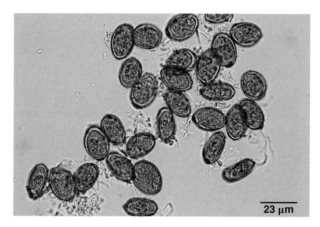

Fig. 1.250 Flukes are also common in amphibians. These eggs of the lung fluke *Haematoloechus* were found in the feces of an American bullfrog. Photo courtesy of Dr. Heather Walden, College of Veterinary Medicine, University of Florida, Gainesville, FL.

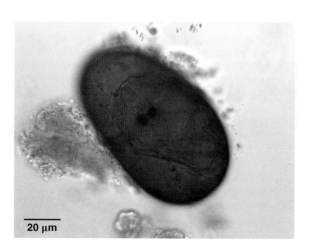

Fig. 1.251 Spirorchid egg detected on sedimentation of feces from a wood turtle. Spirorchids are blood flukes infecting various species of turtles. This large egg lacks an operculum and contains a fully formed miracidium. Note the two black eye spots in this miracidium.

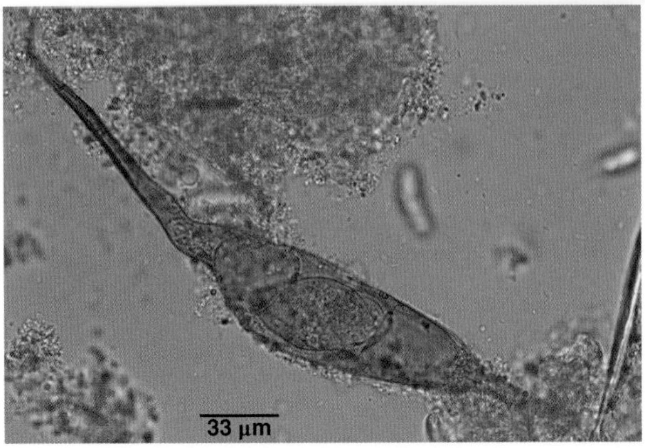

Fig. 1.252   Another spirorchid fluke is *Hapalotrema*. This egg from a green sea turtle has a long filament at each end. Photo courtesy of Dr. Heather Walden, College of Veterinary Medicine, University of Florida, Gainesville, FL.

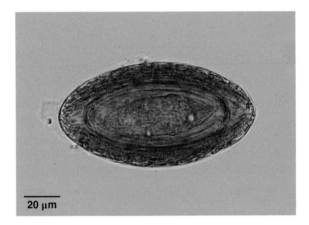

Fig. 1.253   Acanthocephalans (thorny-headed worms) are also common in wild reptiles. This egg was found in mammalian feces but shows the complex layered shell that would also be seen in the eggs of thorny-headed worms of snakes.

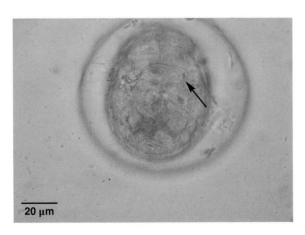

Fig. 1.254   Pentastomid egg in feces from a Boelon's python. This is an unusual group that shows some arthropod characteristics. Adults parasitize the respiratory tract. Large eggs (over 100 μm) in feces are often surrounded by a capsule. Larvae within the eggs have legs bearing hooklets (*arrow*) and could be mistaken for mite eggs. An intermediate host is required for completion of the life cycle. Photo courtesy of Dr. Ellis C. Greiner, College of Veterinary Medicine, University of Florida, Gainesville, FL.

Detection of Protozoan and Helminth Parasites in the Urinary, Reproductive, and Integumentary Systems and in the Eye

TECHNIQUES FOR PARASITE RECOVERY

Parasites of the Urinary System

Several organisms parasitize the urinary tract, and their eggs and cysts can be detected by routine urine sedimentation. Samples collected by cystocentesis are preferred because voided urine samples could be contaminated with fecal material containing parasite eggs or larvae from the intestinal or respiratory systems.

Urine Sedimentation

Centrifuge 5–10 mL of urine in a conical-tip centrifuge tube for 5 minutes at 1500–2000 rpm (approximately $100 \times g$).

1. Decant the supernatant fluid, leaving 0.5 mL. Resuspend the sediment.
2. Transfer a drop of sediment to a slide, add a coverslip, and examine.

Veterinary Clinical Parasitology, Ninth Edition. Anne M. Zajac, Gary A. Conboy, Susan E. Little, and Mason V. Reichard.
© 2021 John Wiley & Sons, Inc. Published 2021 by John Wiley & Sons, Inc.
Companion website: www.wiley.com/go/zajac/parasitology

Parasites of the Reproductive Tract

Organisms that are primary parasites of the reproductive tract are not important pathogens of common domestic species in North America, with the exception of *Tritrichomonas foetus*. In South America, West Asia, and parts of Africa, *Trypanosoma equiperdum* causes serious disease in horses and is transmitted venereally. However, this parasite is difficult to recover from tissue fluids or blood, and immunodiagnostic tests are usually used for confirmation of infection. Several other parasites can affect reproduction as a part of general systematic effects, including *Neospora*, *Toxoplasma*, and *Sarcocystis*. These parasites also would not be recovered and identified in the live animal.

Tritrichomonas foetus is a parasite of cattle found in the uterus and vagina of cows and the prepuce of bulls. Diagnosis of infection is usually by detection of the organism in preputial samples from bulls, although vaginal or cervical secretions from cows can also be tested. A number of U.S. states require testing of bulls for *T. foetus* before interstate movement. A commercial kit is available that provides a plastic pouch containing a medium into which the sample can be inoculated either for culture and microscope examination or for use as a transport medium when the sample is submitted for PCR. (InPouch® TF, Biomed Diagnostics, Inc., White City, OR, www.biomeddiagnostics.com/).

Bovine Preputial Sample Collection

1. Attach a dry 21-in. infusion pipette to a 20-cc syringe and insert into the prepuce of the bull. The tip of the pipette is scraped back and forth across the epithelium while suction is applied.
2. Examine the collected sample microscopically immediately if desired and then inoculate into Ringer's solution (or the commercial InPouch®) and refrigerate for transport to the laboratory for culture.
3. Samples not placed directly into nutritive medium should not be held for more than 48 hours in Ringer's or other balanced salt solution.

Helminth Parasites of the Integumentary System

Several filarial nematode parasites produce microfilariae that are found in the subcutaneous tissue. These larvae can be detected in fresh skin biopsies or on examination of fixed and stained biopsy tissue sections. For recovery of microfilariae from fresh biopsies, the biopsy is macerated and allowed to incubate in saline for several hours at room temperature. Following incubation, the saline is examined microscopically for the presence of microfilariae. Free-living nematodes that occasionally invade the skin may also be seen in fresh or fixed and stained skin biopsies.

Parasite Detection in Urinary and Other Systems

Urinary System Parasites

PARASITE: ***Dioctophyme renale*** (Fig. 2.1)

Common name: Giant kidney worm.

Taxonomy: Nematode (order Enoplida).

Geographic Distribution: North America and Europe.

Location in Host: Kidney and occasionally peritoneal cavity of dogs, mink, and other domestic and wild animals.

Life Cycle: Adult worms in the kidney produce eggs that are passed in the urine. The first intermediate host is an annelid worm; the second intermediate host is a fish. The final host becomes infected when it eats a fish containing infective parasite larvae.

Laboratory Diagnosis: Eggs with a thick, rough shell are detected in the urine.

Size: 60–80 × 39–46 µm

Clinical Importance: The spectacular adult worms (females may reach 100 cm in length) enter the renal pelvis and eventually destroy the kidney, leaving only the capsule. Typically, only one kidney (usually the right) is affected. Most infections are asymptomatic, despite the loss of a kidney, although hematuria and dysuria may occur. *Dioctophyme renale* is a rare finding in dogs in North America.

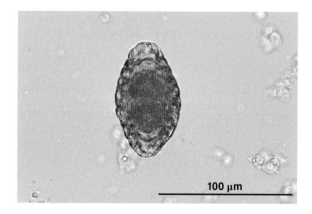

100 µm

Fig. 2.1 *Dioctophyme* eggs are larger than those of *Pearsonema* and have a thicker eggshell with a rougher surface.

Parasite: ***Pearsonema (= Capillaria) plica, P. feliscati*** (Figs. 2.2 and 2.3)

Taxonomy: Nematode (order Enoplida). These parasites were previously included in the genus *Capillaria*.

Geographic Distribution: Worldwide.

Location in Host: Adult worms in the bladder of dogs and foxes (*P. plica*) and cats (*P. feliscati*).

Life Cycle: Parasite eggs passed in the urine become infective in the environment. Although the life cycle is not known with certainty, the final host is probably infected by ingesting an earthworm intermediate host or a transport host, such as a bird.

Laboratory Diagnosis: Typical capillarid eggs are detected in urine sediment. Cystocentesis is preferred for collecting urine samples since fecal material containing similar eggs of other capillarid species may contaminate voided urine samples.

    Size: 51–65 × 24–32 μm

Clinical Importance: Many infections are asymptomatic, although infected animals may develop cystitis.

Parasite: ***Stephanurus dentatus*** (Fig. 2.4)

    Common name: Kidney worm.

Taxonomy: Nematode (order Strongylida).

Geographic Distribution: Tropical and subtropical regions.

Location in Host: Adults are found in the wall of the ureters and the pelvis of the kidney as well as in the peritoneal fat of swine.

Life Cycle: Parasite eggs leave the host via the urine. First-stage larvae hatch from the eggs and develop to the infective third stage. The pig final host is infected by ingestion of infective larvae or an earthworm transport host or by skin penetration by infective larvae. Once in the host, larvae migrate through the liver before moving to the perirenal tissues, where development is completed.

Laboratory Diagnosis: Diagnosis is made by detection of eggs from urine sedimentation tests or from clinical signs. Disease may be present before the infection is patent (prepatent period is 4–6 months).

    Size: 90–114 × 53–65 μm

Clinical Importance: Damage associated with larval migration through the liver is an important component of disease caused by the parasite. Pigs may show reduced growth or weight loss and general loss of condition. *Stephanurus dentatus* is unlikely to occur in modern swine confinement systems.

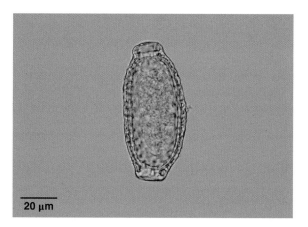

20 µm

Fig. 2.2   *Pearsonema feliscati* egg in urine sediment. Methylene blue stain is often added to these preparations, which will stain the eggs purple. Like other capillarids, *P. feliscati* eggs are elongated and bipolar plugged.

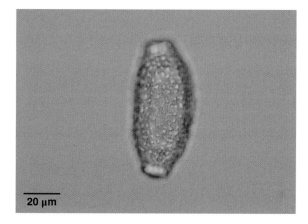

20 µm

Fig. 2.3   If the microscope is focused on the shell wall of the *Pearsonema* egg, a thick globular pattern of ridges can be seen.

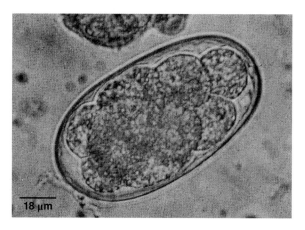

18 µm

Fig. 2.4   *Stephanurus dentatus* adults produce typical strongylid eggs that can be seen in urine. However, disease may develop before the infection becomes patent. Photo courtesy of Dr. T. Bonner Stewart, School of Veterinary Medicine, Louisiana State University, Baton Rouge, LA.

PARASITE: ***Trichosomoides crassicauda*** (Figs. 2.5 and 1.207)

Taxonomy: Nematode (order Enoplida).

Geographic Distribution: Worldwide.

Location in Host: Adult female worms are found in the wall of the bladder of wild and laboratory rats. Male worms exist as hyperparasites in the reproductive tract of the females.

Life Cycle: Eggs leave the host in the urine. Infection occurs when eggs are ingested by the host.

Laboratory Diagnosis: Infection is often detected by identification of adults in the bladder or during histologic examination of bladder sections, but diagnosis may also be made by finding eggs in the urine. *Trichosomoides* eggs are brown with bipolar plugs.

    Size: 60–70 × 30–35 μm

Clinical Importance: Infection is typically subclinical but is undesirable in laboratory rats.

Reproductive System Parasites

PARASITE: ***Tritrichomonas foetus*** (Fig. 2.6)

Taxonomy: Protozoa (flagellate).

Geographic Distribution: Worldwide, but uncommon where artificial insemination is widely practiced.

Location in Host: Preputial cavity of bulls, uterus and vagina of cows.

Life Cycle: Organisms are transmitted during breeding. The trophozoite in the reproductive tract is the only form of the organism.

Laboratory Diagnosis: Organisms are detected in vaginal or uterine discharges or in preputial scrapings. The prepuce is the site most frequently sampled. Organisms may be present in small numbers, and culture is recommended using Diamond's medium or the commercial InPouch® system available in North America. *Tritrichomonas* is easily recognized by its undulating membrane and three anterior flagella. A polymerase chain reaction (PCR) test is also used and may be required before movement of bulls into some U.S. states.

    Size: 10–25 × 3–15 μm

Clinical Importance: The presence of *T. foetus* in a cattle herd produces chronic abortion and infertility and can have a serious economic impact on production.

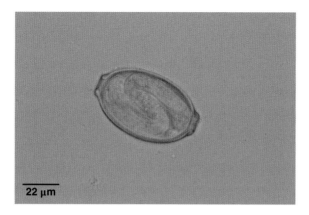

Fig. 2.5 The eggs of *Trichosomoides* have bipolar plugs and are embryonated when passed in the urine. Photo courtesy of Dr. Manigandan Lejeune, Animal Health Diagnostic Center, Cornell University, Ithaca, NY.

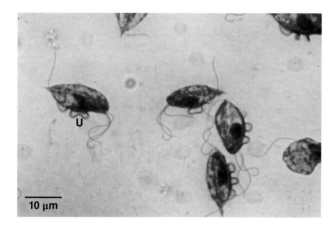

Fig. 2.6 *Tritrichomonas foetus* organisms from culture. The undulating membrane (U) and anterior flagella can be seen in several of the organisms. In culture, living organisms move in a jerky motion, and the rippling undulating membrane can be seen with the 40× objective. Photo courtesy of Dr. Alvin Gajadhar, Centre for Animal Parasitology, CFIA, Saskatoon, Saskatchewan, Canada.

Parasites of Other Systems (Excluding Arthropods)

PARASITE: ***Onchocerca* spp., *Stephanofilaria* spp.** (Figs. 2.7 and 2.8)

Taxonomy: Nematodes (order Spirurida).

Geographic Distribution: *Onchocerca cervicalis* and *O. gutterosa* are found worldwide. Other species have more limited distribution, primarily in Africa but also in the Middle East and Asia. *Stephanofilaria* spp. are found worldwide.

Location in Host: *Onchocerca cervicalis* is found in the equine nuchal ligament. Other species are bovine parasites. *Onchocerca gutterosa* parasitizes the nuchal and gastros-plenic ligament, while *O. gibsoni* is found in subcutaneous and intermuscular nodules and *O. armillata* is found in the wall of the thoracic aorta. *Stephanofilaria* spp. live in the subcutaneous tissue of the ventrum and other areas in cattle.

Life Cycle: Depending on the parasite species, *Culicoides* (midges), *Simulium* (black flies), *Haematobia* (horn flies), and *Musca* species act as the intermediate host and transmit the parasite during feeding.

Laboratory Diagnosis: Diagnosis is made by skin biopsy of affected areas and examination for microfilariae following saline incubation or histopathologic examination. Examination of tissues from lesions caused by *Stephanofilaria* will reveal both adults and microfilariae.

	Size: *Onchocerca* microfilariae	approximately 200 to >300 µm in length, depending on species
	Stephanofilaria microfilariae	approximately 50 µm

Clinical Importance: *Onchocerca* spp. are not generally considered to be highly patho-genic parasites, although equine *O. cervicalis* infection can be associated with dermatitis in horses, and some of the bovine species cause skin or connective tissue lesions that must be trimmed at slaughter. In North America, localized ventral midline dermatitis caused by *Stephanofilaria* is relatively common in adult cattle but has no clinical significance.

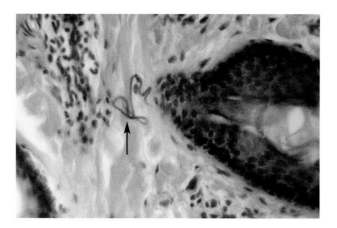

Fig. 2.7   Microfilariae of *Onchocerca gutterosa* (*arrow*) in bovine skin. Diagnosis can be made more rapidly by incubating skin biopsies in saline and examining the fluid several hours later for moving microfilariae that have migrated out of the skin. Photo courtesy of Dr. Fernando Paiva, Universidade Federal de Mato Grosso do Sul, Campo Grande, MS, Brazil.

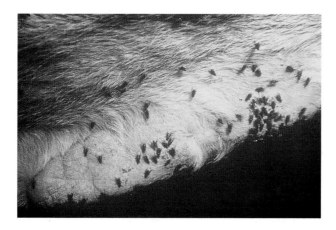

Fig. 2.8   Horn flies (*Haematobia irritans*) feeding on a *Stephanofilaria stilesi* lesion on the ventrum of a bovine host. The flies are the intermediate host of the parasite and ingest microfilariae in the lesion during feeding. *Stephanofilaria stilesi* is common, but clinically unimportant, in North America. Photo courtesy of Dr. Jeffrey F. Williams, Vanson HaloSource, Inc., Redmond, WA.

PARASITE: **Onchocerca lupi** (Fig. 2.9)

Taxonomy: Nematodes (order Spirurida).

Geographic Distribution: Europe, North America.

Location in Host: Adults usually occur in small subconjunctival nodules or cysts in other tissues around the eye in dogs and, more rarely, cats.

Life Cycle: A black fly (Fam. Simulidae) ingests microfilariae during a blood meal. Larvae develop to the infective third larval stage in the fly and are deposited on another host during feeding.

Laboratory Diagnosis: Diagnosis is made by detection of nodules around the eye or skin biopsy of affected areas and examination for microfilariae following saline incubation or histopathologic examination.

Size: microfilariae 110–120 × 5–7 μm

Clinical Importance: *Onchocerca lupi* may cause a variety of signs associated with its location, including exophthalmos, periorbital swelling and discharge. Human cases have also been reported.

PARASITE: **Dracunculus insignis** (Fig. 2.10)

Taxonomy: Nematode (order Spirurida).

Geographic Distribution: North America. Infection with the important human parasite, *Dracunculus medinensis,* has recently been described in dogs and cats in Africa.

Location in Host: Adults occur in the subcutaneous tissue, usually on the limbs, of raccoons and other wild animals. Dogs are occasionally infected. Infection in cats is rare.

Life Cycle: The female worm causes an ulcer on the skin of a limb. When the limb is placed in water, the female extrudes a portion of the uterus, which ruptures, releasing first-stage larvae into the water. Larvae are ingested by a copepod, *Cyclops*, which acts as the intermediate host. The definitive host becomes infected by drinking water containing the infected intermediate host.

Laboratory Diagnosis: Diagnosis is usually made by examination of the skin lesion and removal of the worm.

Size: First-stage larva 596–857 μm

Clinical Importance: *Dracunculus* can cause a chronic ulcer that may develop secondary bacterial infection.

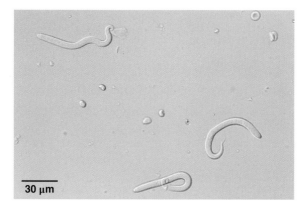

Fig. 2.9   Microfilariae of *Onchocerca lupi* from the uterus of an adult worm. They are present in skin biopsies of infected animals and are the smallest microfilariae found in dogs. Photo courtesy of Dr. Gui Verocai, College of Veterinary Medicine & Biomedical Sciences, Texas A&M University, College Station, TX.

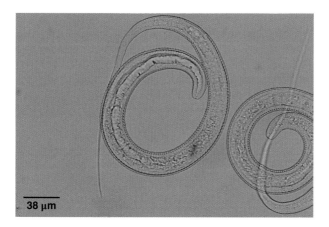

Fig. 2.10   First-stage larvae of *Dracunculus insignis*. These distinctive larvae with their long, thin tails can be teased from the uterus of a worm removed from a skin ulcer and confirm the diagnosis of *Dracunculus* infection.

Parasite: **Pelodera strongyloides** (Figs. 2.11 and 2.12)

Taxonomy: Nematode (order Rhabditida).

Geographic Distribution: Worldwide.

Location in Host: Skin.

Life Cycle: *Pelodera strongyloides* is a free-living nematode that may invade the skin of animals. It is usually seen as a pathogen where animals are confined to areas with moist bedding high in organic material that will support growth and development of the nematodes.

Laboratory Diagnosis: Parasite infection can be diagnosed by finding larvae with a rhabditiform esophagus in skin scrapings from affected areas.

Clinical Importance: *Pelodera* is an uncommon cause of dermatitis in a variety of animal species.

Parasite: **Thelazia spp.** (Fig. 2.13)

Common name: Eye worm.

Taxonomy: Nematode (order Spirurida).

Geographic Distribution: Worldwide.

Location in Host: Conjunctival sac and lacrimal duct of cattle, horses, dogs.

Life Cycle: Muscid flies act as intermediate hosts and ingest first stage larvae released by adult worms into the tears. Development to the third larval stage occurs in the fly, which deposits the infective larvae on the host during feeding.

Laboratory Diagnosis: Laboratory diagnosis is unnecessary since the worms can be seen during examination of the eyes of the host.

Size: Adult worms 1–2 cm

Clinical Importance: Worms may cause tearing and conjunctivitis, but many chronic cases are asymptomatic. Human cases of infection are occasionally reported.

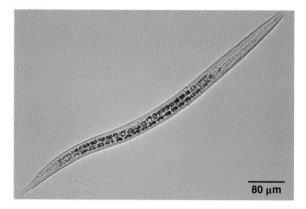

Fig. 2.11   Third-stage larva of *Pelodera strongyloides* recovered from a canine skin lesion. Photo courtesy of Dr. Yoko Nagamori, College of Veterinary Medicine, Oklahoma State University, Stillwater, OK.

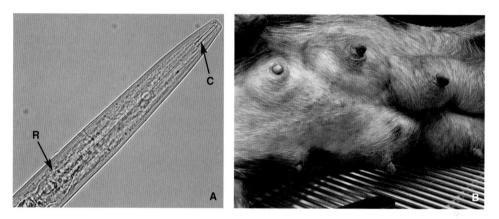

Fig. 2.12   (A) Anterior end of *Pelodera* third-stage larva. The bulb of the rhabditiform esophagus (R) and long buccal tube lined with cuticle (C) are indicated. (B) *Pelodera* dermatitis in a dog. Larvae are recovered in skin scrapings. Photo courtesy of Dr. Yoko Nagamori, College of Veterinary Medicine, Oklahoma State University, Stillwater, OK.

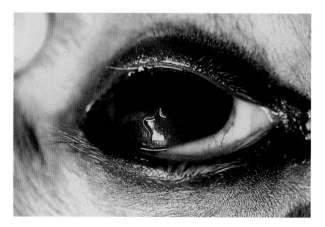

Fig. 2.13   *Thelazia* in the eye of a cow. Photo courtesy of Dr. Jeffrey F. Williams, Vanson HaloSource, Inc., Redmond, WA.

PARASITE: ***Besnoitia* spp.** (Figs. 2.14 and 2.15)

Common name: Elephant skin disease (cattle).

Taxonomy: Protozoa (coccidia).

Geographic Distribution: *Besnoitia besnoiti* (cattle, goats) is found worldwide but is of greatest importance in Africa. *Besnoitia bennetti* (horses and donkeys) occurs primarily in Africa, southern Europe, and South America but is also found in North America.

Location in Host: Cysts are seen in the subcutaneous tissue and scleral conjunctiva of livestock.

Life Cycle: The definitive host of this coccidian parasite is the cat. Oocysts are shed in cat feces and are ingested by the intermediate host (cattle, horses, etc.). Parasites multiply in the endothelial cells and finally form large cysts in the subcutaneous tissue of intermediate hosts.

Laboratory Diagnosis: *Besnoitia* spp. often form cysts ("pearls") in the scleral conjunctiva that can easily be seen with the naked eye. Diagnosis can also be made by examining stained sections of skin biopsies for the presence of subcutaneous cysts.

Clinical Importance: Many cases are asymptomatic. However, an acute febrile illness can develop, followed by thickening and wrinkling of skin that makes the hide unsuitable for leather production. Affected animals may recover slowly. Although *Besnoitia* occurs in North America, its extent is unknown, and it rarely seems to cause clinical disease.

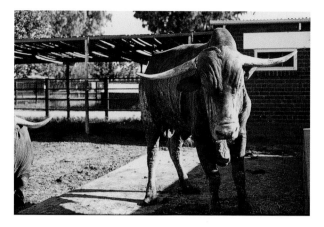

Fig. 2.14   Extensive skin thickening and wrinkling caused by *Besnoitia besnoiti*. This disease is most prevalent in Africa. Photo courtesy of Dr. Jeffrey F. Williams, Vanson HaloSource, Inc., Redmond, WA.

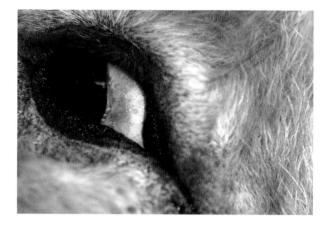

Fig. 2.15   Scleral "pearls," or cysts, of *Besnoitia bennetti* in the eye of a donkey in North America. Photo courtesy of Dr. Hany M. Elsheikha and Dr. Charles Mackenzie, College of Veterinary Medicine, Michigan State University, East Lansing, MI.

CHAPTER 3

Detection of Parasites in the Blood

Various pathogenic and nonpathogenic protozoa and nematodes may be detected in blood samples from domestic animals. Most of these parasites are ingested by arthropod vectors during feeding and are present in the blood of their vertebrate hosts as a normal part of their life cycles.

IMMUNOLOGIC AND MOLECULAR DETECTION OF BLOOD PARASITES

Although the focus of this book is the morphologic diagnosis of parasitism, it is important to recognize that immunologic tests are widely used in conjunction with or in place of microscopic examination of blood smears for some blood-borne parasites, and the use of these tests can be expected to increase in the future. Immunologic and molecular tests offer increased sensitivity compared with morphologic techniques in many cases and are especially valuable in some chronic hemoprotozoan infections and in canine and feline heartworm infection. In both cases, many infections are undetectable by routine microscopic tests. The commercial tests used most widely are the indirect fluorescent antibody (IFA) test, the enzyme-linked immunosorbent assay (ELISA), and polymerase chain reaction (PCR). For additional discussion of the basis and use of immunodiagnostic and molecular diagnostic procedures in veterinary parasitology, see Chapter 4.

MICROSCOPIC EXAMINATION OF BLOOD FOR PROTOZOAN PARASITES

Most hemoprotozoan parasites are intracellular in erythrocytes or white blood cells and may cause anemia. A routine thin blood smear is therefore useful both for assessing erythrocyte abnormalities and for detecting the presence of parasites. Parasites are most likely to be detected in blood smears during acute infection. Once infections become

Veterinary Clinical Parasitology, Ninth Edition. Anne M. Zajac, Gary A. Conboy, Susan E. Little, and Mason V. Reichard.
© 2021 John Wiley & Sons, Inc. Published 2021 by John Wiley & Sons, Inc.
Companion website: www.wiley.com/go/zajac/parasitology

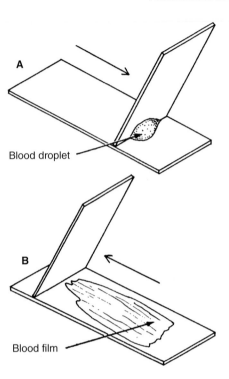

Fig. 3.1   Technique for making a blood smear. (A) Bring a spreader slide back at an angle until it touches the drop of blood; wait until the drop flows laterally. (B) Draw the spreader slide away from the drop, maintaining an angle. The blood will spread into a smooth, thin film.

chronic, immunologic or molecular diagnostic techniques are usually more sensitive as parasitemias can drop below detectable limits by light microscopy.

For microscopic examination of blood smears for hemoprotozoa, Giemsa stain is most effective, but Wright's stain can also be used in most cases. Commercial stain kits used in many veterinary practices (an example is Dip Quick Stain, Jorgensen Laboratories, Loveland, CO, www.jorvet.com) will also stain hemoprotozoa when used as directed, but the stain will be of poorer quality. The following procedure can be used for Giemsa stain.

To prepare a thin blood smear, place a drop of blood on one end of a microscope slide and draw the blood into a thin film as shown in Figure 3.1.

Giemsa Stain

1. Air-dry the blood film, protecting it from flies and other insects if it is not to be stained immediately.
2. Fix in absolute methanol for 5 minutes and air-dry.
3. Dilute stock Giemsa stain 1 : 20 with distilled water and flood the film (or place slide in staining jar). Fresh stain should be prepared at least every 2 days.
4. Stain for 30 minutes.
5. Wash stain away gently with tap water.
6. Air-dry; parasite cytoplasm will stain blue, and nuclei will stain magenta.

Table 3.1. **Average diameters of erythrocytes**

Animal	Erythrocyte diameter (μm)
Horse	5.5
Cattle	5.8
Sheep	4.5
Goat	3.2
Dog	7.0
Cat	5.8
Chicken	7.0 × 12.0

Source: Measurements from Weiss and Wardrop (2010).

The stained blood film can be scanned using the 40× objective of the microscope with use of the oil immersion lens for greater detail when suspected parasites are found.

The dimensions of blood parasites are best determined by means of an ocular micrometer (see Chapter 1). A micrometer is highly recommended for accurate measurement of parasites in blood and fecal samples. If a micrometer is not available, the size of the parasite on a blood film may be approximated by comparison with the dimensions of host erythrocytes (Table 3.1).

MICROSCOPIC EXAMINATION OF BLOOD FOR NEMATODE PARASITES

Many species of parasitic worms enter the bloodstream of the host to reach certain organs, where they develop to maturity. These parasites usually stay in the blood only minutes or hours; thus, they are seldom seen in blood samples taken for diagnostic purposes. There are some filarial nematodes, however, whose larvae (e.g., microfilariae) are normally found in the peripheral blood. The microfilarial stage of these parasite species remains in the circulation until ingestion by the bloodsucking intermediate host. Microfilaria testing is often performed for detection of canine heartworm infection. The following discussion of techniques for microfilaria detection is directed specifically to *Dirofilaria immitis* testing. However, all species of microfilariae in the blood could be detected by the same microscopic techniques.

Although the techniques for microscopic detection of heartworm microfilariae are presented below, the ELISA antigen test for diagnosis of canine heartworm infection is a commonly used screening test. Antigen tests are significantly more sensitive than microfilaria tests because many heartworm infections are amicrofilaremic (occult infections). The absence of microfilariae may be due to low or single-sex worm burdens or immune clearance of microfilariae. Moreover, some heartworm preventives are microfilaricidal and may render infected dogs amicrofilaremic after one or several months of administration.

The American Heartworm Society and the Companion Animal Parasite Council currently recommend annual testing using an antigen test and a microfilaria test to identify *D. immitis* infection in dogs. Dogs testing positive on an antigen test should always be tested for microfilariae to determine if microfilaricidal treatment is necessary. Antigen tests currently available in the United States are available in ELISA and immunochromatographic formats. Differences in sensitivity among these tests have been found experimentally and are particularly evident when only a few adult worms are present. False-negative antigen results can occur, especially when immune complexes have formed, precluding detection. Pre-treatment of the serum or plasma to disrupt immune complexes using heat or chemicals prior to performing the antigen test releases the antigen and allows detection. Because specialized equipment is required, sending a sample to a diagnostic laboratory is recommended when blocked antigen is suspected. Available tests are considered highly specific although false-positive results have been reported both before and after treatment to reveal blocked antigen.

Diagnosis of heartworm infection in cats is more difficult than in dogs. Several of the antigen tests can be used in cats, but false-negative results are common because of immune complex formation as well as the low worm burdens usually found in cats. Similarly, cats are rarely microfilaremic and may develop disease before the adult stage, detectable by antigen testing, is present. To improve the sensitivity of heartworm detection in cats, heartworm antibody tests have been developed. These tests can detect infection earlier than antigen tests but may only indicate exposure to the parasite rather than active infection. Care should be taken in interpreting a feline antibody test, and the results of that test alone should not be used to establish a diagnosis of heartworm infection. In a cat showing clinical signs consistent with heartworm infection, both antigen and antibody tests should be performed as part of the diagnostic workup.

For current recommendations of the American Heartworm Society and the Companion Animal Parasite Council relating to diagnosis and treatment of heartworm infection in dogs and cats, consult the websites of the two organizations: www. heartwormsociety.org and www.capcvet.org.

Tests for Canine Heartworm Microfilariae in Blood Samples

The following techniques can be used to detect microfilariae in blood samples. The canine heartworm, *Dirofilaria immitis*, is found throughout the world. In North America, dogs may also be infected with *Acanthocheilonema* (= *Dipetalonema*) *reconditum* or, rarely, with *Dirofilaria striata*, a parasite of wild felids in North and South America. In parts of Europe, Asia, and Africa, *Dirofilaria repens* and *Acanthocheilonema dracunculoides* parasitize dogs. When a microfilaria test is used for heartworm diagnosis, the microfilariae of other species must be differentiated from those of *D. immitis*.

Staining characteristics can be used in discriminating among species, but are not usually performed in veterinary practices. Measurement of total length, width, and the shape of the head can also aid microfilaria identification (Table 3.2). Sizes should be determined with an eyepiece micrometer (see Chapter 1 for micrometer calibration procedure). The standard measurements of microfilariae in Table 3.2 were determined with formalin-fixed specimens; use of other fixatives or lysing solutions may alter the size of the organisms. Similarly, storage of microfilariae in blood samples for more than 3 days may cause *D. immitis* microfilariae to shrink in length to the size of *A. reconditum*.

Wet Mount

The wet mount is the simplest and most rapid of the procedures for microfilariae detection. It is not a very sensitive technique but can be used in conjunction with an adult heartworm antigen test to determine if microfilariae are present or to evaluate the pattern of movement of microfilariae when attempting to differentiate between *Dirofilaria* and *Acanthocheilonema*

1. Place one drop of anticoagulated venous blood onto a clean microscope slide and coverslip.

Table 3.2. **Characteristics of** *Dirofilaria* **spp. and other microfilariae found in canine blood based on formalin-fixed specimens**

	Dirofilaria immitis	*Dirofilaria repens*	*Dirofilaria striata*	*Acanthocheilonema reconditum*	*Acanthocheilonema dracunculoides*
Length (μm)	295–325	268–360	360–385	250–288	189–230
Width (μm)	5–7.5	5–8	5–6	4.5–5.5	5–6
Head	Tapered	Blunt	Tapered	Blunt	Blunt
Tail	Straight	Variable— straight or hooked	Curved	Variable—hooked (30%) or curved	Sharp and extended
Body shape	Straight		S-shaped	Curved	
Motion (live)	Stationary		Stationary	Progressive	
Relative number	Few to many		Few	Few	
Location of adult	Pulmonary arteries, right heart	Subcutaneous intramuscular tissues	Subcutaneous intramuscular tissues	Subcutaneous tissues	Peritoneum
Geographic location	Worldwide	Europe, Africa, Asia	North and South America	Africa, Europe, North America	Africa, Europe, India

2. Examine the coverslip area under low magnification (10×) of the microscope. Look for undulating movements of larvae, which may retain motility for as long as 24 hours.

Hematocrit Test

This technique is only slightly more sensitive than the wet mount:

1. Draw fresh whole blood into a microhematocrit tube.
2. Spin for 3 minutes in a hematocrit tube centrifuge.
3. Examine the plasma portion of the separated blood, while still in the tube, under low magnification (10×). Moving microfilariae will be present in the plasma above the buffy coat (Fig. 3.2).

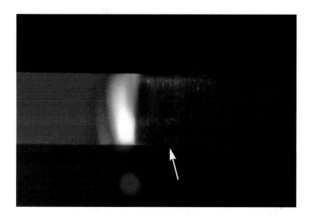

Fig. 3.2   Results of a hematocrit test using a blood sample containing *D. immitis* microfilariae. The microfilariae can be seen as a hazy layer to the right of the buffy coat layer (arrow). Closer microscopic examination would show individual moving microfilariae.

The wet mount and microhematocrit techniques may not detect infections with only small numbers of microfilariae. Therefore, if a microfilariae test is used as a screening procedure for heartworm infection, one of the following concentration techniques should be used.

Modified Knott's Test

The modified Knott's technique is the preferred concentration method for the detection and identification of microfilariae in blood:

1. Draw a sample of blood into a syringe containing anticoagulant such as EDTA or heparin.
2. Mix 1 mL of the blood with 9 mL of a 2% formalin solution. If not well mixed, the red cells will not be thoroughly lysed by the hypotonic formalin solution, making the test much more difficult to read. Microfilariae, but not red cells, will be fixed by 2% formalin. If 10% formalin is used (the concentration used for fixation of tissues), red cells will also be fixed and not lysed.
3. Centrifuge the mixture at 1200 rpm for 5 minutes (or as for fecal flotation procedures) and discard the supernatant.
4. Add one drop of 0.1% methylene blue to the sediment, mix well, and transfer the entire stained sediment to a microscope slide using a Pasteur pipette.
5. Examine using the 10× microscope objective. Microfilariae will be fixed in an extended position with nuclei stained blue.

An alternative procedure using the same amount of blood is the filter test, which traps microfilariae on a filter that is examined with the microscope. This technique can be performed more quickly than the modified Knott's test, but microfilariae are not easily measured for identification. Materials for performing the filter test were sold as a kit (Difil-Test®), which is no longer available. Components of the test can be purchased individually if desired.

Filter Test

1. Mix 1 mL of blood with 9 mL lysing solution (2% formalin) in a syringe.
2. Attach the syringe to a filter holder containing a transparent 25 mm filter with a 5-μm pore size and empty the syringe.
3. Refill syringe with water and pass it through the filter to wash away remaining small debris.
4. Refill syringe with air, reattach to the filter apparatus, and express.
5. Unscrew the filter assembly, remove the filter with forceps, and place the filter on a microscope slide.
6. Add one drop of 0.1% methylene blue, coverslip, and examine at 10×.

BLOOD PARASITES OF DOGS AND CATS

Parasite: **_Hepatozoon_ spp.** (Fig. 3.3)

Taxonomy: Protozoa (hemogregarine).

Geographic Distribution: _Hepatozoon canis_ occurs worldwide, while the distribution of _Hepatozoon americanum_ appears to be limited to the southeastern United States.

Location in Host: Gamonts are found in polymorphonuclear leukocytes (_H. americanum_, _H. canis_) and meronts in skeletal muscle (_H. americanum_) or various organs (_H. canis_) of dogs, cats, and various wild carnivores.

Life Cycle: Ticks acquire infection during feeding. Dogs become infected by ingesting infected ticks. _Hepatozoon americanum_ is transmitted by _Amblyomma maculatum_ (the Gulf Coast tick), and the vector of _H. canis_ is _Rhipicephalus sanguineus_ (the brown dog tick).

Laboratory Diagnosis: Sausage-shaped _Hepatozoon_ gamonts can be detected in polymorphonuclear leukocytes in Wright- or Geimsa-stained blood smears. Although this method of diagnosis readily reveals _H. canis_, _H. americanum_ is rarely found on blood smears, and a molecular diagnostic test may be necessary. Morphologic diagnosis of this species generally occurs by the detection of meronts in skeletal muscle biopsies or on histopathology after necropsy.

Size: Gamonts 8–12 × 3–6 µm

Clinical Importance: _Hepatozoon americanum_ can cause severe disease, with fever, depression, joint pain, myositis, periosteal bone proliferation, and chronic wasting. _Hepatozoon canis_ infections are usually subclinical.

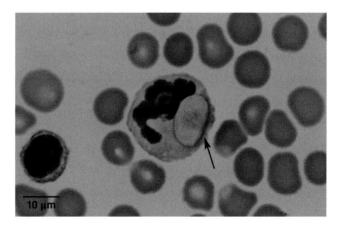

10 µm

Fig. 3.3   _Hepatozoon_ gamont in a polymorphonucleocyte. The parasite is sausage-shaped with a centrally compact nucleus that stains only faintly in this specimen (_arrow_). _Hepatozoon americanum_ is rarely detected in blood films, and muscle biopsies are a more sensitive means of diagnosis.

BLOOD

Parasite: **Large (e.g., *Babesia canis*) and small (e.g., *B. gibsoni*)** *Babesia* spp (Figs. 3.4 and 3.5) ***Babesia* spp.**

Taxonomy: Protozoa (piroplasm). *Babesia* spp. are divided into large (>4 μm) and small (<3 μm). Large species include *B. canis vogeli*, *B. canis rossi*, *B. canis canis*, *Babesia* sp. (Coco), and an unnamed British isolate. Small *Babesia* include *B. gibsoni*, *B. conradae*, and *B. vulpes*.

Geographic Distribution: *Babesia* mostly occurs in the tropical and subtropical regions of the world. *B. canis vogeli* is found worldwide, *B. canis rossi* in Africa, *B. canis canis* in Europe, and *Babesia* sp. (Coco) has been reported sporadically in immunocompromised dogs in various U.S. states. *Babesia gibsoni* is widely distributed throughout most of the world, *B. conradae* in dogs from California and Oklahoma, and *B. vulpes* infects a variety of wild canids (primarily foxes) and occasionally domestic dogs in Europe, North America, and western Asia.

Location in Host: Canine red blood cells. *Babesia* spp. have been described in cats but are not widely distributed and do not appear to be present in North America.

Life Cycle: Ticks are definitive hosts for *Babesia* spp. In North America, dogs acquire *B. canis vogeli* from the brown dog tick, *Rhipicephalus sanguineus*. Other tick vectors include *Dermacentor reticulatus* in Europe and *Haemaphysalis leachi* in Africa. A definitive tick vector for *B. gibsoni* has not been demonstrated in North America and transmission is thought to occur primarily or only through the transfer of blood contaminated with piroplasms. Dog fighting increases the risk of infection with *B. gibsoni*.

Laboratory Diagnosis: Piroplasms can be detected in erythrocytes on Wright- or Giemsa-stained blood smears. Immunologic and molecular diagnostic tests can also be used and are a more sensitive diagnostic technique in chronic infections. *Babesia canis vogeli* is pear-shaped and usually occurs in pairs; *B. gibsoni* is round to oval-shaped.

Size:	Large *Babesia* spp.	4–5 μm
	Small *Babesia* spp.	1–3 μm

Clinical Importance: Severity of clinical disease may range from mild to life threatening. Anemia, hemolytic crisis, and multi-organ failure can occur. North American and European strains appear to be less pathogenic than those infecting dogs in Africa and Asia.

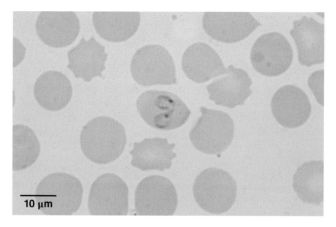

Fig. 3.4   Erythrocyte containing pear-shaped *Babesia canis* piroplasms. The parasite is usually found in pairs; as many as eight piroplasms may be found in a single red blood cell.

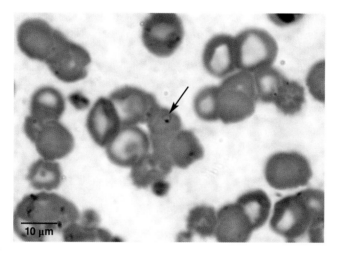

Fig. 3.5   *Babesia gibsoni* (*arrow*) is a smaller organism than *B. canis*. The pear shape seen so clearly with *B. canis* is much less distinct with *B. gibsoni*. Photo courtesy of Dr. Kurt Zimmerman, Virginia-Maryland College of Veterinary Medicine, Virginia Tech, Blacksburg, VA.

PARASITE: **Cytauxzoon felis** (Figs. 3.6 and 3.7)

Taxonomy: Protozoa (piroplasm).

Geographic Distribution: Southern United States.

Location in Host: Merozoites occur in red blood cells, and schizonts occur in histiocytes of bobcats and cats.

Life Cycle: Transmission occurs through the blood-feeding activities of the tick vectors. *Amblyomma americanum* and *Dermacentor variabilis* have been shown to transmit infections experimentally.

Laboratory Diagnosis: Merozoites are detected in red blood cells (1–4 merozoites/erythrocytes) in Wright- or Giemsa-stained blood smears. Schizonts are detected in mononuclear cells in spleen, lymph nodes, and bone-marrow aspirates. PCR diagnostic tests are also available.

Size: 1–2 µm

Clinical Importance: *Cytauxzoon felis* is highly pathogenic in cats. Infections are usually fatal; cats die within a few days of the onset of clinical signs. In the last 20 years, more cats have been found to survive cytauxzoonosis and treatment should be initiated if possible. Anemia, depression, high fever, icterus, hepatomegaly, and splenomegaly occur.

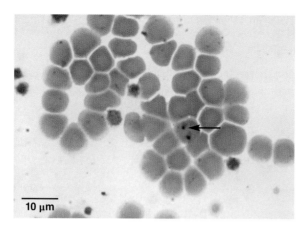

Fig. 3.6   Small *Cytauxzoon felis* merozoites in infected erythrocytes (*arrow*) have a dark nucleus and a light-blue cytoplasm on Wright- or Giemsa-stained blood smears. Photo courtesy of Dr. Karen F. Snowden, College of Veterinary Medicine, Texas A&M University, College Station, TX.

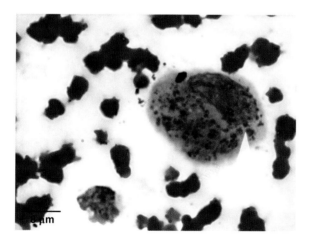

Fig. 3.7   Mononuclear cell containing a *Cytauxzoon felis* schizont. Photo courtesy of Dr. Kurt Zimmerman, Virginia-Maryland College of Veterinary Medicine, Virginia Tech, Blacksburg, VA.

PARASITE: ***Leishmania* spp.** (Figs. 3.8 and 3.9)

Common name: Visceral and cutaneous leishmaniasis.

Taxonomy: Protozoa (hemoflagellate). Species include *L. donovani, L. tropica, L. infantum, L. chagasi, L. braziliensis, L. mexicana.*

Geographic Distribution: Worldwide.

Location in Host: Amastigotes occur in macrophages and cells of the reticuloendothelial system of various organs (skin, spleen, liver, bone marrow, lymph nodes).

Life Cycle: Blood-feeding sand flies (*Lutzomyia, Phlebotomus*) serve as vector.

Laboratory Diagnosis: Diagnosis occurs by detection of amastigotes in macrophages in stained smears made from needle aspirate biopsies of lymph node, bone marrow, or spleen or in impression smears of skin lesions. Amastigotes are rarely seen in stained peripheral blood smears. Serologic and polymerase chain reaction (PCR) techniques are also used in diagnosis.

Size: 2.5–5.0 × 1.5–2.0 μm

Clinical Importance: Infection in dogs is often subclinical. However, disease may develop involving various visceral organs and skin, resulting in cutaneous lesions, lethargy, progressive weight loss, and anorexia that may end in death. Infection with *L. infantum* is common in foxhounds in the United States. Cats are rarely infected. Leishmaniasis is a serious, potentially fatal disease in humans. Dogs serve as an important reservoir host of the parasite in some parts of the world.

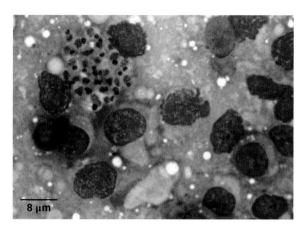

Fig. 3.8 *Leishmania* sp. amastigotes in a lymph node impression smear. Photo courtesy of Dr. Karen F. Snowden, College of Veterinary Medicine, Texas A&M University, College Station, TX.

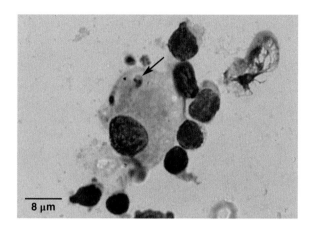

Fig. 3.9 *Leishmania* amastigote (*arrow*) in a macrophage from a canine lymph node. The small round kinetoplast can be seen adjacent to the nucleus in this amastigote. Photo courtesy of Dr. Bernard Feldman, Virginia-Maryland College of Veterinary Medicine, Virginia Tech, Blacksburg, VA.

PARASITE: ***Trypanosoma cruzi*** (Fig. 3.10)

   Common name: Chagas disease.

Taxonomy: Protozoa (hemoflagellate). Dogs and cats can also be infected with *T. brucei*, *T. congolense*, and *T. evansi*, trypanosome species more commonly associated with large animals (see below).

Geographic Distribution: North and South America.

Location in Host: Trypomastigotes occur in the blood; amastigotes and epimastigotes occur in skeletal muscle, reticuloendothelial cells, and various other tissues of humans, dogs, cats, and many wildlife mammalian species.

Life Cycle: Triatomids (kissing or assassin bugs) pass trypomastigotes in the feces during blood feeding on the vertebrate definitive host. Parasites enter the definitive host through mucous membranes or through the triatomid bite-wound site.

Laboratory Diagnosis: Trypomastigotes are detected on Wright- or Giemsa-stained blood smears early in infection. Diagnosis in chronic or light infections may require serologic tests, culture, or xenodiagnosis.

  Size: 16–20 µm

Clinical Importance: Infection with *T. cruzi* is highly pathogenic, causing acute and chronic cardiac disease. Lymphadenopathy, pale mucous membranes, lethargy, ascites, hepatomegaly, splenomegaly, anorexia, diarrhea, and neurologic signs may be seen. In North America infection is most common in the south central United States, particularly in Texas.

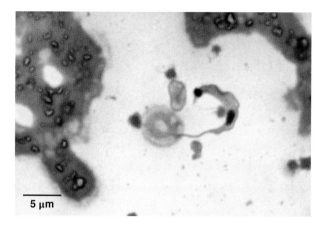

Fig. 3.10   Stained trypomastigote of *Trypanosoma cruzi* in a blood smear from an infected dog. The organisms often assume a C shape in blood smears. The dark-staining kinetoplast can easily be seen in this specimen. Photo courtesy of Dr. Karen F. Snowden, College of Veterinary Medicine, Texas A&M University, College Station, TX.

PARASITE: ***Dirofilaria immitis*** (Figs. 3.11–3.13)

Common name: Heartworm.

Taxonomy: Nematode (order Spirurida).

Geographic Distribution: Worldwide. *Dirofilaria striata* is a rare parasite of dogs in the southeastern United States.

Location in Host: Adult worms are found in the pulmonary arteries and right ventricle of dogs, wild canids, and ferrets. Cats are much less likely than dogs to become infected, and feline infections are rarely patent.

Life Cycle: Mosquitoes serve as intermediate hosts, acquiring microfilariae and transmitting infective third-stage larvae while blood feeding. The prepatent period in dogs is about 6–9 months.

Laboratory Diagnosis: The most sensitive technique for heartworm diagnosis is detection of antigen using one of the various commercial antigen kits for use with serum, plasma, and/or whole blood. Less sensitive is testing for microfilariae in blood samples using the Knott's test or a filter test, which is equal in ability to detect microfilariae. However, the Knott's test should be used for specific identification of microfilariae (on the basis of size and morphology).

Size: 295–325 × 5–7.5 μm

Clinical Importance: Heartworm infection is highly pathogenic and is an important medical health issue in both canine and feline medicine. Chronic heartworm infection in dogs can lead to fatal right-sided congestive heart failure. Caval syndrome occurs in some dogs with heavy worm burdens (>100) that, without prompt surgical removal, leads to a rapidly fatal hemolytic crisis. Heartworm infection in cats can be subclinical or result in severe chronic disease (respiratory or vomiting/gastrointestinal) or cats may die acutely.

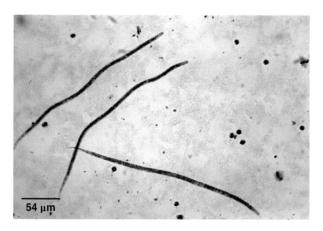

Fig. 3.11   Microfilariae of *Dirofilaria immitis* recovered from a blood sample using the modified Knott's technique. Photo courtesy of Dr. Thomas Nolan, School of Veterinary Medicine, University of Pennsylvania, Philadelphia, PA.

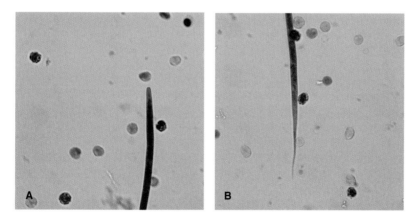

Fig. 3.12   Microfilariae of *Dirofilaria immitis* have gently tapered heads (A) and relatively straight tails (B).

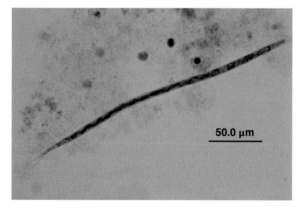

Fig. 3.13   Microfilariae are at an earlier developmental stage than first-stage larvae. Dark-staining cell nuclei can be seen in this *D. immitis* microfilaria. Photo courtesy of Megan Lineberry, Oklahoma State University, Stillwater, OK.

PARASITE: *Acanthocheilonema (= Dipetalonema) reconditum* (Figs. 3.14 and 3.15)

Taxonomy: Nematode (order Spirurida).

Geographic Distribution: United States, South America, Africa, southern Europe, Asia.

Location in Host: Subcutaneous tissues of dogs and various wild canids.

Life Cycle: Dogs acquire infections from fleas (*Ctenocephalides*, *Pulex*) and lice (*Linognathus*, *Heterodoxus*). Arthropods ingest microfilariae in the blood (*Ctenocephalides*, *Pulex*, *Linognathus*) or skin (*Heterodoxus*) of infected canids.

Laboratory Diagnosis: Diagnosis is by detection of microfilariae as for *D. immitis*. Canine heartworm antigen tests do not give a positive reaction in the presence of *Acanthocheilonema* infection. Microfilariae of *A. reconditum* have a blunt anterior end, and the tails of some individuals may form a small hook or U shape, usually referred to as a "buttonhook."

Size: 250–288 × 4.5–5.5 μm

Clinical Importance: Infections with *A. reconditum* are subclinical. The accurate diagnosis of *A. reconditum* infections in dogs is important in order to prevent misdiagnoses of heartworm infection.

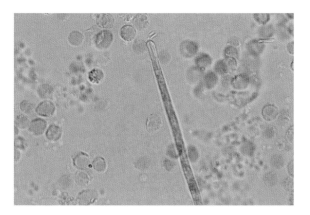

Fig. 3.14 Microfilariae of *Acanthocheilonema* (*Dipetalonema*) *reconditum* in a modified Knott's test. The anterior end is blunter than that of *D. immitis.*

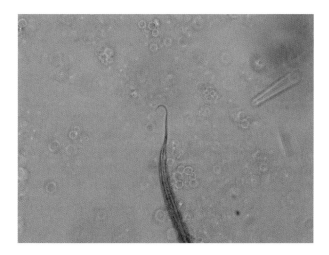

Fig. 3.15 The tails of some individual microfilariae of *Acanthocheilonema reconditum* and *Dirofilaria repens* may form a buttonhook shape when fixed. See Table 3.2 for a comparison of morphologic characteristics of microfilariae found in dogs.

PARASITE: ***Dirofilaria repens*** (Figs. 3.15–3.17)

Taxonomy: Nematode (Spirurida)

Geographic Distribution: Various countries in Europe, Asia, and Africa. Introduction into North America is considered a possibility.

Location in Host: Subcutaneous tissues of canids, felids, and various other carnivores.

Life Cycle: Transmission occurs by introduction of infective third-stage larvae through the bite of culicid mosquito intermediate hosts. After a prepatent period of 6–8 months, microfilariae are produced and circulate in the blood of infected hosts.

Laboratory Diagnosis: Microfilariae are detected in circulating blood by the modified Knott's test or by the use of filter tests. PCR tests have also been used. When detected by the modified Knott's examination, the *D. repens* microfilariae have a relatively blunt anterior end, and the tail may show the buttonhook preservation artifact as occurs with *A. reconditum*. The larger *D. repens* microfilariae may be differentiated from *D. immitis* and *A. reconditum* based on size (see Table 3.2). *Dirofilaria repens* can produce false-positive canine heartworm antigen tests, both before and after treatment to disrupt immune complexes.

    Size: 268–360 × 5–8 μm

Clinical Importance: Infection in dogs and cats is usually subclinical. Infection can result in dermatitis with focal alopecia, pruritus, erythema, and crusting. Human infection can also occur.

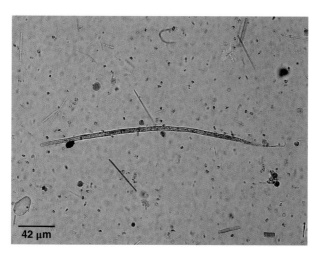

42 µm

Fig. 3.16   *Dirofilaria repens* microfilaria. This species is expanding its range in Europe, and microfilariae can be difficult to distinguish from those of *Dirofilaria immitis*.

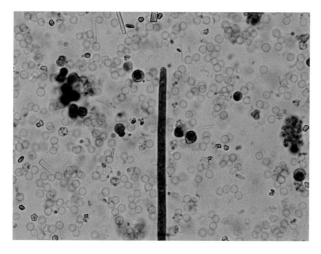

Fig. 3.17   The head of *Dirofilaria repens* is blunt in comparison to the tapering head of *D. immitis* (Fig. 3.12).

BLOOD PARASITES OF LIVESTOCK AND HORSES

Parasite: ***Babesia* spp. of ruminants** (Fig. 3.18)

Common name: Redwater, Texas cattle fever, tick fever.

Taxonomy: Protozoa (piroplasm).

Geographic Distribution: Worldwide, particularly in tropical regions.

Location in Host: Red blood cells of cattle (at least six species, including *B. bovis*, *B. divergens*, *B. bigemina*, *B. major*) and sheep and goats (*B. motasi*, *B. ovis*).

Life Cycle: A variety of tick genera, including *Ixodes* and *Rhipicephalus*, transmit *Babesia* spp. to ruminants. Ticks acquire the parasite during feeding.

Laboratory Diagnosis: In acute infection, blood smears stained with Giemsa or Wright's stain can be examined for parasites in red blood cells. In chronic infection, parasites are difficult to find in peripheral blood, and therefore, antibody tests, including IFA and ELISA tests, are used for diagnosis. *Babesia* typically appears as pairs of organisms in red blood cells, although erythrocytes may also contain single organisms.

Size: 1.5–4.5 × 0.4–2.0 µm, depending on species (*B. bigemina*: 4.5 × 2.5 µm; *B. bovis*: 2.4 × 1.5 µm)

Clinical Importance: In susceptible animals, infection can lead to the development of anemia, hemoglobinuria, and fever, with death often occurring during the acute phase of infection. Unlike many parasitic diseases, young animals are less likely to develop disease than adults. Bovine babesiosis has been eradicated from the United States.

Parasite: ***Babesia caballi, Theileria (Babesia) equi*** (Figs. 3.19 and 3.20)

Taxonomy: Protozoa (piroplasm). *Theileria equi* was previously named *Babesia equi*.

Geographic Distribution: Equine piroplasmosis is endemic in Central and South America, Africa, southern Europe, and parts of Asia.

Location in Host: Equine erythrocytes. Infection is acquired from ticks in the genera *Rhipicephalus*, *Hyalomma*, *Amblyomma* and *Dermacentor*.

Life Cycle: Similar to ruminant *Babesia* spp.

Laboratory Diagnosis: Blood smears are examined in acute infection. Chronic carriers are unlikely to show parasites in the peripheral blood. ELISA and IFA tests are used for detecting antibody to parasites in chronic infection.

Size:		
	T. equi	2 µm
	B. caballi	2.5–4 µm

Clinical Importance: Equine piroplasmosis can cause anemia, hemoglobinuria, and edema. *Babesia caballi* may cause incoordination and paralysis.

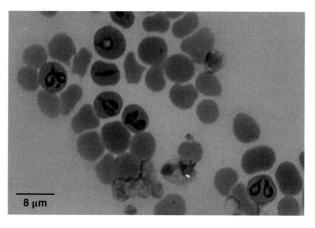

Fig. 3.18 *Babesia bigemina* can be seen in this bovine blood smear. The teardrop-shaped organisms are present in pairs in several erythrocytes. *Babesia trautmanni*, a cause of porcine babesiosis in parts of Europe and Africa, has a similar morphology. Photo courtesy of Dr. Alvin Gajadhar, Centre for Animal Parasitology, CFIA, Saskatoon, Saskatchewan, Canada.

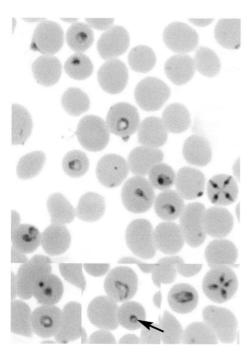

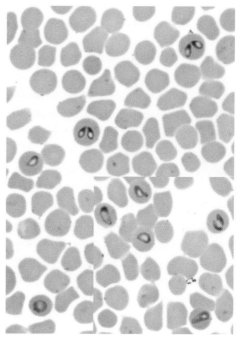

Fig. 3.19 Composite photo showing *Theileria equi* in equine red blood cells. The definitive diagnostic tetrad form is seen in the top right. Also shown in the photo are the small rings (*arrow*) that are most commonly seen in low parasitemia (carrier state). Photo courtesy of Dr. Patricia Holman, College of Veterinary Medicine and Biomedical Sciences, Texas A&M University, College Station, TX.

Fig. 3.20 Composite photo of *Babesia caballi*. The definitive diagnostic form is the joined pair form, in contrast to the tetrad form of *Theileria equi* (Fig. 3.18). Also shown are other forms of the organism. The different large forms of the two species demonstrate the difficulty of distinguishing *B. caballi* from *T. equi* in the absence of paired piriforms in the former and tetrads in the latter. Photo courtesy of Dr. Patricia Holman, College of Veterinary Medicine and Biomedical Sciences, Texas A&M University, College Station, TX.

PARASITE: **_Theileria_ spp.** (Figs. 3.21 and 3.22)

Common name: East Coast fever, corridor disease, African Coast fever, oriental theileriosis.

Taxonomy: Protozoa (piroplasm).

Geographic Distribution: _Theileria parva_ in East Central and South Africa and _T. annulata_ in North Africa and southern Europe. _Theileria orientalis_ has been described worldwide and has recently been detected in the United States.

Location in Host: Bovine erythrocytes and lymph nodes.

Life Cycle: _Rhipicephalus_ (_T. parva_), _Hyalomma_ (_T. annulata_), and _Haemaphysalis_ (_T. orientalis_) ticks are infected when they ingest host red blood cells. Following development in the tick, sporozoites are passed to cattle during feeding and enter lymphocytes, where schizogony occurs, releasing merozoites that infect red blood cells.

Laboratory Diagnosis: Schizonts can be seen in smears of lymph node biopsies and, in the case of _T. annulata_ and _T. orientalis_, infected red blood cells may be seen in a blood smear. _Theileria parva_ is unlikely to be present in blood smears except in advanced cases. IFA and ELISA tests are available, but may not detect acute infection and are of greater use in assessing host response in recovered animals. PCR can also be performed on blood samples, but may be negative in chronic infections.

| Size: | Piroplasms in red blood cells | $1.5–2.0 \times 0.5–1.0$ μm |
| | Schizonts in lymphocytes | approximately 8 μm |

Clinical Importance: In African theileriosis, susceptible animals develop fever, lymphadenopathy, depression, and nasal discharge; there is high mortality in nonimmune animals. Chronic disease signs are variable, including diarrhea and reduced production. _Theileria orientalis_ is less pathogenic, but has been associated with anemia and mortality in Australia and New Zealand.

PARASITE: **_Trypanosoma_ spp.** (Figs. 3.23–3.28)

Common name: Nagana, sleeping sickness, surra, dourine.

Taxonomy: Protozoa (flagellate).

Geographic Distribution: Clinically important livestock species, including _T. congolense_, _T. brucei brucei_, _T. simiae_, _T. vivax_, and _T. evansi_, are all found in Africa. _Trypanosoma evansi_ and _T. vivax_ are also found in South America and parts of Asia. _Trypanosoma theileri_ (cattle only) and _T. melophagium_ (sheep only) occur worldwide. Another species, _T. equiperdum_ (horses), is found in tropical and subtropical regions.

Location in Host: Bloodstream of ruminants, horses, swine, and other domestic animals. _Trypanosma brucei_ can also be found in other tissues, including the heart and central nervous system and _T. equiperdum_ is found in the urethra of stallions and vagina of mares.

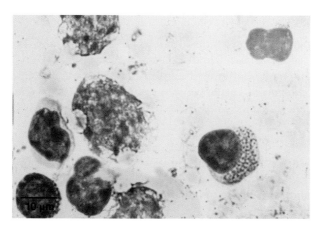

Fig. 3.21 *Theileria parva* multinucleated schizont in a lymphocyte. The species of *Theileria* are difficult to differentiate morphologically. Photo courtesy of Dr. Andrew Peregrine, Ontario Veterinary College, University of Guelph, Guelph, Ontario, Canada.

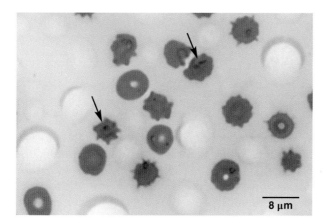

Fig. 3.22 *Theileria orientalis* in a bovine blood smear (*arrows*). Photo courtesy of Dr. Katie Boes, Virginia-Maryland College of Veterinary Medicine, Virginia Tech, Blacksburg, VA.

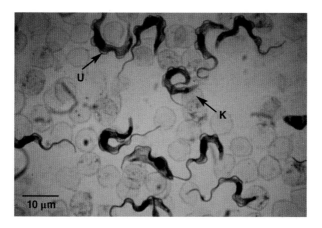

Fig. 3.23 *Trypanosoma brucei* and *T. congolense* are found in domestic mammals in Africa. *Trypanosoma brucei* has a prominent undulating membrane (U) and a kinetoplast that is located subterminally (K). Photo courtesy of Dr. Andrew Peregrine, Ontario Veterinary College, University of Guelph, Guelph, Ontario, Canada.

Trypanosoma (*continued*)

Life Cycle: Trypanosomes are transmitted to the host by biting flies. The vector of *T. congolense*, *T. vivax*, *T. brucei*, and *T. simiae* is the tsetse fly (*Glossina*) in Africa. In other areas, tabanid and other biting flies transmit *T. vivax* and *T. evansi*. Tabanid flies also transmit *T. theileri* in cattle, while the sheep ked (*Melophagus ovinus*) vectors *T. melophagium*. The exception to fly transmission is *T. equiperdum*, which is transmitted venereally.

Laboratory Diagnosis: In acute infection, most trypanosome species can usually be detected in stained smears of blood. Species of trypanosomes can be differentiated based on size, presence or absence of a free flagellum, location and size of the kinetoplast, and characteristics of the undulating membrane. An ELISA antigen test and DNA probes have been developed for detection of African trypanosomiasis in cattle. *Trypanosoma equiperdum* infection is diagnosed by a complement fixation test.

Size:		
	T. vivax	20–26 μm
	T. brucei	12–35 μm
	T. congolense	9–18 μm
	T. evansi	15–35 μm
	T. theileri	60–70 μm, may be up to 120 μm
	T. melophagium	50–60 μm
	T. simiae	13–18 μm

Clinical Importance: The principal clinical signs of trypanosomiasis are anemia accompanied by fever, edema, and loss of condition. Mortality may be high, especially if other disease agents are also present. *Trypanosoma equiperdum* produces the disease known as dourine in horses, which is marked by genital and ventral edema, abortion, nervous system disease, and emaciation. *Trypanosoma melophagium* and *T. theileri* are widespread nonpathogenic species that may occasionally be seen in blood smears.

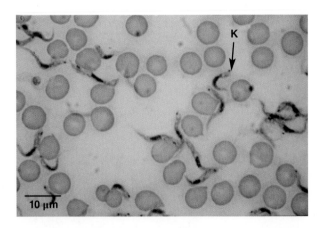

Fig. 3.24　*Trypanosoma congolense* has a subterminal kinetoplast that is on the margin of the trypanosome (K). Its undulating membrane is not distinctive. Photo courtesy of Dr. Andrew Peregrine, Ontario Veterinary College, University of Guelph, Guelph, Ontario, Canada.

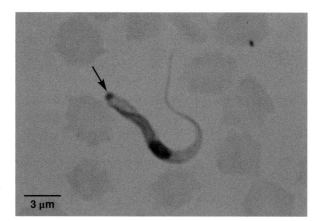

Fig. 3.25 *Trypanosoma vivax* is found in Africa and other parts of the world. Its kinetoplast is at the end of the organism (*arrow*), and its undulating membrane is not distinctive. Photo courtesy of Dr. Andrew Peregrine, Ontario Veterinary College, University of Guelph, Guelph, Ontario, Canada.

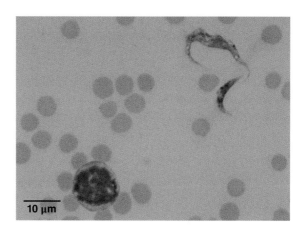

Fig. 3.26 *Trypanosoma theileri* is found worldwide in cattle, and a similar parasite, *T. melophagium*, occurs in sheep. Parasites are occasionally seen in blood smears but rarely are of clinical importance. These species can be distinguished from the pathogenic trypanosome species by their large size (50 μm or more). This blood smear from a calf demonstrates the wide size variation that can occur with *T. theileri*.

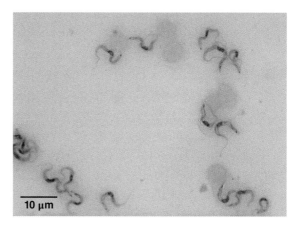

Fig. 3.27 *Trypanosoma evansi* is an important pathogen of horses and camels in parts of Africa, Asia, and Latin America. It is difficult to distinguish from *T. brucei* microscopically. Photo courtesy of Dr. Jeffrey F. Williams, Vanson HaloSource, Inc., Redmond, WA.

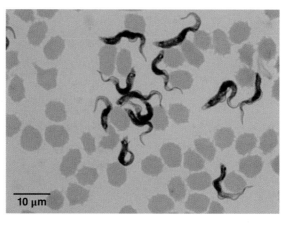

Fig. 3.28 *Trypanosoma simiae* is a parasite of African warthogs that is transmitted by the tsetse fly to domestic pigs and camels. Swine may also be infected with other trypanosome species. Photo courtesy of Dr. Andrew Peregrine, Ontario Veterinary College, University of Guelph, Guelph, Ontario, Canada.

Parasite: *Setaria* **spp.** (Fig. 3.29)

Taxonomy: Nematode (order Spirurida).

Geographic Distribution: Worldwide.

Location in Host: Adult worms are found primarily in the peritoneal cavity of ruminants and equids.

Life Cycle: Microfilariae in the blood are ingested by mosquitoes. The infective third larval stage develops in the mosquito; transmission to the definitive host occurs during feeding.

Laboratory Diagnosis: Detection of sheathed microfilariae in blood smears.

Size: Approximately 200–300 μm in length

Clinical Importance: *Setaria* has no clinical importance, with the exception of rare cases of abnormal migration of parasites in the nervous system.

BLOOD PARASITES OF BIRDS

Parasite: *Leucocytozoon* **spp.** (Figs. 3.30 and 3.31)

Taxonomy: Protozoa (hemosporozoa).

Geographic Distribution: Important species include *L. simondi*, which is found worldwide in domestic and wild ducks and geese; *L. smithi* in North American and European domestic and wild turkeys; and *L. caulleryi* in chickens in Asia.

Location in Host: Gamonts (microgamonts and macrogamonts) occur in leukocytes and erythrocytes.

Life Cycle: Black flies (*Simulium* spp. and other simulids) transmit infections to birds during blood feeding.

Laboratory Diagnosis: Gamonts are detected in white and red blood cells on Wright- or Giemsa-stained blood smears. Meronts are detected in stained tissue sections.

Size: Gamonts 14–22 μm

Clinical Importance: *Leucocytozoon* is pathogenic in ducks, geese, and turkeys, especially in younger birds. Clinical signs vary somewhat with species but can include lethargy, emaciation, and acute or chronic fatalities.

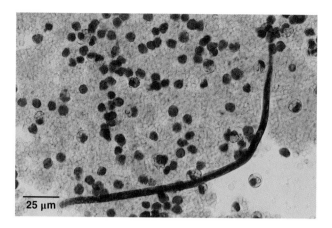

Fig. 3.29 Microfilariae of *Setaria* spp. may occasionally be seen in ruminant or equine blood samples but have no clinical significance. A clear sheath can often be seen projecting beyond the end of the larva, although it is not evident in this specimen. Photo courtesy of Dr. Jeffrey F. Williams, Vanson HaloSource, Inc., Redmond, WA.

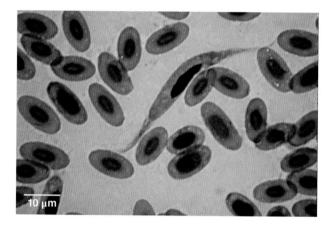

Fig. 3.30 Host leukocytes and erythrocytes containing the sausage-shaped *Leucocytozoon* gamonts appear elongated, with the remnants of the nucleus pushed to one side and the cytoplasm extending beyond the parasite and forming "horns." Photo courtesy of Dr. David Baker, School of Veterinary Medicine, Louisiana State University, Baton Rouge, LA.

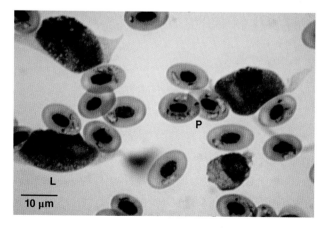

Fig. 3.31 Birds may be infected with more than one species of protozoa. Both *Leucocytozoon* (L) and *Plasmodium* (P) are present in this hawk. Photo courtesy of Dr. David Baker, School of Veterinary Medicine, Louisiana State University, Baton Rouge, LA.

PARASITE: ***Haemoproteus* spp.** (Fig. 3.32)

Taxonomy: Protozoa (hemosporozoa).

Geographic Distribution: Worldwide (except *H. meleagridis*, which occurs only in North America).

Location in Host: Gamonts (microgamonts and macrogamonts) occur in erythrocytes of pigeons and doves (*H. columbae*, *H. sacharovi*), wild and domestic turkeys (*H. meleagridis*), and wild and domestic ducks and geese (*H. nettionis*).

Life Cycle: Birds acquire infections from blood-feeding hippoboscid flies, midges (*Culicoides*), and deer flies (*Chrysops* spp.).

Laboratory Diagnosis: Gamonts are detected in red blood cells on Wright- or Giemsa-stained blood smears. The gamonts of *Haemoproteus* may vary in size and contain pigment granules. They appear morphologically identical to those of *Plasmodium* spp.

Size: Approximately 7 μm

Clinical Importance: Infections are usually subclinical.

PARASITE: ***Plasmodium* spp.** (Figs. 3.31 and 3.33)

Common name: Malaria.

Taxonomy: Protozoa (hemosporozoa).

Geographic Distribution: Worldwide.

Location in Host: Erythrocytes and various other tissues in a wide variety of birds.

Life Cycle: Mosquitoes transmit *Plasmodium* during feeding.

Laboratory Diagnosis: Gamonts, merozoites, and meronts are detected in red blood cells on Wright- or Giemsa-stained blood smears. Gamonts of *Plasmodium* appear morphologically identical to those of *Haemoproteus* spp.

Size: Gamonts 7–8 μm

Clinical Importance: Most species are nonpathogenic. Exceptions are *P. cathemerium* and *P. matutinum* in canaries; *P. gallinaceum* and *P. juxtanucleare* in chickens; *P. hermani* in turkeys; and *P. relictum* in pigeons. Birds infected with these species may become anemic, with high fatality rates possible.

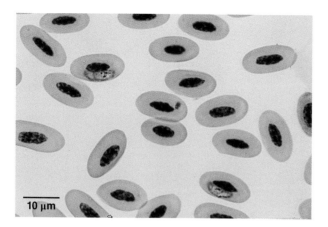

Fig. 3.32   Gamonts of *Haemoproteus* in a Swainson's hawk. The gamonts are often crescent-shaped and wrapped around the nucleus of the host erythrocyte. Pigment granules can be seen inside the gamont. Photo courtesy of Dr. Robert Ridley, College of Veterinary Medicine, Kansas State University, Manhattan, KS.

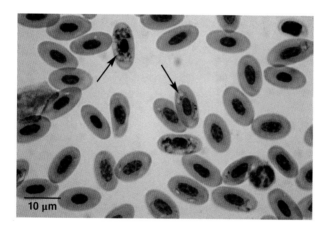

Fig. 3.33   The appearance of multiple stages of the parasite (signet-ring stage, meronts, and gamonts) in infected erythrocytes differentiates *Plasmodium* infection from *Haemoproteus* (in which only gamonts are found). In this sample from a cockatoo, several stages of the parasite are present (*arrows*). Photo courtesy of Dr. David Baker, School of Veterinary Medicine, Louisiana State University, Baton Rouge, LA.

BLOOD

CHAPTER 4

Immunodiagnostic and Molecular Diagnostic Tests in Veterinary Parasitology

Karen F. Snowden

OTHER TESTS

IMMUNODIAGNOSTIC METHODS IN PARASITOLOGY

Immunodiagnostic methods for a range of parasitologic infections are selectively available at fee-for-service diagnostic laboratories and as point-of-care tests that can be conducted in a clinical setting.

There are two basic approaches in designing an immunologic test. **Antigen detection** tests identify specific parasite-associated compounds in blood, serum or fecal suspensions that indicate the presence of the organism in the host. Alternatively, **antibody detection** tests show the host immune response to a parasite through the production of specific antibodies. In order to have a positive test result, it is assumed that the host animal is immunologically competent to react to the pathogen and that a sufficient time of exposure has occurred for the animal to produce detectable antibodies.

There are a variety of test formats for immunodiagnostic tests. The enzyme-linked immunosorbent assay (ELISA) is designed with a series of wells in a plate or tray with an end result indicated colorimetrically (Fig. 4.1). The lateral flow immunochromatographic assay uses similar principles and reagents in a cassette format, and works by capillary action with a series of reagents moving along a membrane with the end result indicated as a colored dot or line on the membrane (Fig. 4.2). Both of these test formats can be designed as antigen or as antibody detection assays, and both test formats have been developed for use with blood, serum, or feces. Most ELISA tests are designed for processing sample batches in a diagnostic lab setting. One benefit of this test format is that the intensity of color generated in the reaction is measurable using a spectrophotometer and is generally proportional to the antigen/antibody that is being detected. Therefore the ELISA may be used as a quantitative measure in a carefully calibrated test. The immunochromatographic tests are designed to give

Veterinary Clinical Parasitology, Ninth Edition. Anne M. Zajac, Gary A. Conboy, Susan E. Little, and Mason V. Reichard.
© 2021 John Wiley & Sons, Inc. Published 2021 by John Wiley & Sons, Inc.
Companion website: www.wiley.com/go/zajac/parasitology

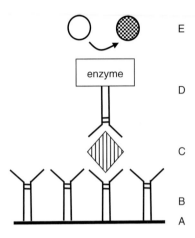

Fig. 4.1 Schematic ELISA antigen detection procedures: (A) test surface: polystyrene well; (B) parasite-specific capture antibody (may be monoclonal or polyclonal); (C) parasite antigen in serum of the animal patient; (D) detecting reagent parasite-specific antibody labeled with an enzyme; (E) visualizing step: if enzyme is present, it acts on soluble substrate to produce color, which can be evaluated visually or measured spectrophotometrically.

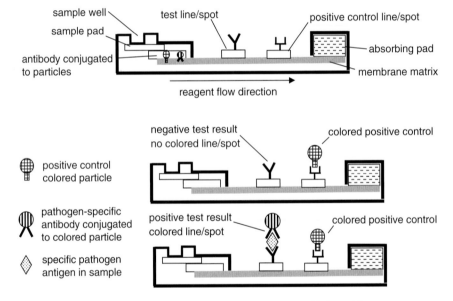

Fig. 4.2 Schematic of antigen detection using an immunochromatographic lateral flow test.

positive/negative results and are not generally designed to be quantitative; therefore the intensity of the colored dot/line is not necessarily proportional to the amount of antigen/antibody detected.

Immunochromatographic tests and selected ELISA assays are available as point-of-care tests that can be performed in a clinical setting on one or several samples in a relatively rapid time frame. Two of the most widely used parasitologic immunochromatographic or ELISA tests in companion animal medicine are the heartworm antigen test, which detects antigens primarily produced by adult female *Dirofilaria immitis* and

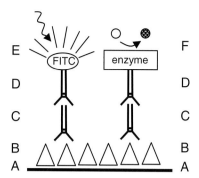

Fig. 4.3   Comparison of common antibody detection procedures: indirect fluorescent antibody (IFA, *left*) test and enzyme-linked immunosorbent assay (ELISA, *right*). A, test surface: glass slide (IFA) or polystyrene well (ELISA); B, parasite antigen: whole parasite, such as cultured tachyzoites and promastigores (IFA), or soluble parasite antigen, which can be a crude homogenate, a purified protein, or a recombinant protein (ELISA); C, serum of the animal patient, which may contain parasite-specific antibodies; D, detecting reagent for host-specific antibody: host-specific antibody labeled with a fluorochrome such as fluorescein (IFA) or host-specific antibody labeled with an enzyme (ELISA); E, visualizing step: specific UV wavelight from microscope causes fluorescein (FITC) to emit yellow-green fluorescence (IFA); F, visualizing step: if enzyme is present, it acts on soluble substrate to produce color, which can be evaluated visually or measured spectrophotometrically.

detected in blood, serum, or plasma, and the fecal antigen test for *Giardia duodenalis*. Since these types of assays are convenient, generally inexpensive, and relatively easy to perform in a clinical setting, it is likely that more point-of-care tests for additional parasites may become commercially available in the future.

Another commonly used format is the indirect immunofluorescent assay (IFA), which is an **antibody detection** test designed for use with serum or plasma (Fig. 4.3). These tests are routinely performed in the diagnostic lab setting because a compound microscope equipped with appropriate barrier filters and a UV light source is needed to conduct the test. The test result is typically expressed as a "titer" and the IgG antibody isotype is usually the immunoglobulin that is detected in the test. The titer value is the reciprocal of the highest dilution of serum/plasma where the test remains positive. Different test formats (ELISA vs. IFA most commonly) have different thresholds of antibody detection. Therefore, the positive/negative cutoff value for each standardized assay should be provided by the laboratory performing the test in order to adequately interpret the meaning of the antibody titer as positive/negative or high/low. For example, the cutoff value for an IFA test might be a 1 : 10 dilution, while a similar test in an ELISA format might have a 1 : 100 dilution cutoff value as positive.

Other less common immunodiagnostic test formats include direct or indirect hemagglutination (HA or IHA), complement-fixation tests (CF) and western blot tests for antibodies that react to selected parasites/pathogens. These tests are conducted at fee-for-service labs since reagents and equipment to conduct these assays are not routinely available in a clinical setting.

It is important to have an understanding of the life cycle and pathogenicity of a specific parasite in order to interpret antibody titers in a specific test. A helpful memory tool is the acronym, "PIE,", which represents Protected, Infected, or Exposed. For some pathogens (usually viruses, but parasites in a few cases), having a high antibody titer is considered protective. For instance, if a cat has a significant antibody titer against

Toxoplasma gondii, that animal is very unlikely to shed oocysts, and it is a low-risk animal as a pet for an immunocompromised or pregnant owner. However, having antibodies against a parasite is not protective in most cases. With most parasites, having a positive titer may indicate current infection or previous exposure without current active infection. Having a measurable antibody titer can be of significant diagnostic value in confirming a parasite infection as the cause of clinical disease. For example, if a dog has chronic dilated cardiac disease with a titer to *Trypanosoma cruzi*, a probable diagnosis is Chagas disease. Alternatively, having an antibody titer may indicate exposure, but not necessarily an active parasite infection. An example of this situation is a domestic cat with an antibody titer to *Dirofilaria immitis*. The cat can produce detectable antibodies to the parasite after exposure to larvae from an infected mosquito bite, but those parasites do not necessarily develop successfully to adult worms causing a patent infection. In summary, interpretation of serologic results is diagnostically helpful in the context of understanding the role that antibodies play in the host–pathogen relationship for each parasite.

In a clinical setting, the veterinarian must interpret the diagnostic test results in the context of the clinical data available for an individual patient or on a group basis for a herd/flock. The diagnostic accuracy of immunodiagnostic tests has traditionally been framed in the context of **sensitivity** and **specificity**). Sensitivity is defined as the probability that an animal that has the infection/disease will test positive, and a sensitive test indicates few false negative results in an infected population (Table 4.1). Specificity is defined as the probability that an animal that does not have the disease will have a negative test result, and a specific test yields few false positive test results in an infection-free population. Typically, commercial point-of-care tests will make sensitivity and specificity data available for each type of test/kit, which provides overall information on the accuracy of the test. However, the use of these terms may have limited applications in a clinical setting when dealing with a problematic or confusing test result for an individual patient.

Other terms that may aid in test result interpretation are **positive and negative predictive values**. These values correspond to the probability that an individual truly is or is not infected, given a positive or negative test result (Table 4.1). These values differ from sensitivity and specificity since predictive values are dependent on the prevalence of infection/disease in the population of interest. The positive predictive values increase as the prevalence of infection increases in the tested population. Conversely, negative predictive values increase as the prevalence of infection decreases in the tested population.

Table 4.1. **Calculation of the diagnostic accuracy of a test (sensitivity, specificity, predictive values)**

Test result	True infection status		Total
	Infection present	Infection absent	
positive	a	b	a + b
negative	c	d	c + d
total	a + c	b + d	a + b + c + d

sensitivity = a / (a + c)
specificity = d / (b + d)
positive predictive value = a / (a + b)
negative predictive value = d / (c + d)
Source: Modified from table in Timsit et al., 2018.

MOLECULAR DIAGNOSTIC METHODS IN PARASITOLOGY

The advent of molecular diagnostic methods has resulted in an expanding selection of sensitive and specific tests for a range of infectious organisms and genetic diseases. Experimental molecular diagnostic tests for parasitic infections are frequently reported in the scientific literature, and an increasing number of specific tests are commercially available to detect parasitic pathogens. Generally, molecular diagnostic tests are able to detect pathogen DNA at very low concentrations when compared with typical antigen detection immunodiagnostic tests. The high sensitivity of these molecular tests makes them especially attractive in cases of low parasite burden.

Molecular diagnostic assays detect DNA (or sometimes RNA) from a specific parasite/pathogen generally indicating active infection. Assays can be performed with many types of samples including blood, urine, tissues, feces, and other body fluids as well as environmental samples. Regardless of the sample matrix, the first step in a protocol is to isolate the nucleic acid for testing. The polymerase chain reaction (PCR) technique is a widely used molecular technique that amplifies and detects a specific short piece of target nucleic acid (such as from a parasite) (Fig. 4.4). In a well-validated assay, the test may be considered positive if the appropriately sized DNA amplicon is visualized by gel electrophoresis. In other cases, in order to confirm the identity of the parasite/pathogen, the amplified DNA fragment must be further analyzed by nucleic acid sequencing for comparison with previously determined target gene sequences from a known pathogen.

Currently, the most popular version for molecular diagnostic tests is the quantitative PCR (qPCR, sometimes called "real-time" or rtPCR), which is a rapid test that is sensitive and reliable for the detection of molecular targets. The technique is quantitative

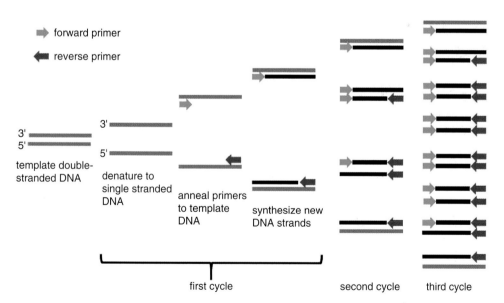

Fig. 4.4   Schematic of a conventional PCR assay. PCR is a process used to selectively amplify a targeted section of double-stranded DNA in a sequence of repeated steps. Double-stranded template DNA is first heated to denature to single-stranded DNA, and then cooled so that pathogen-specific short DNA primers can anneal to their complementary targets on the template DNA. By adding dNTP nucleotides and a DNA polymerase enzyme, new strands of DNA are synthesized. By repeating the cycles of heating and cooling the target DNA segment is amplified in an exponential manner.

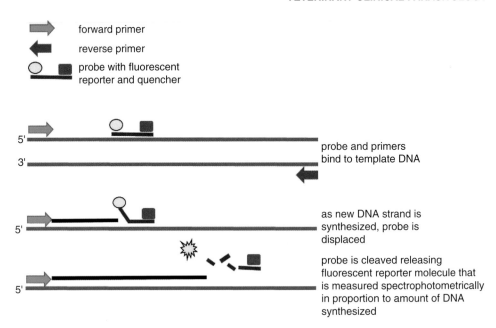

Fig. 4.5 Simplified illustration of how a qPCR assay differs from a conventional PCR assay. The qPCR uses primers to amplify a targeted section of template DNA similar to conventional PCR (see Fig. 4.4), but it also adds a sequence-specific DNA probe with a fluorescent reporter molecule and a quencher molecule that bind to the single-stranded DNA template. As the new strand of DNA is synthesized, the probe is cleaved releasing the fluorescent reporter molecule. The fluorescence intensity is measured spectrophotometrically at each cycle indicating the amount of DNA synthesized. Since a larger amount of template DNA in the starting sample will result in greater fluorescence in fewer cycles, the method is called "real-time" PCR or "quantitative" PCR.

and real-time because the DNA amplification product is measured repeatedly after each cycle of DNA amplification through the detection and quantification of a fluorescent reporter molecule (Fig. 4.5). An advantage of the qPCR assay is that it can be performed in a shorter time period than a conventional PCR. Also, the technique can be designed to simultaneously detect several pathogens by using a mixture of pathogen-specific primers along with sequence-specific probes that are labeled with fluorochromes of various detection wavelengths (Fig. 4.6). The accuracy of the test depends on the quality and quantity of DNA or RNA extracted as well as the presence/absence of inhibitors that can negatively impact the assay. A detractor to PCR methodology is that very small samples of a few microliters of fluid or a few milligrams of tissue or feces are processed for this assay, so it is possible that parasite DNA is not included in the tested sample. Therefore, a positive PCR test result indicates the presence of parasite DNA, while a negative test does not rule out possible infection with the target pathogen.

A parasitologic molecular diagnostic test widely used at this time detects the venereal protozoan of cattle, *Tritrichomonas foetus*, in preputial swabs or specialized short-term *in vitro* cultures. Since this parasite has become a regulatory issue in many states, the validation and comparison of molecular and *in vitro* culture methods has become a topic of interest to many diagnostic laboratories, and to veterinary practitioners and their clients as well. New test offerings, particularly in companion animal medicine, are also becoming available from an expanding number of commercial labs. Illustrating the potential for multi-pathogen molecular tests, canine vector-borne disease agent panels

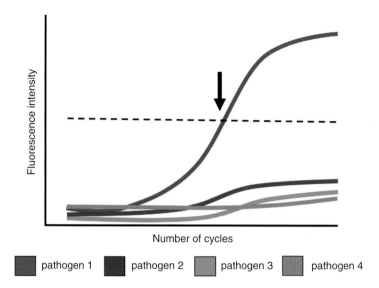

Fig. 4.6   Simple schematic of fluorescence plot of results from a multiplex qPCR assay that potentially detects four pathogens in a single test. For each pathogen, specific primers and probes labeled with fluorescent reporter molecules that emit light at different wavelengths are included in a single assay (see Fig. 4.5). If pathogen template DNA is present in the test sample, then an increasing amount of fluorescence at a specific wavelength is detected as the number of heating/cooling cycles increases. Based on previous standardization of the test with known pathogen DNA, a sample (blue pathogen 1) is considered positive if the fluorescence intensity reaches a minimum threshold at the completion of a pre-determined number of cycles (arrow). If no pathogen template DNA is included in the test sample, then no new DNA is synthesized and no fluorescence is produced for those pathogens, and the test is considered negative (pathogens 2, 3, and 4).

are offered by a number of commercial and university-associated diagnostic laboratories on a fee-for-service basis. These panels may include *Ehrlichia* spp., *Anaplasma* spp., *Rickettsia* spp., *Trypanosoma cruzi*, *Leishmania* spp., and sometimes hemoprotozoan parasites such as *Babesia canis*, *B. gibsoni*, *Cytauxzoon felis*, or *Hepatozoon* spp. Similarly, diarrheal disease molecular panels for a variety of animal hosts that are readily available commercially sometimes include *Giardia duodenalis* or *Cryptosporidium* spp. In the future, it is likely that molecular tests for additional parasites will be available as individual assays or as part of clinically relevant panel screens from commercial laboratories based on clinical demands and the need to develop better diagnostic techniques for problematic parasitic pathogens. At this time, molecular diagnostic tests are conducted in fee-for-service labs or research labs due to the expense of the necessary equipment and the technical expertise used in conducting the tests. However, it is likely that in the foreseeable future, simplified benchtop PCR equipment and pathogen-specific reagent kits will be available for diagnostic use in a clinical setting.

As with any diagnostic testing, false positive or false negative results may occur for any individual immunodiagnostic or molecular diagnostic test. To minimize the likelihood of errors and to ensure accurate results it is important that all involved personnel are well trained and are monitored for consistent performance in following procedures and/or performing assays. When sending out samples for testing remember to: (1) collect samples in appropriate, accurately labeled containers, (2) store/ship/submit samples at the correct temperature using packaging containment appropriate for biological samples, (3) include appropriate submission forms with adequate clinical

OTHER TESTS

history and patient information, (4) when test results are received, promptly enter information into the appropriate medical record. Similarly, best practices for point-of-care tests should include: (1) carefully collect, label, handle, and store samples correctly, (2) only use nonexpired, properly stored and handled reagents and kit/assay contents, (3) follow a standard written protocol for collecting samples and performing each assay according to the manufacturer's instructions, (4) promptly and accurately record test results in appropriate medical records.

CHAPTER 5

Diagnosis of Arthropod Parasites

The phylum Arthropoda contains many parasitic species, including ticks and mites (class Arachnida, subclass Acari) and insects (class Insecta). Crustaceans that parasitize aquatic animals also belong to this phylum (see Chapter 6). Arthropods are characterized by jointed appendages in the adult, and sometimes immature, stages as well as the presence of exoskeletons. This chapter presents a selection of arthropods that are common or important in domestic animals; we are grateful to Dr. Ellis Greiner, University of Florida (retired), who provided the original text.

SUBCLASS ACARI (MITES AND TICKS)

Mites and ticks are divided into two parts: the gnathosoma, which bears the mouthparts (pedipalps, chelicerae), and the idiosoma, where the jointed appendages (legs) and reproductive structures are found. Upon larval emergence from the egg, mites and ticks develop through simple metamorphosis to subsequent nymphal and adult stages. Larvae of ticks and mites have six legs; nymphs and adults have eight legs. Nymphal ticks and mites usually closely resemble the adults but are smaller and lack a genital opening.

Mite Identification

The majority of parasitic mites are microscopic, rarely exceeding 1 mm in length. Female mites are usually larger than males. All stages are covered by a soft integument. Respiration may occur directly across the integument (astigmata) or through spiracular openings (stigmata) associated with tracheal ducts; stigmata are often used in identification. Scales, spines, or setae (hairs) on the body and claws or suckers on the legs (Fig. 5.1) are also used in identifying the organisms. Many common sarcoptiform (round-bodied) mites resemble one another, but they can be differentiated on the basis of the characteristics outlined in Table 5.1.

Veterinary Clinical Parasitology, Ninth Edition. Anne M. Zajac, Gary A. Conboy, Susan E. Little, and Mason V. Reichard.
© 2021 John Wiley & Sons, Inc. Published 2021 by John Wiley & Sons, Inc.
Companion website: www.wiley.com/go/zajac/parasitology

ARTHROPODS

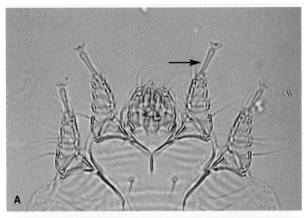

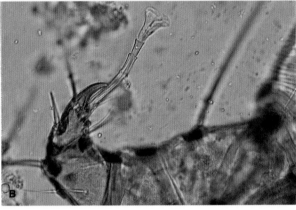

Fig. 5.1   Important characteristics for identification of a number of common mites are length and segmentation of the stalk (pedicle) connecting a terminal sucker to the leg. In *Sarcoptes scabiei* (A) the stalk is long and unjointed (*arrow*) whereas *Psoroptes* spp. mites have a long, jointed pedicle (B).

Table 5.1.   Microscopic characteristics of some mites important in veterinary medicine

	Leg characteristics		
Genus	Egg-laying female	Male	Anus
Sarcoptes	Suckers on long, unsegmented stalks on legs 1, 2; many pointed scales on dorsum	Suckers on long unsegmented stalks on legs 1, 2, 4; few pointed scales on dorsum	Terminal
Notoedres	Suckers as above; many prominent rounded scales on dorsum	Suckers as above; few rounded scales on dorsum	Dorsal
Knemidokoptes	No suckers	Suckers on unsegmented stalks on legs 1, 2, 3, 4	Terminal
Psoroptes	Suckers on long, segmented stalks on legs 1, 2, 4	Suckers on long, segmented stalks on legs 1, 2, 3	Terminal
Chorioptes	Suckers on short, unsegmented stalks on legs 1, 2, 4	Suckers on short, unsegmented stalks on legs 1, 2, 3, 4; legs 4 rudimentary	Terminal
Otodectes	Suckers on short, unsegmented stalks on legs 1, 2; legs 4 rudimentary	Suckers on short, unsegmented stalks on legs 1, 2, 3, 4	Terminal

Most common mite infestations are diagnosed by deep or superficial skin scrapings. For a deep skin scraping, a dulled, rounded scalpel blade (#10) is coated with mineral oil. The site selected for scraping should be at the periphery of a lesion or the predilection site of the suspected parasite. The blade should be scraped back and forth over the skin until capillary bleeding is evident (a shallower scraping can be done for surface-dwelling mites). For collection of *Demodex*, the follicle mite, a fold of skin should be gently compressed between the fingers to express the mites before scraping. The debris collected on the scalpel blade is then placed on a microscope slide, a coverslip applied, and the material examined using the 10× microscope objective. Several slides may need to be examined before mites are found, especially in cases of *Sarcoptes* infestation.

To recover surface mites, such as *Cheyletiella* spp., a superficial scraping that does not cause bleeding is made with a scalpel blade coated in mineral oil. Alternatively, scurf can be combed from animals and examined directly, or clear tape can be used to collect material. The tape is pressed to the hair coat in an affected area and then placed on a microscope slide, trapping skin debris and mites against the slide and allowing microscopic examination.

If mites are shipped to a veterinary diagnostic laboratory for identification, they should be stored in 70% alcohol. Storing skin scrapings and mites dry may prevent successful identification.

ARTHROPODS

Parasite: **Sarcoptes scabiei** (Figs. 5.2–5.5)

      Common name: Itch mite or scabies mite.

Taxonomy: Mite (family Sarcoptidae).

Host: Host-specific varieties of *Sarcoptes scabiei* are found on a wide range of hosts including dogs, pigs, humans, ruminants, horses, rodents, and camelids. Traditionally, each mite is referred to according to the host on which it was found (*S. scabiei* var *canis*, *S. scabiei* var *suis*, *S. scabiei* var *hominis*, etc.).

Geographic Distribution: Worldwide.

Location on Host: On dogs, the margins of the ear, lateral elbows, and lateral hocks are most commonly affected. In pigs, the ears, neck, and back are infested. Over time, large portions of the skin can be involved.

Life Cycle: Transmission of *Sarcoptes scabiei* occurs following direct contact with an infested animal or fomites (e.g., clippers). Mites burrow deep into the epidermis, depositing eggs and feces. The life cycle from egg to adult requires approximately 3 weeks to complete.

Laboratory Diagnosis: To confirm the diagnosis, examine multiple, deep skin scrapings from the margins of affected areas. When mites are not detected, patients may be treated presumptively and the diagnosis confirmed upon resolution of pruritus. Fecal examination is also useful in revealing mites and mite eggs ingested during grooming. In pigs, *S. scabiei* is found in hyperkeratotic crusts on the margins of the pinnae. On the farm, this crusted material can be removed and crumbled over dark paper to reveal the tiny, motile mites. Digesting crusts with 10% sodium hydroxide may also reveal mites.

      Size: Females approximately 400 µm; males approximately 250 µm

Clinical Importance: Mange caused by *Sarcoptes scabiei* is extremely pruritic and often accompanied by alopecia, hyperkeratosis, and dermal thickening. In North America, infestations occur most commonly in dogs and pigs; mites from animals readily transfer to humans and cause self-limiting pruritus.

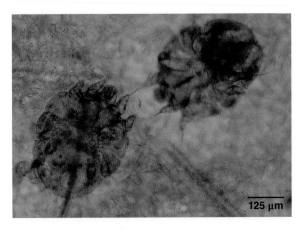

Fig. 5.2   Pruritic mite infestations may stimulate intense grooming by the host, resulting in the presence of both mites and eggs (not shown) in the feces.

ARTHROPODS

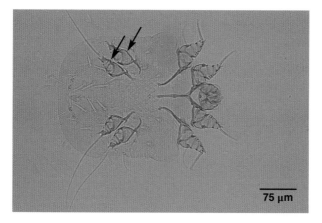

Fig. 5.3 *Sarcoptes* and related mites are typically round bodied. The third and fourth pairs of legs (*arrows*) are short and often do not project beyond the margin of the body. Photo courtesy of Dr. Heather Walden, College of Veterinary Medicine, University of Florida, Gainesville, FL.

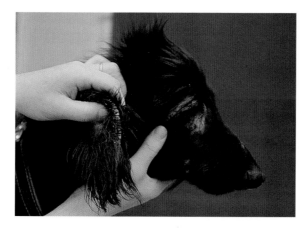

Fig. 5.4 *Sarcoptes scabiei* var *canis* causes "scabies" or "sarcoptic mange" in dogs. Lesions commonly occur on the face and along the margin of the ear as well as on the lateral elbows and hocks of infested dogs. Photo courtesy of Dr. Jeffrey F. Williams, Vanson HaloSource, Inc., Redmond, WA.

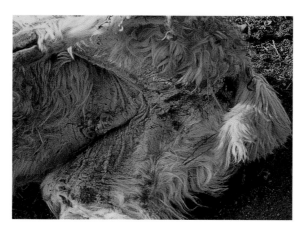

Fig. 5.5 Sarcoptic mange in an alpaca. In chronic sarcoptic mange, affected skin is hairless, thickened, and wrinkled. These nonspecific changes also occur in other chronic skin diseases. Photo courtesy of Dr. Jeffrey F. Williams, Vanson HaloSource, Inc., Redmond, WA.

ARTHROPODS

PARASITE: *Notoedres* **spp.** (Fig. 5.6)

Common name: Feline mange mite, Ear mange mite (rodents).

Taxonomy: Mite (family Sarcoptidae).

Host: *Notoedres cati* occurs on cats. Other species occur on bats, rodents, and other small mammals.

Geographic Distribution: Worldwide.

Location on Host: The head is usually infested first, but mites may spread to other regions of the body.

Life Cycle: Similar to *Sarcoptes scabiei*.

Laboratory Diagnosis: Mites are observed in deep skin scrapings.

Size: *Notoedres cati* approximately 200–225 µm

Clinical Importance: Feline notoedric mange is usually confined to the head and neck. Infestations are rarely seen in North America.

PARASITE: *Knemidokoptes* **spp.** (Figs. 5.7 and 5.8)

Common name: Scaly leg or scaly face mite.

Taxonomy: Mite (family Knemidokoptidae).

Host: Birds, including domestic poultry and pet birds.

Geographic Distribution: Worldwide.

Location on Host: Nonfeathered portions of the body, including feet, legs, and face.

Life Cycle: Like *Sarcoptes scabiei*, transmission occurs by direct contact with infested birds or fomites, and all stages of the mite are found on the host.

Laboratory Diagnosis: Mites can be found in skin scrapings collected from the periphery of lesions. Typically, the exudative lesions produced by the mites contain numerous small holes, giving them a honeycombed appearance.

Size: Approximately 400 µm

Clinical Importance: *Knemidokoptes* species burrow under the scales on the legs or nonfeathered portions of the face, inducing a serous exudate that hardens into crusts. These proliferative lesions eventually may cause trauma and disfigurement leading to the death of the host.

ARTHROPODS

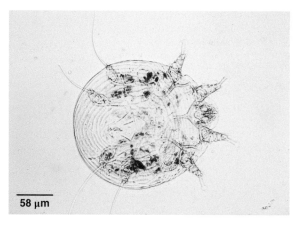

Fig. 5.6 *Notoedres* mites are similar in appearance to *Sarcoptes*. However, the anus of *Notoedres* is located on the dorsal surface rather than the ventral. *Notoedres* also has scalloped scales on the dorsum rather than the sawtooth scales on *Sarcoptes*. The suckers on the front legs of both *Notoedres* and *Sarcoptes* are attached to the legs by long, unjointed stalks.

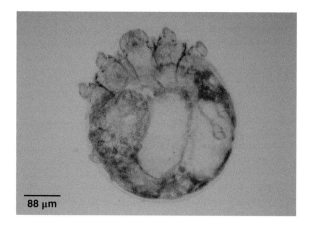

Fig. 5.7 *Knemidokoptes* is a round-bodied mite, generally similar in appearance to sarcoptiform mites.

ARTHROPODS

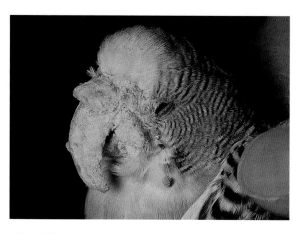

Fig. 5.8 Budgerigar with a deformed beak resulting from the proliferative lesion produced by *Knemidokoptes* infestation. Photo courtesy of Dr. Jeffrey F. Williams, Vanson HaloSource, Inc., Redmond, WA.

PARASITE: *Trixacarus* **spp.** (Fig. 5.9)

Taxonomy: Mite (family Sarcoptidae).

Host: Guinea pigs (*Trixacarus caviae*) and rats (*T. diversus*).

Geographic Distribution: Europe and North America.

Location on Host: Lesions begin on the head, neck, and back but can spread to other areas.

Life Cycle: Similar to *Sarcoptes scabiei*. Mites are readily transferred from the dam to young animals in the neonatal period.

Laboratory Diagnosis: Mites are identified in skin scrapings.

   Size: Approximately 200 μm

Clinical Importance: *Trixacarus* is the sarcoptic mange mite of guinea pigs. Infestation is associated with pruritus, alopecia, and hyperkeratosis and can become a serious problem in guinea pig colonies. Humans in contact with infested guinea pigs may develop transient lesions.

PARASITE: *Chorioptes bovis* (Figs. 5.10 and 5.11)

   Common name: Foot mange, leg mange, itchy heel.

Taxonomy: Mite (family Psoroptidae).

Host: Varieties of *C. bovis* are found on ruminants, horses, and rabbits.

Geographic Distribution: Worldwide.

Location on Host: *Chorioptes* are found primarily on the lower body of the host. In horses, the mites are seen more often in breeds with feathered legs. In cattle, the rear legs, base of the tail, and back of the udder are most often affected.

Life Cycle: Transmission is by direct contact or fomites. *Chorioptes* mites spend their entire life cycle on the skin surface. The life cycle can be completed in about 3 weeks.

Laboratory Diagnosis: Mites are observed in skin scrapings. *Chorioptes* has short, unsegmented stalks bearing the suckers on the legs (Table 5.1).

   Size: Approximately 400 μm

Clinical Importance: Infestation may be asymptomatic or cause only mild lesions in some animals. As mite populations increase, pruritus, alopecia, and crusting may develop.

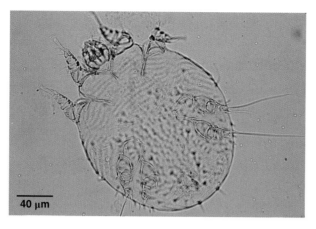

Fig. 5.9   Like other sarcoptiform mites, *Trixacarus* is a round-bodied mite with short legs. *Trixacarus caviae* causes mange in guinea pigs.

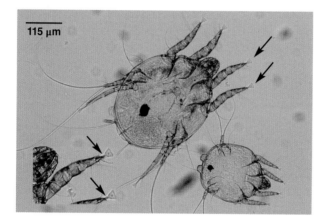

Fig. 5.10   *Chorioptes* mites are more elongated, with longer legs than the sarcoptiform mites. Suckers are evident on short, unsegmented stalks (*arrows*) at the end of the legs. Photo courtesy of Dr. Yoko Nagamori, College of Veterinary Medicine, Oklahoma State University, Stillwater, OK.

ARTHROPODS

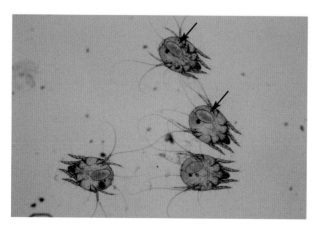

Fig. 5.11   Female *Chorioptes* mites with eggs present (*arrows*). Mite eggs are large, ~200 μm long, and may be seen retained within mites or found on fecal flotation from infested animals. Photo courtesy of Dr. Yoko Nagamori, Oklahoma State University, Stillwater, OK.

PARASITE: ***Psoroptes* spp.** (Figs. 5.12–5.15)

Common name: Scab mite (ruminants).

Taxonomy: Mite (family Psoroptidae).

Host: *Psoroptes ovis* is the cause of psoroptic mange in ruminants; *P. ovis cuniculi* (formerly referred to as *P. cuniculi*) is found on rabbits and ruminants. *Psoroptes* spp. can also be found on horses and some wildlife hosts.

Geographic Distribution: Worldwide.

Location on Host: *Psoroptes ovis cuniculi* is found in the ears of rabbits, sheep, goats, and horses. Other *Psoroptes* infestations are often first detected on the dorsum of the host but may spread to other areas.

Life Cycle: Transmission is by direct contact or fomites. Unlike sarcoptiform mites, *Psoroptes* spp. do not burrow, and all stages are found on the skin surface. The life cycle can be completed in as little as 10 days. Mites may survive for several days off the host.

Laboratory Diagnosis: Superficial skin scrapings should be collected from the periphery of skin lesions. Alternatively, skin scabs can be broken apart or digested and the residue examined microscopically. Crusts from the ears can be treated similarly when infestations of *P. ovis cuniculi* are suspected. Psoroptic mites are more oval in shape and have longer legs than sarcoptiform mites.

Size: Approximately 750 μm

Clinical Importance: *Psoroptes* is a highly contagious, economically important cause of skin disease in ruminants worldwide. Infestation leads to exudative dermatitis and hair loss. In the United States, the strain of *P. ovis* affecting sheep has been eradicated, and the bovine strain has diminished in importance since the introduction of macrocyclic lactone endectocide drugs. In severe cases, *P. ovis cuniculi* lesions on rabbits may extend beyond the ears to the face, neck, and back.

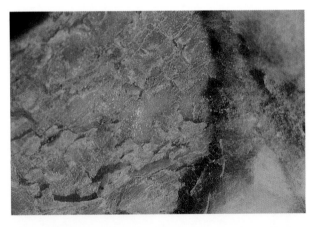

Fig. 5.12   Psoroptic mange or "scab" can be a serious infestation in ruminants. In sheep, mite activity causes an exudate that forms a crust on the surface of the skin, with the resulting loss of the fleece over affected areas.

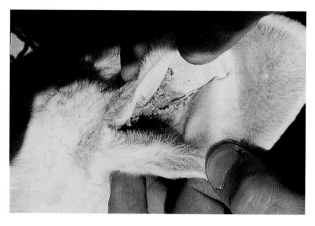

Fig. 5.13   Psoroptic ear mange in a rabbit. Photo courtesy of Dr. Jeffrey F. Williams, Vanson HaloSource, Inc., Redmond, WA.

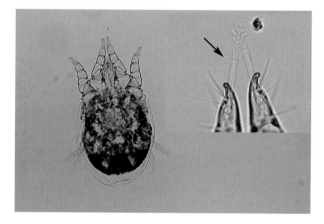

Fig. 5.14   *Psoroptes* sp. mites have a more oval shape and longer legs than round-bodied, sarcoptiform mites. This morphology is sometimes referred to as "psoroptiform." Terminal suckers are connected to the legs by long, segmented stalks (*arrow*). Photo courtesy of Dr. Manigandan Lejeune, Animal Health Diagnostic Center, Cornell University, Ithaca, NY.

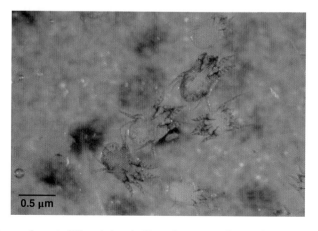

Fig. 5.15   *Psoroptes* may be up to 800 μm in length. Shown here are specimens of *Psoroptes cuniculi* from rabbit ears. Figures 5.1B and 5.14 show a closer view of the jointed pedicle on some of the legs of *Psoroptes*. Photo courtesy of Dr. David Baker, School of Veterinary Medicine, Louisiana State University, Baton Rouge, LA.

Parasite: ***Otodectes cynotis*** (Figs. 5.16–5.19)

Common name: Ear mite.

Taxonomy: Mite (family Psoroptidae).

Host: Dogs, cats, and ferrets.

Geographic Distribution: Worldwide.

Location on Host: Ear canal.

Life Cycle: Mites complete their life cycle in the ear. Transmission occurs by direct contact or fomites. Kittens and puppies are easily infested by contact with the dam.

Laboratory Diagnosis: Routinely diagnosed by otoscope or microscopic examination of aural exudate collected with cotton swabs.

Size: Approximately 300 μm

Clinical Importance: These mites are a common cause of otitis externa. Bacterial decomposition of otic secretions and exudate leads to the formation of black, waxy cerumen. Infested animals often suffer severe pruritus that may lead to self-inflicted trauma. Heavy infestations may spread outside the ear to the face, neck, and back.

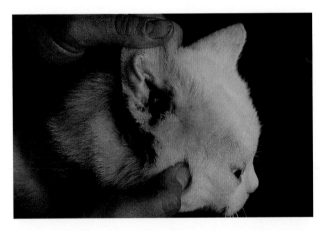

Fig. 5.16 *Otodectes cynotis* infestation in a cat. The mites cause the production of black, waxy exudate in the ear canal. Photo courtesy of Dr. Jeffrey F. Williams, Vanson HaloSource, Inc., Redmond, WA.

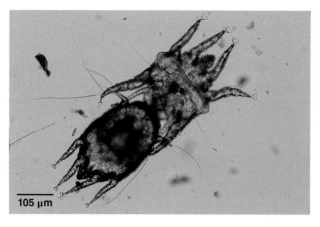

Fig. 5.17 Mating *Otodectes cynotis* mites from a ferret. *Otodectes* is another psoroptiform mite with an oval-shaped body and long legs. They are similar in size and appearance to *Chorioptes*. In heavy infestations, it is common to find copulating mites in ear swab preparations. The short unsegmented stalks carrying the suckers can be seen in this photo.

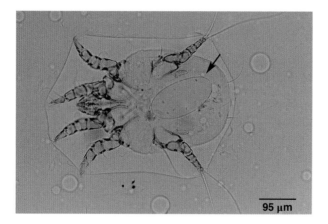

Fig. 5.18 Gravid female of *Otodectes cynotis* with egg present (*arrow*). Photo courtesy of Dr. Heather Walden, College of Veterinary Medicine, University of Florida, Gainesville, FL.

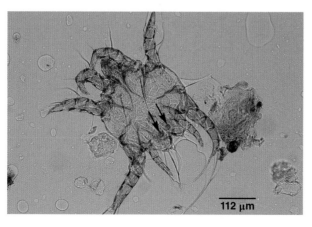

Fig. 5.19 Male *Otodectes cynotis*. The pair of distinct circular structures evident on the posterior end (*arrows*) are copulatory suckers. Photo courtesy of Dr. Manigandan Lejeune, Animal Health Diagnostic Center, Cornell University, Ithaca, NY.

ARTHROPODS

PARASITE: ***Demodex* spp.** (Figs. 5.20–5.23)

Common name: Follicle mite, red mange.

Taxonomy: Mite (family Demodicidae).

Host: Species of *Demodex* are host-specific and have been identified from many animals, including dogs, cats, pigs, horses, cattle, goats, sheep, laboratory animals, and humans.

Geographic Distribution: Worldwide.

Location on Host: Sebaceous glands and hair follicles.

Life Cycle: Mites are usually transferred from the dam to offspring in the neonatal period. All stages of the life cycle are found on the host.

Laboratory Diagnosis: Deep skin scrapings are required for diagnosis. Compressing a skin fold before scraping aids in expressing mites from follicles and sebaceous glands. A high proportion of eggs and immature mites on skin scraping is considered indicative of a more severe infestation. *Demodex* mites and eggs are often ingested during grooming and identified by fecal flotation.

Size: 100–400 µm, depending on species

Clinical Importance: Most animals harbor mites but do not develop clinical disease. When the immune system fails to keep mite populations in check, proliferation can occur leading to folliculitis, furunculosis, and secondary bacterial infection. Disease is seen most often in dogs and may be localized and self-limiting or generalized, severe, and potentially fatal.

ARTHROPODS

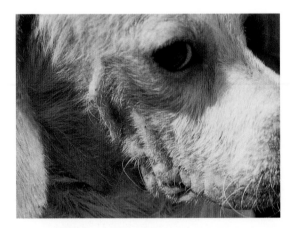

Fig. 5.20 *Demodex* is most often seen as a clinical problem in dogs. Lesions often appear first on the face or forelegs. Photo courtesy of Dr. Jeffrey F. Williams, Vanson HaloSource, Inc., Redmond, WA.

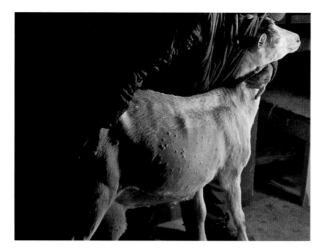

Fig. 5.21   In goats and cattle, clinical demodecosis is usually associated with the formation of nodular pustules. Photo courtesy of Dr. Jeffrey F. Williams, Vanson HaloSource, Inc., Redmond, WA, and Dr. C. Williams, Langley, WA.

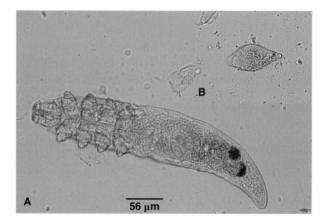

Fig. 5.22   *Demodex* spp. mites (A) have a distinct, elongated appearance and are often described as looking like cigars with legs. *Demodex canis* reaches a length of ~390 μm. Eggs (B) are spindle-shaped (~100 μm). Both may be present on skin scrape or found on fecal flotation from infested animals after self-grooming. Photo courtesy of Dr. Manigandan Lejeune, Animal Health Diagnostic Center, Cornell University, Ithaca, NY.

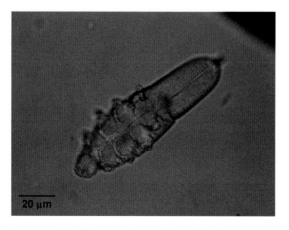

Fig. 5.23   Many animals are parasitized by *Demodex* spp. Shown here is *Demodex* from a gerbil. Hosts rarely show clinical signs of infestation. Photo courtesy of Dr. David Baker, School of Veterinary Medicine, Louisiana State University, Baton Rouge, LA.

PARASITE: *Cheyletiella* **spp.** (Figs. 5.24 and 5.25)

Common name: Walking dandruff.

Taxonomy: Mite (family Cheyletiellidae).

Host: *Cheyletiella parasitovorax*, *C. yasguri*, and *C. blakei* are seen on rabbits, dogs, and cats, respectively.

Geographic Distribution: Worldwide.

Location on Host: *Cheyletiella* infestations are usually seen on the back. In cats, the head is also often affected.

Life Cycle: Transmission is by direct contact or fomites. *Cheyletiella* can be carried from one animal to another by fleas (*Ctenocephalides*). Mites can live up to 10 days in the environment.

Laboratory Diagnosis: *Cheyletiella* is a fur mite and not a skin dweller, so only superficial skin scrapings are required for diagnosis. Alternatively, if material combed from the hair is examined against a dark background, mites can be seen as moving white dots ("walking dandruff"). The distinctive feature of the mite is the large palpal claws.

Size: Approximately 400 µm

Clinical Importance: Many infested animals do not show clinical signs. Young animals are most likely to show evidence of infestation, including crusting, increased skin scurf, and pruritus. In heavy infestations, hair loss may occur. Owners may develop lesions in areas of close contact with their animals.

PARASITE: *Psorobia* (*Psoregates*) **spp.** (Fig. 5.26)

Taxonomy: Mite (family Cheyletiellidae).

Host: Mice (*Psorobia simplex*); related species (e.g. *Psoregates* spp.) are found on ruminants.

Geographic Distribution: *Psorobia simplex* is found on mice worldwide. *Psoregates ovis* of sheep is uncommon and occurs in Australia, New Zealand, South Africa, and South America. *Psoregates bos* of cattle is also uncommon but has been reported from Africa, Australia, Europe, and North America.

Location on Host: *Psorobia simplex* can be found anywhere on the body although lesions often develop in the ears and mite numbers are highest on the head and neck. Lesions of *Psoregates ovis* develop on the neck and shoulders and then spread to the flanks and rump. Cattle with *Psoregates bos* develop lesions on the dorsal head, neck, shoulders, rump, and back.

Life Cycle: Similar to *Sarcoptes scabiei*. Mites readily move between animals in close contact.

Laboratory Diagnosis: Mites are identified in skin scrapings.

Size: 100–200 µm; smaller than *Sarcoptes scabiei*

Clinical Importance: *Psorobia simplex* can cause ear mange as well as small, white, dermal nodules in mice. *Psoregates ovis* causes fleece damage in sheep; Merinos are particularly susceptible. Cattle with psorergatic mange present with pruritus, scaling, and alopecia.

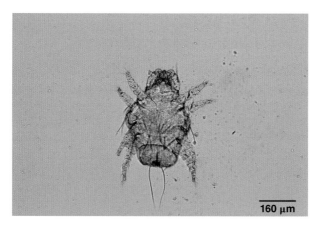

Fig. 5.24 *Cheyletiella* is a surface mite that can be collected by brushing the hair coat or collecting material with sticky tape. In heavy infestations, mites may be found throughout the hair coat. Photo courtesy of Dr. Yoko Nagamori, College of Veterinary Medicine, Oklahoma State University, Stillwater, OK.

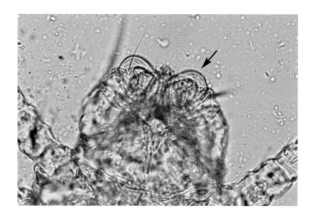

Fig. 5.25 *Cheyletiella* spp. are readily identified microscopically by the presence of large palpal claws (*arrow*). Small combs are present on the legs instead of the suckers seen in some other species of parasitic mites. Photo courtesy of Dr. Yoko Nagamori, College of Veterinary Medicine, Oklahoma State University, Stillwater, OK.

ARTHROPODS

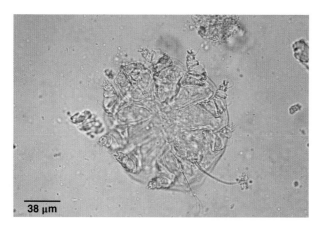

Fig. 5.26 *Psorobia simplex* from a mouse. Note the rounded body, short legs, and presence of small claws or combs rather than suckers on the end of each leg. Photo courtesy of Dr. Yoko Nagamori, College of Veterinary Medicine, Oklahoma State University, Stillwater, OK.

PARASITE: **_Lynxacarus radovskyi_** (Fig. 5.27)

Taxonomy: Mite (family Listrophoridae).

Host: Cats; other species infest bobcats and weasels.

Geographic Distribution: Australia, southern United States, Caribbean, and Hawaii.

Location on Host: Mites clasp the hairs of cats, primarily on the tail head, tail tip, and in the perineal area.

Life Cycle: The entire life cycle is spent on the host. Infestation is by direct contact.

Laboratory Diagnosis: Laterally flattened mites can be seen clinging to cat hairs. Eggs are attached to the hairs.

   Size: Approximately 450 μm

Clinical Importance: Heavy mite infestations can affect the entire body and lead to poor condition of the hair coat. This mite is rare in North America.

PARASITE: **_Leporacarus (= Listrophorus) gibbus_** (Figs. 5.28 and 5.29)

   Common name: Fur mite.

Taxonomy: Mite (family Listrophoridae). This mite formerly belonged to the genus _Listrophorus_.

Host: Rabbits.

Geographic Distribution: Worldwide.

Location on Host: Throughout the fur.

Life Cycle: Transmission is by direct contact. All stages of the life cycle are found on the host.

Laboratory Diagnosis: Mites are large enough to be seen as small specks on the hairs and can be collected by combing and examining hairs with a magnifying glass or microscope.

   Size: Approximately 350–500 μm

Clinical Importance: Mites usually cause no clinical signs even though large numbers may be present.

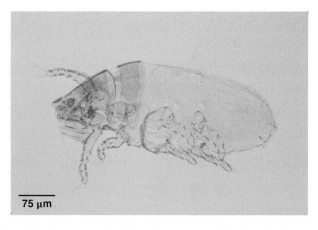

Fig. 5.27 The body of the *Lynxacarus* mite is laterally compressed like that of a flea and has large sternal plates that are used, along with the first two pairs of legs, to encircle the hair.

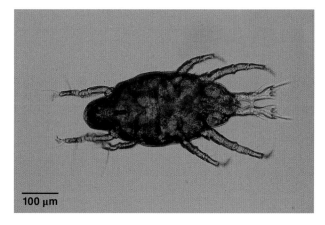

Fig. 5.28 Male *Leporacarus* mites have a brown anterior shield that projects beyond the mouthparts. Males also have distinctive adanal clasping organs.

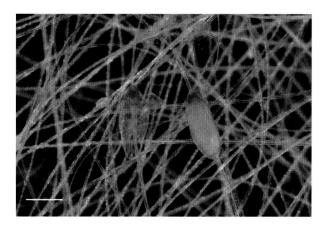

Fig. 5.29 Adult *Leporacarus* on the hair of a rabbit. The female mites also bear an anterior shield. Photo courtesy of Dr. Yoko Nagamori, College of Veterinary Medicine, Oklahoma State University, Stillwater, OK.

PARASITE: ***Chirodiscoides caviae*** (Fig. 5.30)

Common name: Fur mite.

Taxonomy: Mite (family Listrophoridae).

Host: Guinea pigs.

Geographic Distribution: Worldwide.

Location on Host: Attached to hairs.

Life Cycle: Transmission is by direct contact with an infested individual or fomite.

Laboratory Diagnosis: Mites are detected by examining hairs from the host.

  Size: Approximately 350–500 µm

Clinical Importance: This mite is considered generally nonpathogenic.

PARASITE: ***Mycoptes musculinus, Myobia musculi, Radfordia* spp.** (Figs. 5.31 and 5.32)

Common name: Fur mite.

Taxonomy: Mites (families Listrophoridae and Myobidae).

Host: Mice and rats.

Geographic Distribution: Worldwide.

Location on Host: Hair coat.

Life Cycle: Transmission is by direct contact; all stages of the life cycle are found on the host.

Laboratory Diagnosis: Diagnosis is made by detecting mites on host hairs.

  Size: *Radfordia* and *Myobia*   approximately 400–450 µm

                 Mycoptes   approximately 350 µm

Clinical Importance: Some infested animals tolerate large numbers of mites without clinical signs, although pruritus, erythema, hair loss, and thickened skin may occur in others. Secondary bacterial infections may develop.

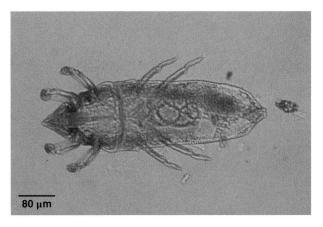

Fig. 5.30 *Chirodiscoides* from a guinea pig. The first two pairs of legs are adapted for wrapping around the hair shafts of the host. Photo courtesy of Dr. David Baker, School of Veterinary Medicine, Louisiana State University, Baton Rouge, LA.

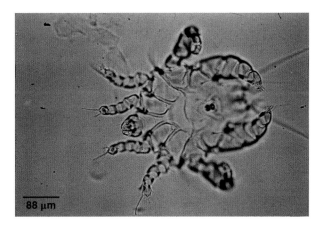

Fig. 5.31 *Mycoptes musculinus* from the hair coat of a mouse. In males, the fourth pair of legs is enlarged and directed backward. Photo courtesy of Dr. David Baker, School of Veterinary Medicine, Louisiana State University, Baton Rouge, LA.

ARTHROPODS

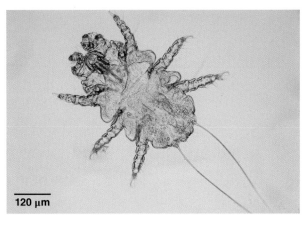

Fig. 5.32 *Radfordia* is found at the base of the hairs. The first pair of legs is modified for feeding and project forward. *Radfordia* is similar in appearance to another rodent fur mite, *Myobia musculi*. However, *Radfordia* has two claws on the second pair of legs, while *Myobia* has only one claw.

Parasite: **Avian Feather Mites** (Figs. 5.33 and 5.34)

Taxonomy: Mites (numerous families and species).

Host: Domestic and wild birds.

Geographic Distribution: Worldwide.

Location on Host: Species specialized for different feather environments.

Life Cycle: Most mites live on the feather surface and feed on secretions and skin and feather debris. Quill mites live in the base of the feathers and feed on host tissue or fluids.

Laboratory Diagnosis: Diagnosis is made by detection and identification of mites on feathers.

   Size: Variable with species

Clinical Importance: Most feather mite infestations appear to cause little damage and are usually considered of minor clinical importance. Occasionally irritation, dermatitis, and feather damage develop.

ARTHROPODS

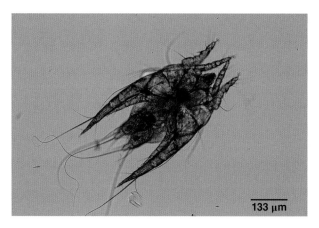

Fig. 5.33   Feather mite from a chicken. Feather mite species show great variation in morphology as a result of specialization for life in different parts of the avian feather environment. Photo courtesy of Dr. Manigandan Lejeune, Animal Health Diagnostic Center, Cornell University, Ithaca, NY.

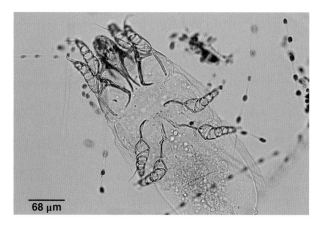

Fig. 5.34   *Megninia*, a feather mite from a finch. Feather mites infest various species of birds, often feeding at the base of feathers. Photo courtesy of Dr. Manigandan Lejeune, Animal Health Diagnostic Center, Cornell University, Ithaca, NY.

ARTHROPODS

Parasite: ***Ornithonyssus sylviarum, O. bursa*** (Figs. 5.35 and 5.36)

Common name: Northern fowl mite, tropical fowl mite.

Taxonomy: Mite (order Mesostigmata).

Geographic Distribution: The northern fowl mite, *O. sylviarum*, is found in temperate regions worldwide. The tropical fowl mite, *O. bursa*, is found in tropical and subtropical climates. Both species are found in the United States.

Location on Host: Mites and egg masses can be found on the skin among the feathers. In poultry, *O. sylviarum* often concentrates around the vent, causing a dark discoloration of the area.

Life Cycle: *Ornithonyssus sylviarum* spends its life on the avian host, whereas *O. bursa* spends greater periods of time off the host. Wild birds can introduce the mites into poultry facilities. Under appropriate conditions, the life cycle of *O. sylviarum* can be completed in a week.

Laboratory Diagnosis: Large, grossly visible mites are observed on birds or in the environment.

Size: Approximately 750 µm

Clinical Importance: Scabbed, matted feathers develop on infested birds. In severe cases, anemia, production loss, and death may occur. Mites can act as vectors of other avian disease agents, including those causing Newcastle disease and fowl pox. Humans in contact with mites may also develop lesions.

Parasite: ***Ornithonyssus bacoti*** (Figs. 5.35 and 5.36), other *Ornithonyssus* spp.

Common name: Tropical rat mite.

Taxonomy: Mite (order Mesostigmata).

Host: Rodents, wild birds; occasionally other animals and humans.

Geographic Distribution: Worldwide.

Location on Host: Skin.

Life Cycle: Adult mites lay eggs in the environment. Mites visit the host only to feed; they spend the rest of the time in the host's bedding or nest. The life cycle can be completed in about 2 weeks.

Laboratory Diagnosis: Large, grossly visible mites are observed on animals or in the environment.

Size: Approximately 750 µm

Clinical Importance: In large numbers, this blood-feeding mite can cause anemia, debilitation, and death. Humans in contact with infested laboratory or pet rodents may develop lesions. Lesions can also develop on pets and people when rodent or bird nests associated with human dwellings are abandoned, leaving mites behind to seek other hosts.

ARTHROPODS

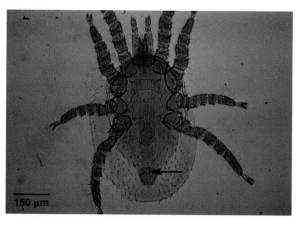

Fig. 5.35 *Ornithonyssus* spp. belong to the mesostigmatid order of mites. These mites are quite large and have long legs in the anterior portion of the body. In *Ornithonyssus* spp., the anus (*arrow*) is at the anterior end of the anal plate. The anus of *Dermanyssus* spp., a morphologically similar mite, is located in the posterior portion of the anal plate. Photo courtesy of Dr. David Baker, School of Veterinary Medicine, Louisiana State University, Baton Rouge, LA.

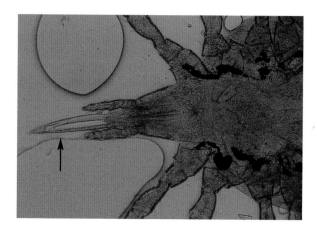

Fig. 5.36 Another characteristic used to differentiate *Ornithonyssus* from the similar genus *Dermanyssus* is the chelicerae (*arrow*). The chelicerae in this *Ornithonyssus* mite are shorter than the long, whip-like chelicerae of *Dermanyssus*.

PARASITE: ***Dermanyssus gallinae*** (Fig. 5.37)

Common name: Red poultry mite.

Taxonomy: Mite (order Mesostigmata).

Host: Wild and domestic birds.

Geographic Distribution: Worldwide.

Location on Host: Mites can occur anywhere on the body.

Life Cycle: Mites visit the host at night only to take blood meals. During the day, the mites are found in crevices in the environment. The life cycle can be completed in as little as 10 days. Adults can survive in the environment for several months without feeding.

Laboratory Diagnosis: Mite infestation may be difficult to diagnose because the mites are not on the host during the day. Close examination of the environment may reveal mites under crusts of manure on perches or in nest boxes. If infestation is suspected in caged birds, the cage can be covered with a white cloth at night. In the morning, mites will be seen as small black or dark red dots clinging to the cloth.

Size: Approximately 750 μm

Clinical Importance: Heavy infestation can cause anemia and death, particularly in hatchlings. Hens may be reluctant to sit on their nests. Other animals and humans in close proximity to infested birds or their nests may also develop lesions.

PARASITE: ***Pneumonyssoides caninum*** (Fig. 5.38)

Common name: Nasal mite.

Taxonomy: Mite (order Mesostigmata).

Host: Dogs. A similar mite, *Pneumonyssus simicola*, is found in the lungs of rhesus macaques.

Geographic Distribution: Worldwide.

Location on Host: Nasal sinuses of dogs.

Life Cycle: The life cycle of this mite is poorly understood, but transmission is thought to be by direct contact since mites are sometimes seen crawling on the nose.

Laboratory Diagnosis: Large mites grossly visible in the nasal sinuses and passages or crawling outside the nostrils.

Size: Approximately 1 mm

Clinical Importance: Infestations are usually asymptomatic but may produce sneezing, rhinitis, sinusitis, and malaise. In captive rhesus macaques, *Pneumonyssus simicola* can cause significant respiratory disease.

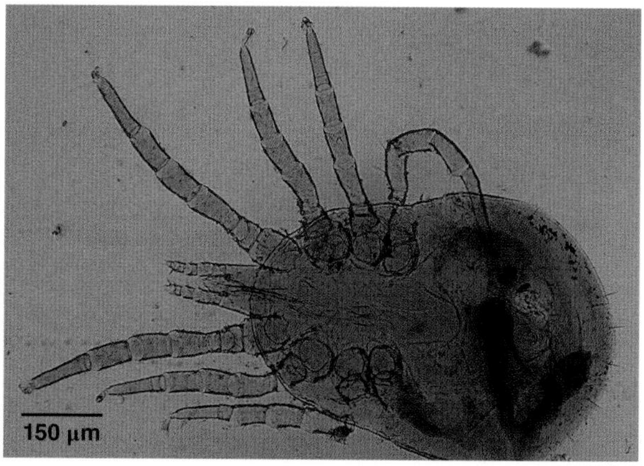

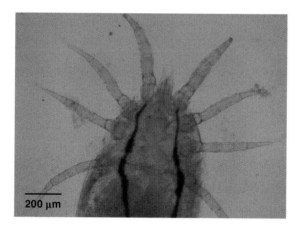

Fig. 5.37 *Dermanyssus gallinae* infests both domestic and wild birds. The anus of this mite is present in a more posterior position on the anal plate than in *Ornithonyssus*. *Dermanyssus* also has long, whip-like chelicerae (not visible in this figure). Differentiating the genera may be helpful in determining appropriate control measures because of differences in life cycles.

Fig. 5.38 *Pneumonyssoides caninum*, the nasal mite of dogs. A related mite, *Pneumonyssus simicola*, is the lung mite of several species of African monkeys. Photo courtesy of Dr. Jeffrey F. Williams, Vanson HaloSource, Inc., Redmond, WA.

ARTHROPODS

PARASITE: ***Ophionyssus natricis*** (Figs. 5.39 and 5.40)

Common name: Snake mite.

Taxonomy: Mite (order Mesostigmata).

Geographic Distribution: Worldwide on captive snakes.

Location on Host: Mites are found on the skin or under the scales of snakes and may also infest lizards.

Life Cycle: *Ophionyssus* nymphs and adults feed and females deposit eggs in the environment after taking a blood meal. Larvae do not feed. The entire life cycle takes about 13–19 days. Infestation occurs by direct contact with an infested snake or its environment.

Laboratory Diagnosis: Identification of large mites collected from snakes. Females that have taken a blood meal are dark colored. A cotton-tipped swab can be dipped in mineral oil and used to collect mites for identification.

Size: Females 0.6–1.3 mm

Clinical Importance: *Ophionyssus* infestations are common in captive snakes. Affected animals may show irritation and depression. Shedding may increase, and snakes may soak themselves more frequently in water.

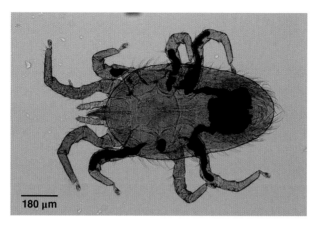

Fig. 5.39 *Ophionyssus* mites are the most common external parasite on captive snakes and may seriously affect the health of the host. Female mites lay eggs off the host, and successful control of infestation requires environmental treatment. Photo courtesy of Dr. Yoko Nagamori, College of Veterinary Medicine, Oklahoma State University, Stillwater, OK.

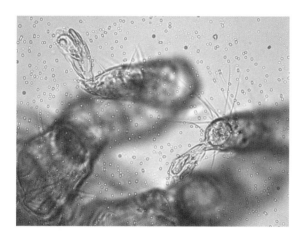

Fig. 5.40 *Ophionyssus*, like other mesostigmatid mites, has claws on the tips of the legs instead of the suckers seen in many other parasitic mites (Fig. 5.1).

ARTHROPODS

PARASITE: **Trombiculid Mites** (Figs. 5.41–5.43)

Common name: Chigger, harvest mite, scrub itch mite.

Taxonomy: Mites (family Trombiculidae).

Host: Wide variety of animals and humans.

Geographic Distribution: Several species parasitize a variety of hosts, including *Eutrombicula alfreddugesi, E. splendens* (North America), and *Neotrombicula autumnalis* (Europe).

Location on Host: Predilection sites include the face, head, and legs.

Life Cycle: Only the larval stage of chigger mites is parasitic. Eggs are laid in the environment. Larvae attach to a host and feed for 3–5 days and then complete development in the environment. Contrary to a commonly held misunderstanding, chiggers do not burrow beneath the skin. Adults are free-living predators of other arthropods.

Laboratory Diagnosis: Small, often orange or red mites are often seen in clusters on the face of the host. The presence of only larval stages is helpful in diagnosing chigger infestations.

Size: Approximately 200–500 µm, depending on species

Clinical Importance: Chigger mites cause intense pruritus. The feeding tube, or stylostome, left behind after mites are dislodged by scratching or detach to complete their development in the environment, is intensely irritating. Humans are also commonly infested by chiggers, with pruritic lesions frequently appearing in areas where clothing is constrictive (e.g., at the waistband of pants or top of socks).

ARTHROPODS

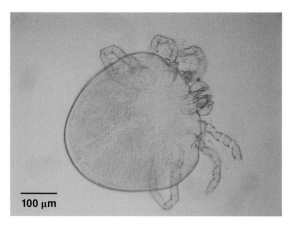

Fig. 5.41   Only the six-legged larvae of chiggers are parasitic, which is helpful in identification of the parasites. This *Blankaartia* sp. chigger was removed from a bird.

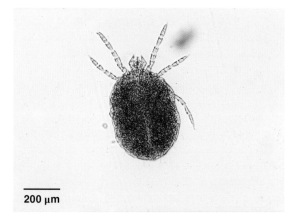

Fig. 5.42   Specimen of trombiculid larvae that cause mammalian chigger infestation. Photo courtesy of Dr. Jeffrey F. Williams, Vanson HaloSource, Inc., Redmond, WA.

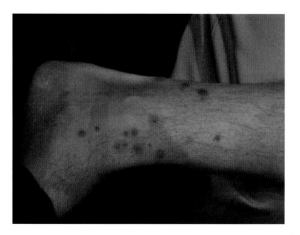

Fig. 5.43   Typical chigger lesions on the leg of a parasitologist. Chiggers may also cause pruritus and irritation on animals.

Tick Identification

Ticks are usually larger than mites, ranging in length from 3 to 12 mm, or more in the case of engorged females. Ticks are divided into two families: Ixodidae (hard ticks) and Argasidae (soft ticks). The Ixodid (hard) ticks are of greatest importance in veterinary medicine. Various hard tick species are vectors of a number of viral, bacterial, protozoal, and nematodal animal and human pathogens. In addition, hard tick species cause tick paralysis and tick toxicosis.

All ticks pass from the egg through larval and nymphal stages before becoming adults and utilize one or more host animals during the developmental cycle. Eggs are always laid in the environment. Hard tick larvae are acquired by the host from the environment. All hard ticks undergo a single molt from the larval to the nymphal stage and a second molt from the nymph to the adult. These molts follow attachment and blood-feeding on the host that usually lasts for several days. Tick species that remain on the host during the two molting periods are known as one-host ticks. In two-host tick species, the molt to the nymphal stage occurs on the host, but the engorged nymph leaves the host, molts in the environment, and then finds a new host. In the three-host tick life cycle, both the larva and nymph leave the host to molt, attaching to a host again after each molt. In some cases, each tick stage prefers the same host species; in others, host preference may vary with the stage of the tick. In much of North America, the most important tick species are three-host ticks. Soft tick life cycles are more variable than those of the hard ticks. Many soft tick species live in the environment and visit the host only briefly to take repeated blood meals.

All stages of ticks are large enough to be grossly visible on animals, although larvae may be only a few millimeters in length and soft ticks usually do not attach for long periods. Hard ticks may attach anywhere on their hosts but are likely to be found attached in areas on the host that cannot be easily groomed, for example, the head, neck, and ears of most host species (Fig. 5.44), and also the tail of horses. Because ticks are important vectors of pathogens that may result in disease (e.g., Lyme disease, Rocky Mountain spotted fever, ehrlichiosis, cytauxzoonosis, anaplasmosis, etc.), they should be removed as quickly as possible using forceps or tweezers instead of fingers to reduce the possibility of contact with tick body fluids containing infectious organisms. The tick should be firmly grasped directly behind the point of attachment to the skin and then pulled off. Often a small portion of skin will also be pulled away.

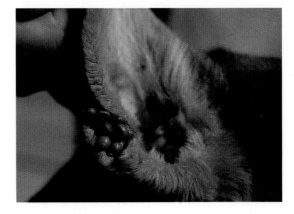

Fig. 5.44   Ticks are often found attached on parts of the body that are difficult for the host to groom. Unidentified ticks are attached to the ear of this dog. Photo courtesy of Dr. Jeffrey F. Williams, Vanson HaloSource, Inc., Redmond, WA.

Hard ticks have a hard dorsal shield called the scutum. The scutum is limited to the anterior, central region of the dorsum in females, whereas in males, the scutum extends over the entire dorsal region. The mouthparts of hard ticks are evident from the dorsal surface. The Argasid (soft) ticks have a leathery integument, which often is spinose or bumpy. The mouthparts of adult soft ticks can be seen only from the ventral aspect of the tick.

Identification of adult hard ticks to the level of genus is not difficult in a veterinary practice. One of the most useful characteristics for identifying the genus of a hard tick is the shape of the basis capituli and mouthparts. Figure 5.45 shows these characteristics on adult females; a magnifying glass or dissecting microscope is useful for looking at the basis capituli. The pigmented markings of the scutum (referred to as "ornamentation") are another useful characteristic. Ticks with ornamentation are called "ornate"; those lacking these markings are "inornate." Additionally, in some genera, the posterior margin of the body has a series of indentations, known as festoons (see adult *Dermacentor*). Features like festoons are much more difficult to appreciate on engorged female ticks. Identification is easiest with non-engorged females or males. Nymphs, like adults, have eight legs but lack the genital pore seen in adults. Larvae have six legs (Fig. 5.46), are smaller than nymphs, and may require the assistance of an expert to identify beyond genus. Figure 5.47 shows adult female ticks of the most common species in the United States. They also represent the most common tick genera found

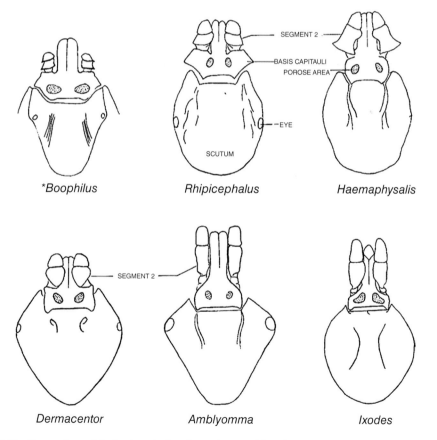

Fig. 5.45 Comparison of the basis capituli and mouthparts of females of the important Ixodid tick genera of domestic animals in North America. The scutum of the adult male hard ticks covers the entire dorsum of the parasite. *Boophilus* ticks have now been incorporated into the genus *Rhipicephalus*. Modified from USDA APHIS Agriculture Handbook No. 485.

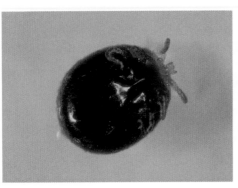
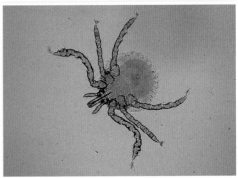

Fig. 5.46   Larval ticks are often called "seed ticks" because of their small size. Tick larvae have only six legs and can be distinguished from nymphs and adults each of which has eight legs. Microscopic examination will likely be necessary to count the number of legs on tick larvae. Left, engorged tick larva. Right, non-engorged or flat tick larva that has been treated with a clearing solution to highlight morphological characteristics.

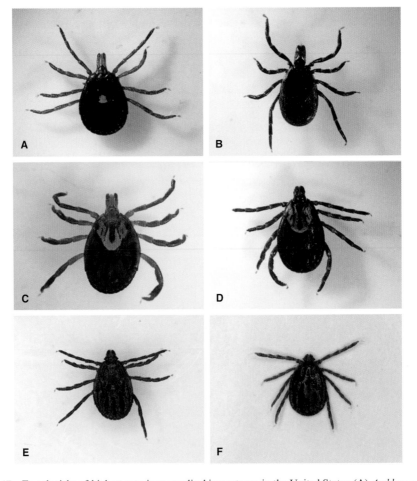

Fig. 5.47   Female ticks of highest veterinary medical importance in the United States. (A) *Amblyomma americanum*, lone star tick; (B) *Ixodes scapularis*, black-legged tick or deer tick; (C) *Amblyomma maculatum*, Gulf Coast tick; (D) *Dermacentor variabilis*, American dog tick; (E) *Rhipicephalus sanguineus*, brown dog tick; (F) *Haemaphysalis longicornis*. More information on these species can be found in the following pages. Photos courtesy of Megan Lineberry, Oklahoma State University, Stillwater, OK.

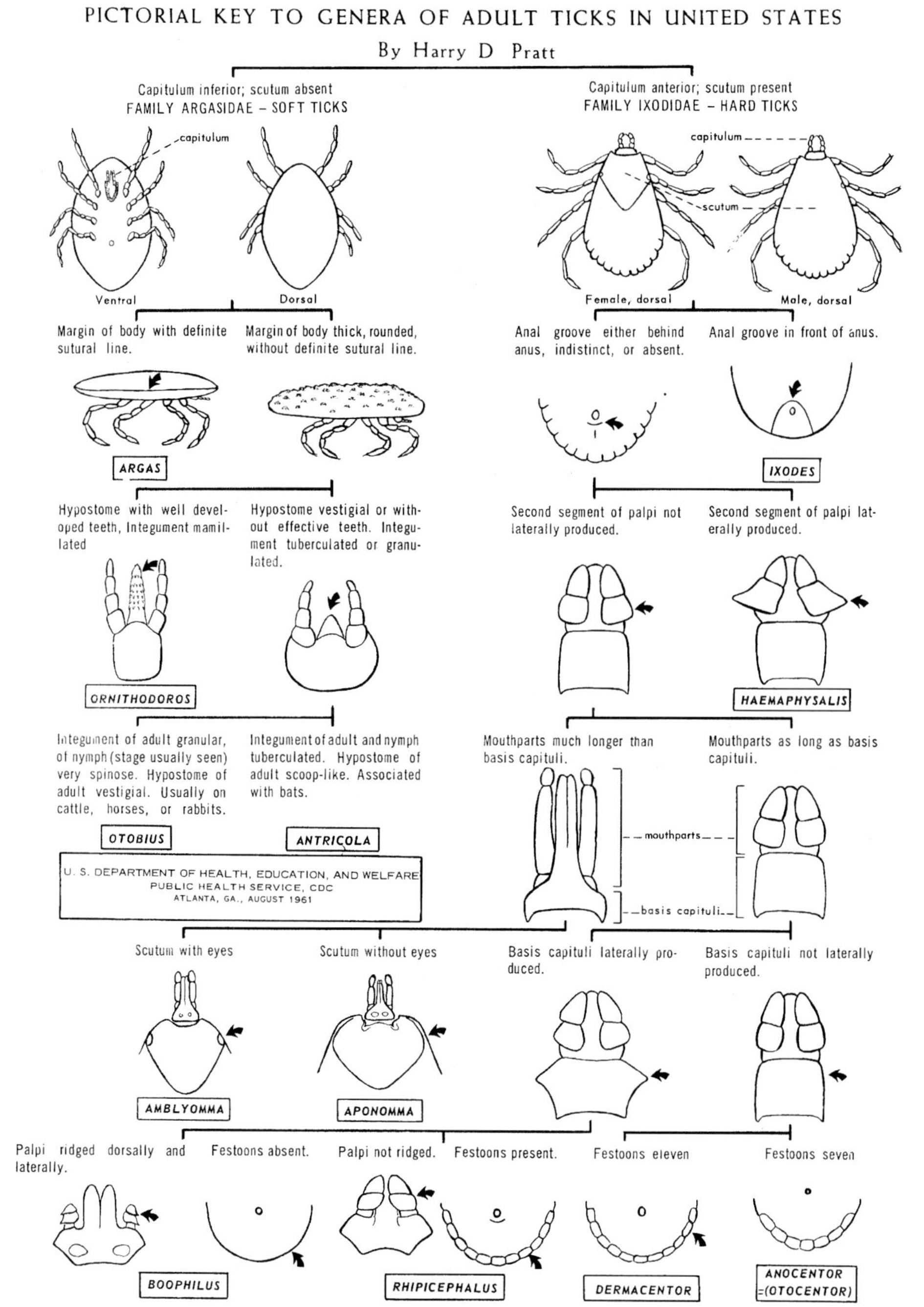

PICTORIAL KEY TO GENERA OF ADULT TICKS IN UNITED STATES
By Harry D Pratt

Capitulum inferior; scutum absent
FAMILY ARGASIDAE – SOFT TICKS

Capitulum anterior; scutum present
FAMILY IXODIDAE – HARD TICKS

capitulum

Ventral   Dorsal

Female, dorsal   Male, dorsal

capitulum
scutum

Margin of body with definite sutural line.

Margin of body thick, rounded, without definite sutural line.

Anal groove either behind anus, indistinct, or absent.

Anal groove in front of anus.

ARGAS

IXODES

Hypostome with well developed teeth, Integument mamillated

Hypostome vestigial or without effective teeth. Integument tuberculated or granulated.

Second segment of palpi not laterally produced.

Second segment of palpi laterally produced.

ORNITHODOROS

HAEMAPHYSALIS

Integument of adult granular, of nymph (stage usually seen) very spinose. Hypostome of adult vestigial. Usually on cattle, horses, or rabbits.

Integument of adult and nymph tuberculated. Hypostome of adult scoop-like. Associated with bats.

Mouthparts much longer than basis capituli.

Mouthparts as long as basis capituli.

OTOBIUS   **ANTRICOLA**

U. S. DEPARTMENT OF HEALTH, EDUCATION, AND WELFARE
PUBLIC HEALTH SERVICE, CDC
ATLANTA, GA., AUGUST 1961

mouthparts
basis capituli

Scutum with eyes

Scutum without eyes

Basis capituli laterally produced.

Basis capituli not laterally produced.

AMBLYOMMA

APONOMMA

Palpi ridged dorsally and laterally.

Festoons absent.

Palpi not ridged.

Festoons present.

Festoons eleven

Festoons seven

BOOPHILUS

RHIPICEPHALUS

DERMACENTOR

ANOCENTOR =(OTOCENTOR)

ARTHROPODS

Fig. 5.48 Key to adult tick genera found in North America. Examination of ticks with low magnification should allow identification of features used in this key. *Boophilus* ticks have now been incorporated into the genus *Rhipicephalus*. Courtesy of U.S. Public Health Service, CDC.

throughout the world. If assistance is needed with specific identification of ticks, they should be preserved and submitted to a diagnostic laboratory in 70%–80% alcohol. A dichotomous key for the genera of adult ticks (Fig. 5.48) can be followed for identification of most tick specimens in North America.

PARASITE: ***Amblyomma* spp.** (Figs. 5.49–5.54; see also Fig. 5.47)

Common names: Lone star tick, Gulf Coast tick, Cayenne tick, tropical bont tick.

Taxonomy: Tick (family Ixodidae).

Host: A wide variety of domestic and wild animals serve as hosts.

Geographic Distribution: Approximately 100 species are found predominantly in tropical and subtropical areas. *Amblyomma americanum* (lone star tick) and *A. maculatum* (Gulf Coast tick) are common species in the United States. *Amblyomma cajennense* (Cayenne tick) and other species are also found on a variety of wild and domestic animals in the United States, Mexico, Central and South America. *Amblyomma hebraeum* and *A. variegatum* are important species in Africa.

Location on Host: Various, prefer ventral aspect of many hosts.

Life Cycle: *Amblyomma* spp. are three-host ticks, meaning that each stage of the life cycle must find a new host following a molt in the environment. Larvae and nymphs feed on a wide variety of hosts; adults are often found on ruminants and other domestic animals and humans.

Laboratory Diagnosis: Long mouthparts are an important diagnostic feature of *Amblyomma*. The scutum is usually ornamented.

Clinical Importance: The long mouthparts of *Amblyomma* make attachment particularly painful and susceptible to secondary infection. *Amblyomma americanum* is a vector of several notable pathogens (e.g., *Ehrlichia* spp., *Francisella tularensis*, *Cytauxzoon felis*, *Phlebovirus*) that cause disease in animals and humans. *Amblyomma maculatum* transmits *Hepatozoon americanum* and *Rickettsia parkeri*. Infestations with *A. maculatum* can cause permanent damage to the ears of cattle known as "gotch ear." The lesions caused by *A. cajennense* are particularly painful. It serves as a vector of *R. rickettsia* and agents of equine piroplasmosis. In Africa, *A. hebraeum* and *A. variegatum* transmit *Ehrlichia ruminantium*, *R. conori*, and *Nairovirus*. In the Caribbean, *A. variegatum* also transmits *E. ruminantium*.

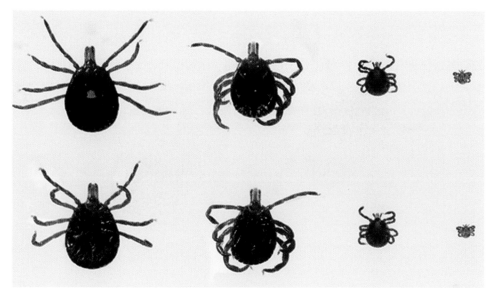

Fig. 5.49 Dorsal (top row) and ventral (bottom row) aspects of all motile stages of *Amblyomma americanum* (lone star tick), demonstrating the considerable variation in size of life stages. From left to right are adult female, adult male, nymph, larva. This tick is a generalist and all stages may infest medium- and large-sized animals within its range. The female of this common U.S. tick is easily recognized by the presence of the large white spot at the posterior margin of the scutum. Males do not have conspicuous ornamentation on the scutum, although with closer inspection, some iridescent markings can be seen on the margin of the scutum and festoons. Photo courtesy of Megan Lineberry, Oklahoma State University, Stillwater, OK.

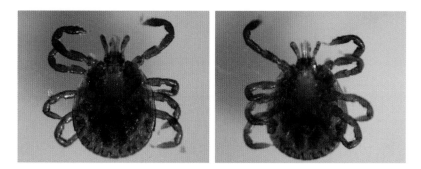

Fig. 5.50 Dorsal (*left*) and ventral (*right*) views of *Amblyomma americanum* nymph. Like adults, nymphs have eight legs, but are smaller and lack a genital opening. The nymphs of *A. americanum* lack the dramatic "lone star" of adult females. Photos courtesy of Megan Lineberry, Oklahoma State University, Stillwater, OK.

ARTHROPODS

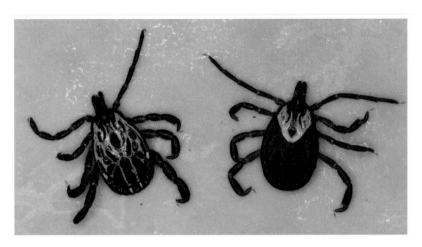

Fig. 5.51   *Amblyomma maculatum*: (*left*) male; (*right*) female. The Gulf Coast tick is found in the southeastern United States, Mexico, and South and Central America. It feeds primarily on the head and neck of birds and mammals. Note the long mouthparts typical of this genus.

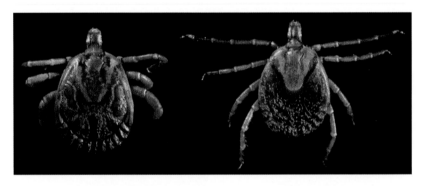

Fig. 5.52   *Amblyomma cajennense*: (*left*) male; female (*right*). The Cayenne tick is found in Texas, Mexico, Central and South America. It parasitizes a wide variety of mammals and birds. Photo courtesy of James Gathany and Christopher Paddock, Centers for Disease Control and Prevention (Public Health Image Library).

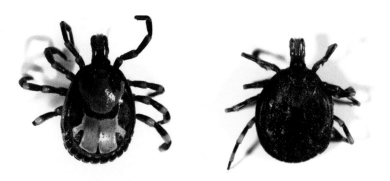

Fig. 5.53 *Amblyomma variegatum*: (*left*) male; (*right*) female. The tropical bont tick is an important vector of heartwater in cattle. This tick is also found in the Caribbean.

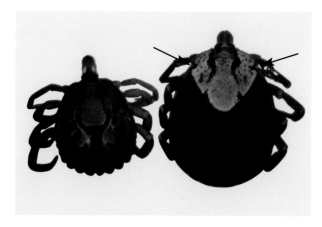

Fig. 5.54 *Amblyomma* spp. are common in the tropics and subtropics. They are often highly ornamented with iridescent markings like these African *Amblyomma*. Some tick genera, like *Amblyomma*, have simple eyes on the margin of the scutum (*arrows*).

Parasite: **Hyalomma spp.** (Fig. 5.55)

Common name: Bont-legged tick, camel tick, tortoise tick.

Taxonomy: Tick (family Ixodidae).

Host: Many host species, including domestic animals. One species, *H. aegyptium*, is a parasite of tortoises.

Geographic Distribution: Asia, Europe, North Africa.

Location on Host: Various.

Life Cycle: *Hyalomma* species are usually two-host ticks, which leave the host after nymphal and adult blood meals.

Laboratory Diagnosis: Ticks of the genus *Hyalomma* have eyes and long mouthparts like those of *Amblyomma*, but lack the ornamentation usually seen on *Amblyomma* spp.

Clinical Importance: *Hyalomma* species cause tick toxicosis and serve as vectors of *Babesia*, *Theileria*, and *Rickettsia* spp.

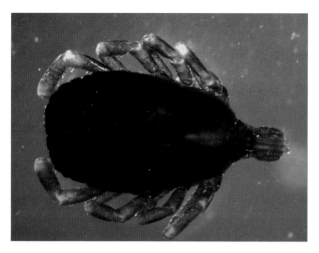

Fig. 5.55   *Hyalomma* spp. ticks are important disease vectors in Africa, Asia, and Australasia, although they are not found in the Western Hemisphere. They have long mouthparts, eyes, and festoons like *Amblyomma* but are not highly ornamented.

Parasite: ***Ixodes* spp.** (Figs. 5.56–5.58; see also Figs. 5.47, 5.67)

Common name: Black-legged tick, deer tick, European sheep tick (castor bean tick), hedgehog tick, British dog tick, Australian and South African paralysis ticks.

Taxonomy: Tick (family Ixodidae). *Ixodes* is the largest genus of hard ticks, containing more than 200 species. Approximately 35 species of *Ixodes* are found in North America.

Host: Many host species, including domestic animals and humans.

Geographic Distribution: Some of the most important species in domestic animals include *I. scapularis* (black-legged or deer tick) and *I. pacificus* (western black-legged tick) in North America; *I. ricinus* (sheep or castor bean tick), *I. canisuga* (British dog tick), and *I. hexagonus* (hedgehog tick) in Europe; *I. rubicundus* (South African paralysis tick); and *I. holocyclus* (Australian paralysis tick).

Location on Host: Various.

Life Cycle: *Ixodes* species are three-host ticks.

Laboratory Diagnosis: The most helpful characteristic for identification of *Ixodes* ticks is an anal groove that runs from the posterior margin of the body to just anterior to the anus. A magnifying glass or dissecting-type microscope may be needed to identify this feature.

Clinical Importance: *Ixodes* spp. in North America and Europe are vectors of *Borrelia* spp., *Babesia* spp., *Ehrlichia* spp., and *Flavivirus*. *Ixodes ricinus* transmits *Flavivirus* and *Babesia* spp. in Europe. *Ixodes* spp can also cause dermatitis and tick worry and are major causes of tick paralysis in Australia and South Africa.

ARTHROPODS

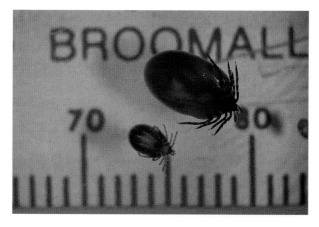

Fig. 5.56   Engorged nymph and engorged adult female *Ixodes scapularis*, the deer tick. This species is the primary vector of the agent of Lyme disease in the United States and is smaller than other common ticks (see Fig. 5.47 for comparison).

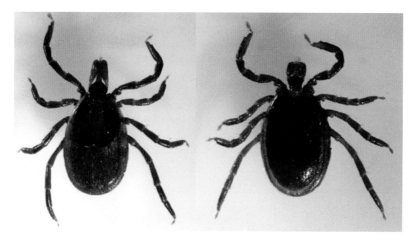

Fig. 5.57   Unfed adult female (*left*) and male (*right*) *Ixodes scapularis* viewed dorsally. The scutum of *Ixodes scapularis* is not ornamented and both legs and scutum are a dark brown-black color. Photo courtesy of Megan Lineberry, Oklahoma State University, Stillwater, OK.

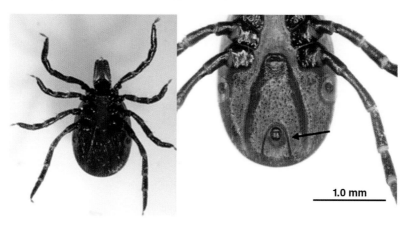

Fig. 5.58   A distinctive morphologic detail of the *Ixodes* ticks is the groove that runs anterior to the anus (*arrow*). In other tick genera, this groove is either posterior to the anus or absent. *Ixodes* ticks also have long mouthparts. Photos courtesy of Parna Ghosh, Oklahoma State University, Stillwater, OK.

ARTHROPODS

PARASITE: ***Dermacentor* spp.** (Figs. 5.59–5.62; see also Fig. 5.47)

Common name: American dog tick, Rocky Mountain wood tick, winter tick, tropical horse tick.

Taxonomy: Tick (family Ixodidae).

Host: Depending on the species, a wide variety of wild and domestic hosts can be used.

Geographic Distribution: Primarily Europe, Asia, and North America. *Dermacentor variabilis* (American dog tick), *D. andersoni* (Rocky Mountain wood tick), *D. albipictus* (winter or elk or horse tick), and *D. occidentalis* (Pacific Coast tick) are found in North America and parasitize a variety of animals. *Dermacentor (= Anocentor) nitens* is a parasite of equids in Florida, the Caribbean, Central and South America. In Europe, *D. reticulatus* is an important species.

Location on Host: Various.

Life Cycle: Most *Dermacentor* spp. are three-host ticks that prefer small rodents in larval and nymphal stages and larger vertebrates in the adult stage. *Dermacentor nitens* and *D. albipictus* are one-host ticks.

Laboratory Diagnosis: *Dermacentor* spp. are usually ornamented with relatively short mouthparts and a rectangular basis capituli.

Clinical Importance: *Dermacentor* spp. in the United States are the most common vectors of *Rickettsia rickettsii* and can also transmit *Anaplasma marginale* to cattle. *Dermacentor (Anocentor) nitens* is the vector of *Babesia caballi* and *Theileria equi* in the United States. In Europe, *D. reticulatus* is the vector of *Babesia* spp. to horses and dogs. Several species of *Dermacentor* are known to cause tick paralysis.

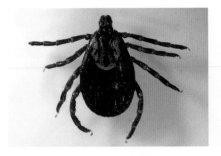 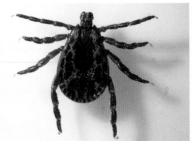

Fig. 5.59 *Dermacentor variabilis*: female (*left*); male (*right*). Like many members of this genus, *D. variabilis* (the American dog tick) is an ornamented tick. The short mouthparts, rectangular shape of the basis capituli, and presence of festoons are used in identifying the genus. Photos courtesy of Megan Lineberry, Oklahoma State University, Stillwater, OK.

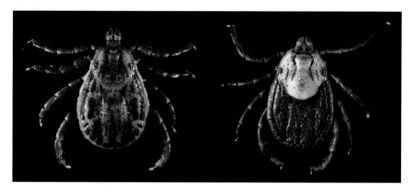

Fig. 5.60 *Dermacentor andersoni*: (*left*) male; (*right*) female; the Rocky Mountain wood tick. This tick is found in the central and western United States and Canada. Photo courtesy of James Gathany and Christopher Paddock, Centers for Disease Control and Prevention (Public Health Image Library).

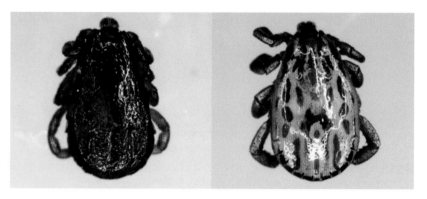

Fig. 5.61 *Dermacentor albipictus*, the winter or moose tick, is a one-host tick most active in winter. Both the brown variant (*left*) and ornamented (*right*) strains of *D. albipictus* occur widely in North America. Photo courtesy of Dr. Manigandan Lejeune, Animal Health Diagnostic Center, Cornell University, Ithaca, NY.

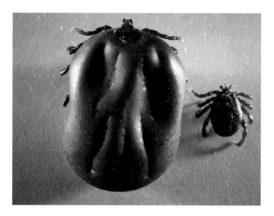

Fig. 5.62 *Dermacentor* (*Anocentor*) *nitens* engorged female (*left*) and male (*right*). Unlike most important hard ticks, this is a one-host tick species that prefers horses as host but will attach to many mammals. It is important as a vector of equine piroplasmosis in Central and South America, the Caribbean, Mexico, Texas, and Florida.

ARTHROPODS

Parasite: ***Rhipicephalus* spp.** (Figs. 5.63–5.66; see also Figs. 5.47, 5.67)

Common name: Brown dog tick or kennel tick, brown ear tick, red-legged tick, cattle fever tick, blue tick, tropical cattle tick.

Taxonomy: Tick (family Ixodidae). Important parasites of domestic animals include *R. sanguineus* (brown dog tick), *R. appendiculatus* (brown ear tick), and *R. evertsi* (red-legged tick). Ticks previously classified in the genus *Boophilus* are now included in *Rhipicephalus*, including the former *B. microplus* (tropical cattle tick), *B. annulatus* (cattle fever tick), and *B. decoloratus* (blue tick).

Host: This genus is most important in livestock and dogs.

Geographic Distribution: *Rhipicephalus sanguineus* is found worldwide. *Rhipicephalus appendiculatus* and *R. evertsi* are found on livestock in Africa. *Rhipicephalus* (*Boophilus*) *microplus* (tropical cattle tick) is found worldwide; *R. annulatus* (cattle fever tick) is found in the Western Hemisphere and parts of Africa; *R. decoloratus* (blue tick) is an African tick.

Location on Host: Various.

Life Cycle: *Rhipicephalus sanguineus* is a three-host tick that uses a dog host for each stage of the life cycle. *Rhipicephalus appendiculatus* is also a three-host tick, while *R. evertsi* is a two-host tick and *R. microplus*, *R. annulatus*, and *R. decoloratus* are one-host ticks. After hatching from the egg in the environment, ticks locate the host, where they remain through the subsequent nymphal and adult stages. Females leave the host to lay their eggs in the environment.

Laboratory Diagnosis: *Rhipicephalus* spp. have a hexagonally shaped basis capituli. The members of the genus that were formerly called *Boophilus* have ridged palps.

Clinical Importance: *Rhipicephalus sanguineus* transmits *Babesia canis vogeli* and *Ehrlichia canis* to dogs. *Rhipicephalus* species infesting livestock, including *R. appendiculatus*, *R. evertsi*, *R. microplus*, and *R. annulatus* are the primary vectors of bovine *Theileria* spp., *Babesia* spp., *Anaplasma* spp., and *Nairvirus* to livestock.

ARTHROPODS

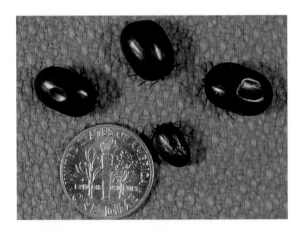

Fig. 5.63   Engorged female *Rhipicephalus sanguineus* (brown dog tick). This species is not ornate. In the United States, it is most common in southern states but can also be a pest in kennels in other areas since dogs are used as hosts for every stage of the life cycle. Photo courtesy of Dr. Jeffrey F. Williams, Vanson HaloSource, Inc., Redmond, WA.

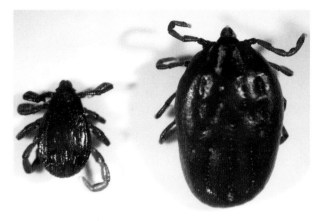

Fig. 5.64   *Rhipicephalus sanguineus* male (*left*) and engorged female (*right*). There are no markings on the scutum.

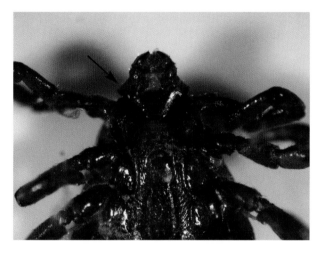

Fig. 5.65   The brown dog tick, *Rhipicephalus sanguineus*. Members of this tick genus have a basis capituli that is hexagonal in shape with flared sides (*arrow*; see also Fig. 5.45).

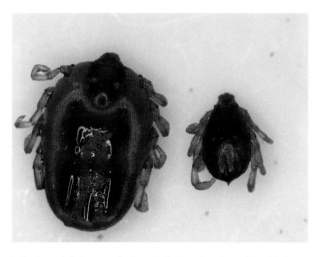

Fig. 5.66   *Rhipicephalus* (*Boophilus*) *microplus* female (*left*) and male (*right*). This is a one-host tick of cattle and the vector for bovine babesiosis.

PARASITE: **Haemaphysalis spp.** (Figs. 5.67–5.70; see also Fig. 5.47)

Common name: Rabbit tick, yellow dog tick, bush tick, longhorned tick.

Taxonomy: Tick (family Ixodidae).

Host: *Haemaphysalis* ticks parasitize a wide range of mammals and birds, depending on the species.

Geographic Distribution: Worldwide. *Haemaphysalis leporispalustris* (rabbit tick) is found in the Western Hemisphere; *H. leachi* (yellow dog tick) is found in Africa and parts of Asia; and *H. longicornis* (longhorned tick) is found primarily in Asia but was identified in the United States in 2017. Several other species parasitize livestock in Europe, Africa, Asia, and Australasia.

Location on Host: Various.

Life Cycle: *Haemaphysalis* spp. are three-host ticks and leave the host after each blood meal. Larvae and nymphs typically feed on small mammals and birds, and adult ticks feed on larger mammals. *Haemaphysalis longicornis* females are capable of reproduction through parthenogenesis. Introduction with only one or a few female ticks may result in massive infestations.

Laboratory Diagnosis: Ticks of this genus have festoons, and the second segment of the palps flares out on the lateral margin.

Clinical Importance: Large numbers of *Haemaphysalis* ticks contribute to poor condition and "tick worry." *Haemaphysalis punctata* can transmit several species of *Babesia* and *Anaplasma* to livestock. *Haemaphysalis leachi* is a vector of canine babesiosis. *Haemaphysalis longicornis* is capable of producing severe clinical disease impacting the health and production of infested animals. *Haemaphysalis longicornis* is a vector for *Phlebovirus* and infected with various species of *Anaplasma*, *Babesia*, *Borrelia*, *Ehrlichia*, and *Rickettsia* of animals and humans. At the time of this writing, it is unknown if any exotic pathogens were introduced with *H. longicornis* into the United States.

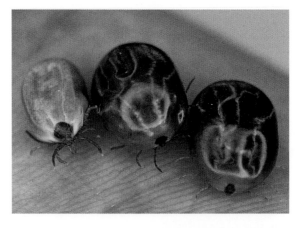

Fig. 5.67   From left to right, engorged *Ixodes*, *Haemaphysalis*, and *Rhipicephalus* females. Photo courtesy of Dr. Nick Sangster, Charles Sturt University, Wagga Wagga, NSW, Australia and Ms. Sally Pope, Faculty of Veterinary Science, University of Sydney, Sydney, NSW, Australia.

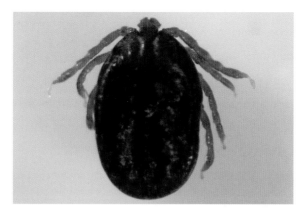

Fig. 5.68   *Haemaphysalis longicornis*, the longhorned tick, was recently discovered in North America. These ticks are inornate with festoons and short mouthparts. The second segment of the palps project laterally and are wider than the rectangular basis capituli. Photo courtesy of Megan Lineberry, Oklahoma State University, Stillwater, OK.

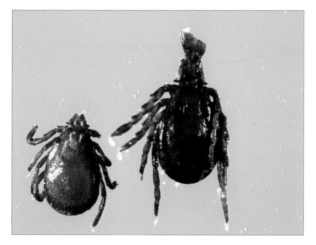

Fig. 5.69   *Haemaphysalis leporispalustris*, the rabbit tick, is found in North America and can carry the bacterial agent of tularemia, *Francisella tularensis*. Other members of this tick genus are vectors of *Babesia* and *Theileria* in Africa, Asia, and Australasia. The female tick in this photo (*right*) has host skin tissue attached to the mouthparts.

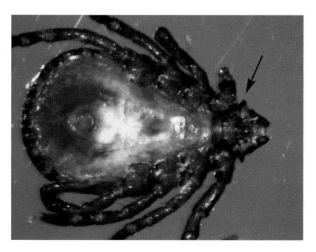

Fig. 5.70   The palps of *Haemaphysalis* ticks are wider than they are long, and in most species, the second segment of the palps flares laterally (*arrow*).

PARASITE: *Otobius megnini* (Figs. 5.71–5.73)

Common name: Spinose ear tick.

Taxonomy: Tick (family Argasidae).

Host: Ruminants and horses primarily, also camelids and small animals.

Geographic Distribution: North and South America, Africa, India.

Location on Host: External ear canal.

Life Cycle: Eggs hatch in the environment. Larvae enter the ear of the host and may remain for several months until the nymphal stage is completed. There are one larval and two nymphal stages. Nymphs leave the host after feeding and molt to the adult stage, which does not feed.

Laboratory Diagnosis: These ticks are easily diagnosed based on host location and recognition of specimens as soft ticks. *Otobius* is covered with short spines, leading to the name spinose ear tick. Hard ticks may also attach in the ears, but they have a distinctive hard, enameled appearance compared with soft ticks like *Otobius*. Also, any adult-stage ticks found in the ears will not be *O. megnini*, since spinose ear ticks are parasitic only as larvae and nymphs.

Clinical Importance: Large numbers can cause severe inflammation and rupture the ear drum.

ARTHROPODS

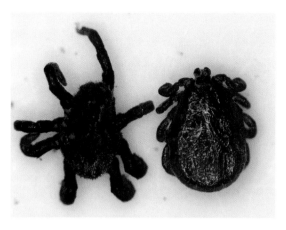

Fig. 5.71   *Otobius*, the spinose ear tick, and *Dermacentor andersoni*. This picture demonstrates the difference between soft and hard ticks. The soft tick, *Otobius* (*left*), does not have the hard enamel-like surface of the ixodid tick, *Dermacentor* (*right*). The capitulum of soft ticks is also not always visible from the dorsal surface. Hard ticks are much more common than soft ticks on domestic animals in North America.

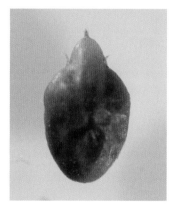

Fig. 5.72   Partially engorged larva of *Otobius megnini*, the spinose ear tick. The integument is striated with a few bristle-like hairs. In fed larvae (above), the capitulum extends from a conical anterior projection. They are found clustered in the ears of the host. Photo courtesy of Megan Lineberry, Oklahoma State University, Stillwater, OK.

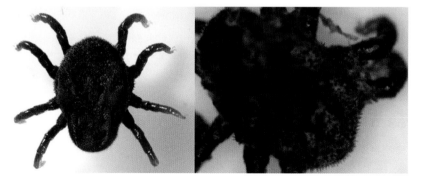

Fig. 5.73   This closer view of *Otobius megnini* nymphs shows the spines that cover the surface. The hypostome is well developed and more commonly viewed from the ventral aspect. The second nymphal stage is the one most often encountered. Photos courtesy of Megan Lineberry, Oklahoma State University, Stillwater, OK.

ARTHROPODS

Parasite: ***Argas* spp.** (Fig. 5.74)

        Common name: Fowl tick.

Taxonomy: Tick (family Argasidae). Important species include *Argas persicus* and *Argas reflexus*.

Host: Poultry and wild birds.

Geographic Distribution: Worldwide.

Location on Host: Various.

Life Cycle: *Argas* is a soft tick that lives in the environment, attacking birds only to feed, usually during the night. Several blood meals are taken by larval and adult ticks.

Laboratory Diagnosis: As their name suggests, soft ticks lack the hard "enameled" appearance of hard ticks. The mouthparts of soft ticks cannot be seen from the dorsal surface, which also helps to distinguish them from hard ticks. *Argas* spp. have a flattened body margin.

Clinical Importance: Heavy burdens can cause loss of production and death. *Argas* spp. act as vectors for *Borrelia anserine* and can cause fowl paralysis. They are uncommon in total-confinement poultry systems.

Parasite: ***Ornithodoros* spp.** (Fig. 5.75)

        Common name: Tampan.

Taxonomy: Tick (family Argasidae). *Ornithodoros moubata* is the African tampan; *O. hermsi* is one of the species found in the United States.

Host: Domestic livestock and humans.

Geographic Distribution: Africa, Asia, North and South America.

Location on Host: Various.

Life Cycle: These ticks are often nocturnal and are found in animal or human habitations, including dens, nests, or crevices of buildings.

Laboratory Diagnosis: In contrast to *Argas* spp. ticks, *Ornithodoros* spp. do not have a lateral sutural line and there is no distinct body margin.

Clinical Importance: Large numbers of these soft ticks can cause significant blood loss. *Ornithodoros* transmits endemic relapsing fever in humans. In the United States, *Ornithodoros* ticks are most common in the western and southwestern states.

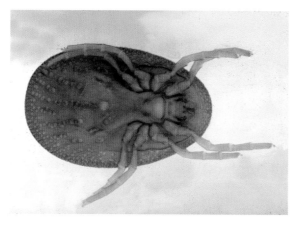

Fig. 5.74   *Argas* sp., the fowl tick, is a soft tick. The ventral location of the mouthparts is clearly seen in this specimen. The surface of *Argus* is granulated. Photo courtesy of Dr. Dwight Bowman, College of Veterinary Medicine, Cornell University, Ithaca, NY.

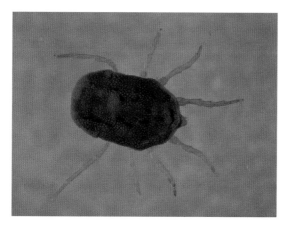

Fig. 5.75   The surface of the soft tick *Ornithodoros* is covered with mammillae (small bumps) and there is no distinct margin to the body.

CLASS INSECTA

Like ticks and mites, insects also belong to the phylum Arthropoda. All insects have bodies composed of three parts: the head, the thorax (which bears the legs), and the abdomen. Adult insects have six legs and some have wings. Life cycles of parasitic insects may be quite simple, in which larval stages are similar in appearance to the adults, or very complex, involving transformation from a worm-like maggot through a pupal stage to the adult. The insects of greatest veterinary importance are the lice, fleas, and flies.

Lice (Order Phthiraptera)

Lice are wingless, dorsoventrally flattened insects ranging in length from about 1 to 8 mm. They are common ectoparasites of mammals and birds. Louse infestations in domestic animals are most commonly observed in the winter and are referred to as "pediculosis," a term derived from a genus of lice important to humans. Lice are highly species-specific and the entire life cycle is completed on the host; stages only survive off the host for 2–3 days. Immature lice resemble adults but are smaller. Eggs (nits) are white or yellow in color and may be observed attached individually to hair shafts and sometimes at the base of feathers on birds. Lice and nits can usually be seen with the unaided eye although magnification aids recovery.

    Lice are traditionally divided into two groups based on how they feed: anopluran (sucking lice) and mallophagan (chewing lice). Both sucking and chewing lice are found on mammals, but birds are parasitized only by chewing lice. Sucking lice (anopluran) feed on blood, move slowly compared to chewing lice, and may be seen with their head pointed downward, close to the skin surface, or actually feeding. Sucking lice are generally larger than chewing lice (Fig. 5.76) and are gray to dusky red, depending on the quantity of blood ingested (Fig. 5.77). The head of sucking lice is narrower than the thorax and has elongated protrusible piercing mouthparts. Chewing lice (mallophagan) are smaller (Fig. 5.76, 5.78) and feed on skin scurf and other organic material on the skin. Chewing lice move rapidly and have blunt heads that are wider than the thorax and mandible-like mouthparts. Chewing lice are often a yellow color. While species

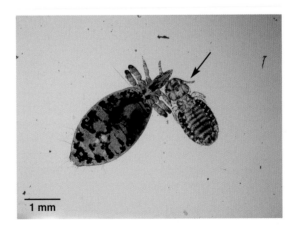

1 mm

Fig. 5.76   Chewing lice of domestic animals are usually smaller than sucking lice. *Bovicola bovis* (*arrow*) is pictured here with one of the bovine sucking lice, *Linognathus*. Photo courtesy of Dr. Robert Ridley, College of Veterinary Medicine, Kansas State University, Manhattan, KS.

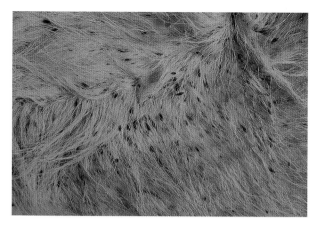

Fig. 5.77   Sucking louse infestation on a calf. Note the reddish-brown color of these blood-feeding lice. Photo courtesy of Dr. Jeffrey F. Williams, Vanson HaloSource, Inc., Redmond, WA.

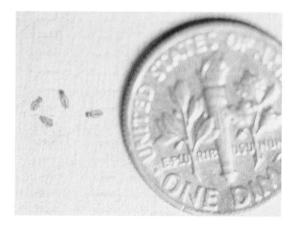

Fig. 5.78   *Bovicola ovis* is a small white or tan chewing louse that can be very difficult to detect on a heavily fleeced sheep. Photo courtesy of Dr. Jeffrey F. Williams, Vanson HaloSource, Inc., Redmond, WA.

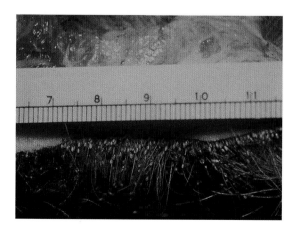

Fig. 5.79   Section of bovine skin with louse eggs (nits) attached to the hairs. "Nits" refers to insect eggs adhered to the hair and is used to describe the eggs of lice or bot flies on animals. Photo courtesy of Dr. Jeffrey F. Williams, Vanson HaloSource, Inc., Redmond, WA.

ARTHROPODS

identification of lice is usually not required in veterinary practice, recognition of an organism as a chewing or sucking louse may be helpful when selecting treatment.

Lice or their eggs (nits, Fig. 5.79) can be recovered from animals with a fine-toothed comb or by examining hair coat brushings. A magnifying lens or dissecting microscope may be useful if lice are very small. Specimens may be transferred to saline, mineral oil, or Hoyer's solution and placed on a microscope slide with fine forceps to facilitate viewing. If shipping to a laboratory, lice should be placed in 70% ethanol.

PARASITE: ***Haematopinus* spp.** (Fig. 5.80)

Common name: Pig louse, short-nosed cattle louse, cattle tail louse.

Taxonomy: Insect (Order Phthiraptera, anopluran or sucking lice).

Host: Species important in domestic animals include *H. suis* (pigs), *H. asini* (horses), *H. eurysternus* (short-nosed sucking louse of cattle), and *H. quadripertusus* (tail louse of cattle). Sucking lice are also found on camelids (genus *Microthoracius*).

Geographic Distribution: Worldwide. *Haematopinus quadripertusus* is found primarily in the tropics and subtropics.

Location on Host: *Haematopinus* spp. are often found on the head, neck, and back of the host. *Haematopinus quadripertusus* is usually found around the tail.

Life Cycle: Transmission is by direct contact or fomites. Eggs are glued to the hairs of the host.

Laboratory Diagnosis: Members of this genus are large, about 4–5 mm in length, with the elongated heads typical of the sucking lice.

Clinical Importance: *Haematopinus* infestations can produce alopecia and pruritus, leading to self-inflicted trauma and production losses. Heavy infestations can produce anemia. *Haematopinus suis* is a common and important ectoparasite of swine; *H. eurysternus* is considered the most important cattle louse worldwide. Infestation of horses is uncommon in well-managed stables.

PARASITE: ***Linognathus* spp.** (Figs. 5.81 and 5.82)

Common name: Face louse and foot louse of sheep, long-nosed cattle louse.

Taxonomy: Insect (Order Phthiraptera, anopluran or sucking lice).

Host: *Linognathus pedalis* (ovine foot louse), *L. ovillus* (ovine face louse), *L. vituli* (long-nosed cattle louse), *L. africanus* (bovine African blue louse), *L. setosus* (dogs).

Geographic Distribution: Worldwide.

Location on Host: The face and foot lice of sheep are found primarily in those locations; other species are less restricted in distribution.

Life Cycle: Transmission is by direct contact or fomites.

Laboratory Diagnosis: Detection of lice and eggs on the host by gross observation.

Clinical Importance: As with other lice, infested animals show pruritus and dermatitis, and severe infestations can lead to production losses and anemia.

ARTHROPODS

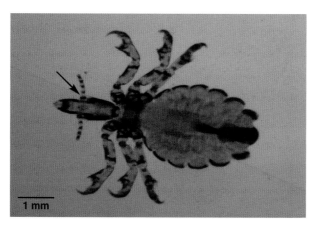

Fig. 5.80   *Haematopinus* spp. have prominent ocular points (*arrow*, partially obscured by antenna) and legs of equal size. *Haematopinus suis*, shown here, is the largest louse found on domesticated animals. Photo courtesy of Dr. Alvin Gajadhar, Centre for Animal Parasitology, CFIA, Saskatoon, Saskatchewan, Canada.

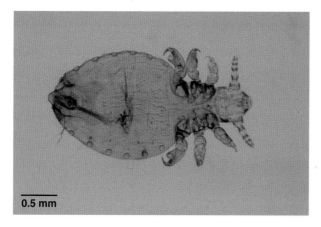

Fig. 5.81   *Linognathus* spp. have no ocular points. Unlike *Haematopinus*, the second and third pairs of legs are larger than the first pair. The louse shown here is *L. setosus*, the sucking louse of dogs. Members of this genus are usually 2–3 mm in length.

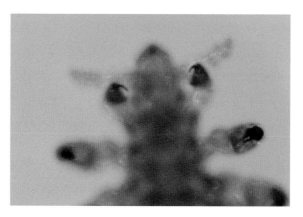

Fig. 5.82   Each sucking louse leg ends in a prominent claw. Shown are the claws of *L. africanus* from a goat. Photo courtesy of Dr. Manigandan Lejeune, Animal Health Diagnostic Center, Cornell University, Ithaca, NY.

ARTHROPODS

Parasite: **Solenopotes capillatus** (Fig. 5.83)

Common name: Little blue cattle louse.

Taxonomy: Insect (Order Phthiraptera, anopluran or sucking lice).

Host: Cattle.

Geographic Distribution: Worldwide.

Location on Host: Usually found concentrated on the face, neck, shoulders, back, and tail.

Life Cycle: The entire life cycle is spent on the host with transmission by direct contact or fomites.

Laboratory Diagnosis: *Solenopotes capillatus* is similar in appearance to *Linognathus*, but *Solenopotes* has tubercles carrying spiracles that project from abdominal segments.

Clinical Importance: Large numbers of lice may cause production loss from dermatitis and anemia.

Parasite: **Pediculus spp.** (Fig. 5.84), **Pthirus pubis** (Fig. 5.85)

Common name: Human head louse, body louse, crab louse.

Taxonomy: Insects (Order Phthiraptera, anopluran or sucking lice). *Pediculus humanus humanus* is the body louse; *Pediculus humanus capitis* is the head louse; and *Pthirus pubis* is the pubic or crab louse.

Host: Humans.

Geographic Distribution: Worldwide.

Location on Host: Head lice are found on the scalp, while body lice live principally in clothing and visit the skin to feed. Crab lice are found in the pubic area or on other coarse body hair.

Life Cycle: Transmission of all human lice infestations is by direct contact or fomites. Head and crab lice glue their eggs to host hair, while body lice deposit their eggs in clothing.

Laboratory Diagnosis: Observation of lice and eggs (nits).

Clinical Importance: Humans are the only hosts of these parasites. Their veterinary importance lies in the occasional detection of a human louse on a pet and resulting confusion about who gave what to whom. In these cases, the family pet has lice only because of close contact with infested humans. Human lice do not survive or reproduce on domestic animals.

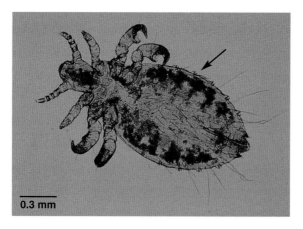

Fig. 5.83 *Solenopotes capillatus*, the little blue cattle louse, is less common than *Linognathus* spp. The projecting tubercles carrying spiracles on the abdominal segments of *Solenopotes* (*arrow*) are helpful in identification of this louse. Photo courtesy of Merial.

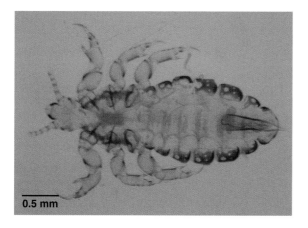

Fig. 5.84 *Pediculus humanus* has well-developed eyes, no ocular points, and three large pairs of legs.

ARTHROPODS

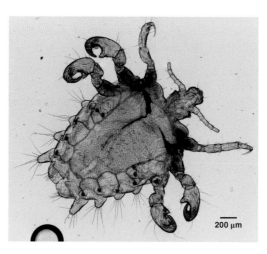

Fig. 5.85 The human crab louse, *Pthirus pubis*, has a distinctive crab-shaped body. Photo courtesy of Dr. Brian Herrin, College of Veterinary Medicine, Kansas State University, Manhattan, KS.

PARASITE: ***Polyplax spinulosa*** (Figs. 5.86 and 5.87)

Common name: Spiny rat louse.

Taxonomy: Insect (Order Phthiraptera, anopluran or sucking lice)

Host: Rats. Other species of *Polyplax* spp. are found on mice and other rodents, and other sucking lice are found on rabbits.

Geographic Distribution: Worldwide.

Location on Host: Predilection sites variable, depending on species.

Life Cycle: As with other lice, transmission is by direct contact with an infested animal or fomites.

Laboratory Diagnosis: Detection of eggs and lice on hair and morphologic identification of lice.

Clinical Importance: Large numbers of lice may cause loss of condition and possibly anemia.

PARASITE: ***Gliricola porcelli*** (Fig. 5.88)

Common name: Slender guinea pig louse.

Taxonomy: Insect (Order Phthiraptera, mallophagan or chewing lice).

Host: *Gliricola porcelli* is the most common louse of guinea pigs. Two other species of chewing lice, *Gyropus ovalis* and *Trimenopon jenningsi*, are also found on guinea pigs.

Geographic Distribution: Worldwide.

Location on Host: *Gliricola porcelli* prefers the fine hair around the back legs and anus, whereas *Gyropus ovalis* is found around the head and face.

Life Cycle: Transmission is by direct contact.

Laboratory Diagnosis: Detection and identification of lice and eggs. *Gyropus ovalis* is a broader louse than *Gliricola* and has a wide head. Eggs of *Gyropus ovalis* can be found most easily around the back of the ears. *Trimenopon jenningsi* is a dark brown louse that is less common than the other two species.

Clinical Importance: Light infestations are usually asymptomatic. Heavier infestations may be associated with hair loss, unthriftiness, and pruritus, especially at the back of the ears. Louse infestation may not be evident until the death of the host, when lice move up to the hair tips as the body temperature declines.

ARTHROPODS

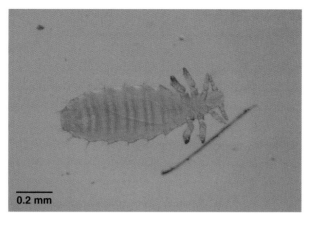

Fig. 5.86   Sucking lice (*Polyplax*) species from a rat. Typical of sucking lice, the head is narrower than the thorax in this specimen.

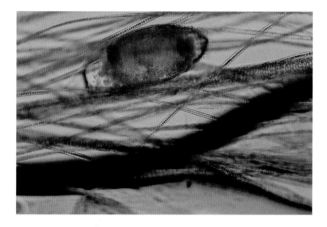

Fig. 5.87   *Polyplax* egg glued to a rat hair. The presence of lice eggs ("nits") on the hairs is helpful in diagnosis of infestation.

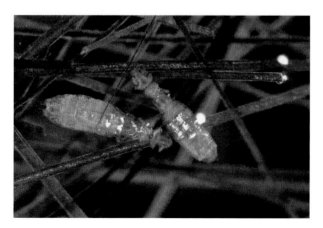

Fig. 5.88   *Gliricola porcelli*, a chewing louse of guinea pigs, is one of three species of lice infesting guinea pigs. Photo courtesy of Dr. Yoko Nagamori, College of Veterinary Medicine, Oklahoma State University, Stillwater, OK.

ARTHROPODS

Parasite: **Bovicola spp.** (Figs. 5.89)

Common name: Chewing louse.

Taxonomy: Insect (Order Phthiraptera, mallophagan or chewing lice); formerly *Damalinia* spp.

Host: *Bovicola bovis* (cattle), *B. ovis* (sheep), *B. caprae* (goats), *B. breviceps* (camelids).

Geographic Distribution: Worldwide.

Location on Host: In general, preferred sites include the neck, shoulder, and back, but lice can be found anywhere on the body.

Life Cycle: Like the sucking lice, all stages of chewing lice are found on the host, and transmission is by direct contact with an infested animal or fomites.

Laboratory Diagnosis: Infested animals should be closely observed for nits and lice, although *Bovicola* spp. are only a few millimeters in length and may be difficult to see. A fine-toothed comb may be useful in recovering lice, and hair coat brushings can also be examined with a magnifying glass.

Clinical Importance: These common external parasites cause pruritus and dermatitis and are associated with production losses and secondary infections in heavy infestations.

Parasite: **Werneckiella equi** (Figs. 5.90 and 5.91)

Common name: Chewing louse.

Taxonomy: Insect (Order Phthiraptera, mallophagan or chewing lice); formerly *Damalinia equi*.

Host: Horses.

Geographic Distribution: Worldwide.

Location on Host: Preferred sites include the head, mane, and base of tail.

Life Cycle: Transmission is by direct contact with an infested horse, shared grooming supplies, shared tack, or other fomites. All stages are found on horses.

Laboratory Diagnosis: Lice and associated eggs (nits) are usually identified by close visual examination. A fine-toothed comb may be useful in recovering lice, and hair coat brushings can also be examined with a magnifying glass.

Clinical Importance: *Werneckiella equi* is very allergenic and may cause pruritus, hyperkeratosis, and alopecia. Heavy infestations are most often seen in horses in poor condition and those rarely treated with parasite control products; weight loss and self-trauma may occur.

ARTHROPODS

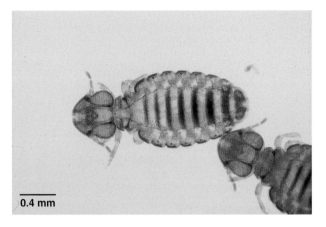

Fig. 5.89   Like other chewing lice, the head of *Bovicola* spp. is broader than the thorax. Pictured here is the bovine parasite *Bovicola bovis*. Photo courtesy of Dr. Robert Ridley, College of Veterinary Medicine, Kansas State University, Manhattan, KS.

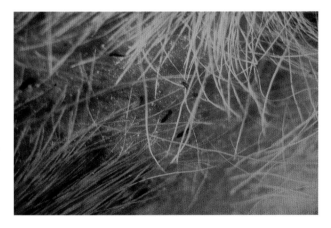

Fig. 5.90   Chewing lice (*Werneckiella equi*) in the hairs of a horse.

ARTHROPODS

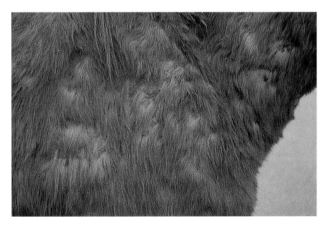

Fig. 5.91   Lesions on the shoulder and neck of a horse with a heavy burden of chewing lice. Photo courtesy of Dr. Jeffrey F. Williams, Vanson HaloSource, Inc., Redmond, WA.

PARASITE: **_Trichodectes canis_** (Fig. 5.93)

Taxonomy: Insect (Order Phthiraptera, mallophagan or chewing lice).

Host: Dogs and other canids.

Geographic Distribution: Worldwide. Another species of chewing louse, _Heterodoxus spinigera_, may also be found on dogs in tropical and subtropical areas.

Location on Host: Predilection sites for _T. canis_ are the head, neck, and tail, but lice will be found throughout the hair coat in heavy infestations.

Life Cycle: Transmission is by direct contact or fomites. Louse eggs are adhered to host hairs.

Laboratory Diagnosis: Recovery and identification of lice. Dogs can be infested with the chewing lice _Trichodectes_ and _Heterodoxus_, as well as the sucking louse, _Linognathus setosus_.

Clinical Importance: Large infestations of lice cause pruritus and poor hair condition. _Trichodectes_ is the most common dog louse seen in the United States and can act as an intermediate host for the tapeworm _Dipylidium caninum_.

PARASITE: **_Felicola subrostratus_** (Figs. 5.92, 5.94–5.95)

Taxonomy: Insect (Order Phthiraptera, mallophagan or chewing lice).

Host: Cats.

Geographic Distribution: Worldwide.

Location on Host: Predilection sites for _F. subrostratus_ include the face, back, and ears although lice can be found anywhere on the body in heavily infested cats.

Life Cycle: Transmission is by direct contact or fomites. Louse eggs are adhered to host hairs.

Laboratory Diagnosis: _Felicola_ is the only louse infesting cats, although infestations on cats may be difficult to diagnose because of the effective grooming habits of the host. Infestations are rare in pet cats but may be seen in kittens or adults in poor condition.

Clinical Importance: Pruritus is variable. When present, self-excoriation from scratching can lead to trauma, alopecia, and crust formation.

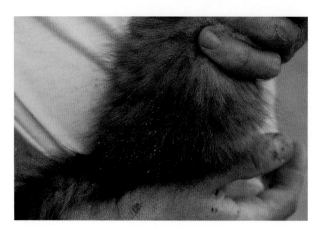

Fig. 5.92   White louse eggs (nits) can be seen attached to the hairs of this infested kitten. Photo courtesy of Dr. Jeffrey F. Williams, Vanson HaloSource, Inc., Redmond, WA.

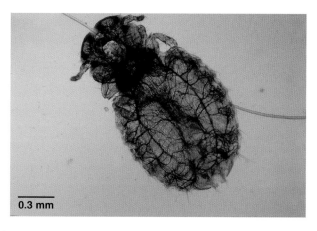

Fig. 5.93   *Trichodectes canis* is the canine chewing louse.

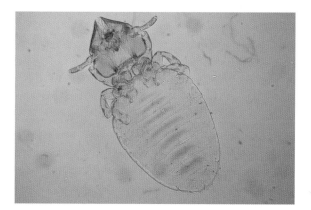

Fig. 5.94   The head of *Felicola subrostratus*, the feline chewing louse, is notched at the tip. Photo courtesy of Dr. Heather Walden, College of Veterinary Medicine, University of Florida, Gainesville, FL.

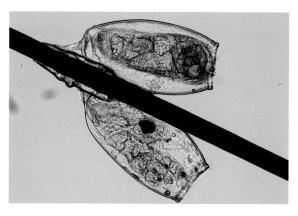

Fig. 5.95   Eggs (nits) of *Felicola subrostratus* adhered to cat hair. Photo courtesy of Dr. Manigandan Lejeune, Animal Health Diagnostic Center, Cornell University, Ithaca, NY.

PARASITE: **Avian Lice** (Figs. 5.96–5.100)

Taxonomy: Insects (Order Phthiraptera, mallophagan or chewing lice).

Host: Lice are common external parasites of birds, and multiple louse species may be found occupying different niches on the same host species. All avian lice are mallophagan or chewing lice.

Geographic Distribution: Worldwide.

Location on Host: Lice can be found on all areas of birds, with different species showing specific predilection sites.

Life Cycle: Similar to other lice; the entire life cycle is spent on the host, and transmission is by direct contact or fomites.

Laboratory Diagnosis: Detection of lice and eggs on the host with morphologic identification of lice.

Clinical Importance: Heavy infestations may cause loss of condition. Sick or malnourished birds often carry large numbers of lice.

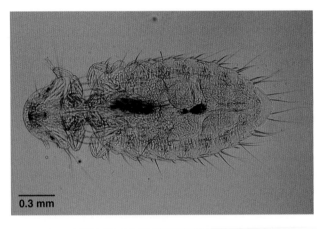

Fig. 5.96   There are more than 700 species of avian lice, all of which are chewing lice. Morphology of the chewing lice of birds is widely variable. Shown here is *Menopon gallinae*, the shaft louse of chickens.

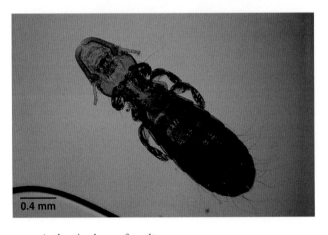

Fig. 5.97   *Lipeurus caponis*, the wing louse of poultry.

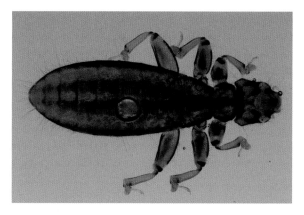

Fig. 5.98 *Laemobothrion* sp. from an eagle. Photo courtesy of Dr. Manigandan Lejeune, Animal Health Diagnostic Center, Cornell University, Ithaca, NY.

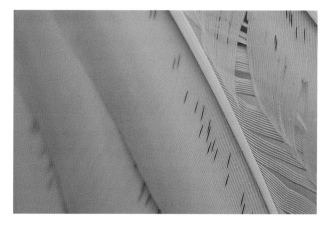

Fig. 5.99 *Columbicula columbae*, the slender pigeon louse, on the flight feathers of a pigeon. Photo courtesy of Dr. Jeffrey F. Williams, Vanson HaloSource, Inc., Redmond, WA.

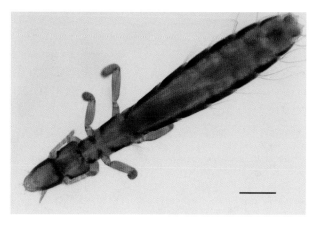

Fig. 5.100 *Columbicula columbae*, the slender pigeon louse. Photo courtesy of Dr. Heather Walden, College of Veterinary Medicine, University of Florida, Gainesville, FL.

ARTHROPODS

Fleas (Order Siphonaptera)

Fleas are laterally compressed, wingless insects, typically medium to dark brown in color. Unlike many insects, they do not demonstrate clear delineations between body regions (head, thorax, and abdomen). The sucking mouthparts are usually seen protruding from the ventral aspect of the head. The three pairs of legs originate on the thorax. The enlarged third pair of legs facilitates the incredible jumping potential of these insects. In veterinary medicine, fleas are most often encountered on dogs and cats; however, they also live on a variety of other animals, including birds. Fleas are more likely than lice to move onto a different host species if the preferred host is unavailable, although they may leave after obtaining a blood meal. The adult flea is the only parasitic stage of the life cycle. The egg, larva, and pupa are found in the environment.

Fleas can be seen with the unaided eye (Fig 5.101). They are most easily collected from the host by using a quick-acting insecticide and then removing individual fleas from the hair coat or combing them out with a flea comb. On birds, fleas may be attached to the unfeathered portions of the host and can be removed with forceps. Fleas should be placed in 70% ethanol for fixation and storage. They may be cleared in 5% potassium hydroxide or mounted in Hoyer's solution to allow visualization of reproductive structures used in identification. The presence of combs on the cheek (genal comb) or at the back of the first thoracic segment (pronotal comb), the shape of the head, and host preference are important characteristics used in identification. Figure 5.102 is a key for identification of some common species in North America. In many cases, a specialist is required for specific identification. When submitting fleas for identification, it is best to submit as many individuals as possible to ensure that both sexes are represented and that structures damaged on one individual are still intact on another.

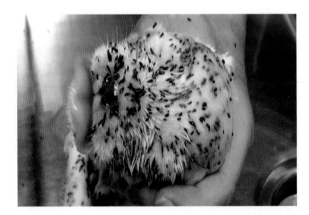

Fig. 5.101   Puppy infested with fleas. This severe level of infestation causes anemia, especially in young animals and small breeds of dogs. Photo courtesy of Dr. Stephen Jones, Lakeside Animal Hospital, Moncks Corner, SC.

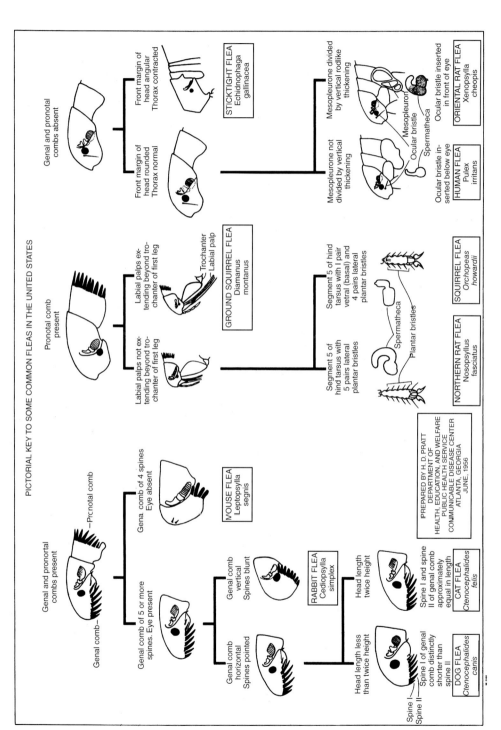

Fig. 5.102   Key to common flea species in the United States. Courtesy of U.S. Public Health Service, CDC.

PARASITE: ***Ctenocephalides felis felis*** (Figs. 5.103–5.105)

Common name: Cat flea.

Taxonomy: Insect (order Siphonaptera). *Ctenocephalides felis felis* is the most common flea that infests dogs and cats. A similar species, *Ctenocephalides canis*, also occurs but is less common than *C. felis felis* on both dogs and cats in the United States.

Host: Cats, dogs, ferrets, and numerous small and medium-sized wild mammals. Occasionally, populations may adapt to living on confined animals, such as goats or calves in a barn.

Geographic Distribution: Worldwide. *Ctenocephalides* is the most common flea of dogs and cats.

Location on Host: Fleas can be found throughout the hair coat, but predilection sites include the tail head, neck, and flanks.

Life Cycle: Adult cat fleas seldom leave the host. Females deposit eggs that fall off the host and hatch in the environment. Flea larvae feed on organic debris and adult flea feces and pupate in the environment. Adults are stimulated to emerge from the pupa by vibration and mechanical compression. Under optimum conditions, the life cycle can be completed in about 2 weeks.

Laboratory Diagnosis: Cat fleas have both pronotal and genal combs.

Size:		
	Adult female	approximately 2.5 mm in length
	Adult male	approximately 1 mm in length
	Larva	approximately 5 mm in length

Clinical Importance: Low levels of flea infestation may be mildly pruritic. Large flea populations can produce severe pruritus, alopecia, and anemia. Animals that develop flea-bite hypersensitivity may suffer severe dermatologic disease even when flea numbers are very low.

ARTHROPODS

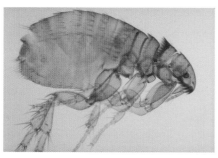
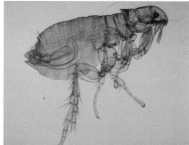

Fig. 5.103   Female (*left*) and male (*right*) *Ctenocephalides felis*. The cat flea is the most common flea found on both dogs and cats. It is difficult to differentiate from the less common *Ctenocephalides canis*. Characteristics helpful in identifying this genus are the genal and pronotal combs. Male cat fleas are smaller than females. Photos courtesy of Dr. Byron Blagburn, College of Veterinary Medicine, Auburn University, Auburn, AL.

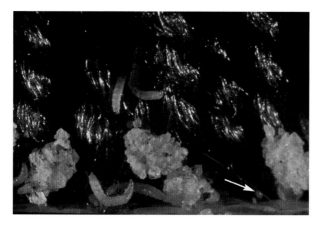

Fig. 5.104   *Ctenocephalides* spp. eggs (*arrow*) are about 0.5 mm long. Larvae and pupae (covered with sand grains) of the cat flea are also shown in this figure. The surface of the pupa is sticky and becomes camouflaged with environmental debris. Photo courtesy of Dr. Byron Blagburn, College of Veterinary Medicine, Auburn University, Auburn, AL.

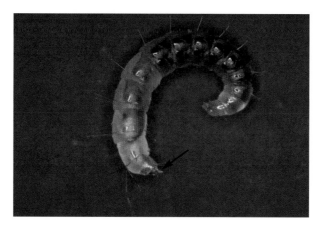

Fig. 5.105   Pet owners may find larvae of the cat flea, *C. felis felis*, in their homes and present them for identification. Mature larvae are about 5 mm long. The two "anal stuts" projecting from the posterior end of the body (*arrow*) are distinctive. Photo courtesy of Dr. Byron Blagburn, College of Veterinary Medicine, Auburn University, Auburn, AL.

ARTHROPODS

Parasite: **Pulex spp.** (Fig. 5.106)

Common name: Human flea.

Taxonomy: Insect (order Siphonaptera). *Pulex irritans* and *P. simulans* are closely related species found on dogs and cats in the New World.

Host: Humans, pigs, dogs, cats.

Geographic Distribution: Worldwide.

Location on Host: General distribution on the host.

Life Cycle: Like *C. felis felis*, only adults are found on the host; other stages are present in the environment.

Laboratory Diagnosis: Adult *Pulex* spp. have no genal or pronotal combs and possess an ocular bristle below the eye. Female *P. irritans* and *P. simulans* have no morphologically distinguishing features and cannot be identified to species morphologically.

Clinical Importance: Worldwide, *P. irritans* is found more often on swine than on humans or cats and dogs. Heavy flea infestations can produce intense irritation and pruritus. *Pulex irritans* is uncommon in North America, although it has been recorded from most states in the United States. *Pulex* spp. can serve as a vector of *Yersinia pestis*, the bubonic plague bacillus, and *Rickettsia typhi*, the agent of murine typhus.

Parasite: **Echidnophaga gallinacea** (Fig. 5.107), **Ceratophyllus spp.**

Common name: Sticktight flea, European chicken flea.

Taxonomy: Insects (order Siphonaptera).

Host: *Echidnophaga gallinacea*, the sticktight flea, is found on poultry, wild birds, and occasionally on dogs, cats, and other animals. *Ceratophyllus* spp. are parasites of wild and domestic birds, especially chickens.

Geographic Distribution: Worldwide. *Echidnophaga* is found primarily in tropical and subtropical regions of the New World.

Location on Host: The sticktight flea is usually found on nonfeathered skin on the head, comb, and wattles of poultry.

Life Cycle: The life cycle of poultry fleas is similar to other fleas, but female *Echidnophaga* attach permanently to the head of the host. Eggs are deposited either onto the ground or into the sore created at the attachment site.

Laboratory Diagnosis: Identification of adult fleas. Female *Echidnophaga* can be identified by their location and attachment. This species also lacks genal and pronotal combs and has a sharply angled head. *Ceratophyllus* has a pronotal comb.

Size: Female *Echidnophaga*   approximately 2 mm in length
             Ceratophyllus   approximately 4 mm in length

Clinical Importance: Sticktight fleas may cause severe irritation by their attachment to birds and other hosts. Heavy infestations can produce anemia. In wild birds, attachment near the eyes may lead to blindness and death. Heavy infestations of *Ceratophyllus* have been associated with anemia, restlessness, and decreased production.

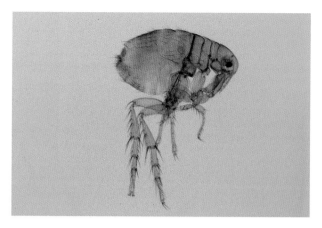

Fig. 5.106 The human flea, *Pulex irritans*, is less common on people in industrialized countries. It may also be found on companion animals and pigs. The absence of genal and pronotal combs and location of the ocular bristle below the eye are helpful in identification.

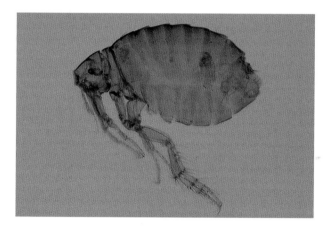

Fig. 5.107 *Echidnophaga gallinacea*, the sticktight flea, has no combs and a sharply angled head. Because this flea attaches to its host, it is most often submitted as a tick for identification.

PARASITE: **Fleas of Rodents and Rabbits** (Figs. 5.108 and 5.109)

Taxonomy: Insects (order Siphonaptera).

Host: A variety of species parasitize rodents and rabbits, including *Xenopsylla cheopsis* (oriental rat flea), an important vector of bubonic plague. *Xenopsylla cheopsis* will also readily feed on dogs, cats, humans, and other animals when normal rodent hosts are unavailable.

Geographic Distribution: Worldwide.

Location on Host: General distribution on the host. *Spilopsyllus cuniculi*, a flea of rabbits, attaches to the skin in the ears for long periods of time in a manner similar to *Echidnophaga gallinacea*, the sticktight flea of birds (see below).

Life Cycle: Similar to other fleas. Some species of rodent flea only visit the host to feed, unlike the common cat flea, which is resident on the host as an adult.

Laboratory Diagnosis: Rodent and rabbit fleas are identified based on morphologic characteristics.

Clinical Importance: *Xenopsylla cheopsis* and some other rodent fleas are vectors of bubonic plague, caused by *Yersinia pestis*, and murine typhus, caused by *Rickettsia typhi*. Because the bacteria interfere with normal flea feeding, fleas rapidly move from host to host, spreading infection. Other rodent fleas can transmit tapeworms, trypanosomes, and myxomatosis to rabbits.

ARTHROPODS

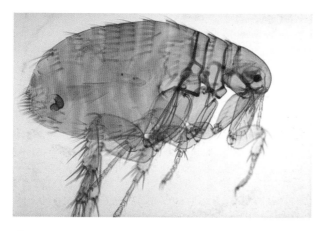

Fig. 5.108   *Xenopsylla cheopsis*, the oriental rat flea. Genal and pronotal combs are absent like *Pulex* spp.; however, the ocular bristle for *X. cheopis* originates in front of the eye. Fleas belonging to several genera are found on rodents and rabbits. Photo courtesy of Dr. Byron Blagburn, College of Veterinary Medicine, Auburn University, Auburn, AL.

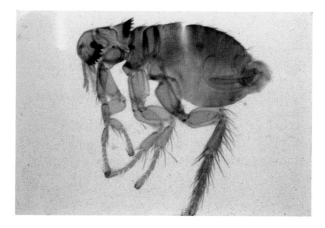

Fig. 5.109   *Cediopsylla simplex*, a rabbit flea. Photo courtesy of Dr. David Baker, School of Veterinary Medicine, Louisiana State University, Baton Rouge, LA.

ARTHROPODS

Flies (Order Diptera)

Flies belong to the order Diptera, and some species feed on animals in the larval or adult stage. Larval flies parasitizing animals are referred to as either "bots" ("grubs" and "warbles" are synonymous terms) or "maggots."

Bots are obligate parasites that develop in various internal locations in the host; adults are free-living, non-feeding, bee-like flies. Mature bot larvae are barrel-shaped and often have rows of spines on the body. The genus of a bot or maggot can be identified by examining the pattern of the spiracular plates surrounding the breathing holes (spiracles) on the posterior end (Fig. 5.110). Spiracles are best examined by positioning the bot on a small amount of modeling clay or sand so that the structures can be examined from the posterior view.

Maggots are fly larvae associated with "fly strike" or "fly blow." In most cases, they are opportunistic parasites. Adult flies attracted to wounds or hair stained with feces or blood lay their eggs on the animal, and larvae feed on debris and necrotic tissue. Maggots are more elongated than bots and are narrower at the anterior than at the posterior end. They are usually present on the surface of the body in conjunction with wounds or hair soiled with feces, urine, blood, or other organic material.

Parasitic adult flies are usually blood feeders. Hematophagy (blood-feeding) has evolved multiple times in flies and a diverse array of diptera feed on blood.

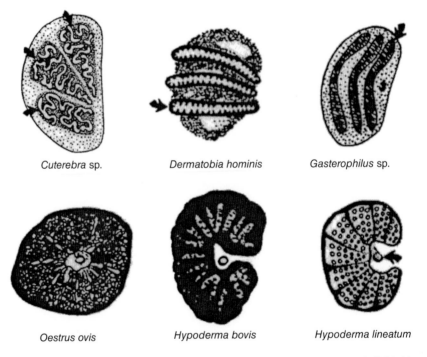

Cuterebra sp.   *Dermatobia hominis*   *Gasterophilus* sp.

Oestrus ovis   *Hypoderma bovis*   *Hypoderma lineatum*

Fig. 5.110   Posterior spiracles of bot fly larvae. Row 1: *Cuterebra* spp. spiracles are each divided into several plates. *Dermatobia hominis* spiracles are sunken in a deep cavity, and *Gasterophilus* spp. spiracles are curved and in a shallow cavity. Row 2: Spiracles of *Oestrus ovis* have a central button that is completely surrounded, whereas *Hypoderma* spp. spiracles have either a narrow opening (*H. bovis*) or a wider opening (*H. lineatum*). Adapted from Pictorial Keys to Arthropods, Centers for Disease Control and Prevention, 1969.

ARTHROPODS

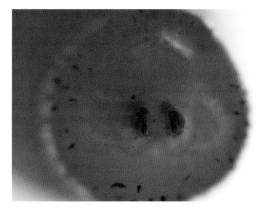

Fig. 5.111   Paired spiracle plates on the posterior end of a bot larvae (*Cuterebra* sp.) Photo courtesy of Dr. Manigandan Lejeune, Animal Health Diagnostic Center, Cornell University, Ithaca, NY.

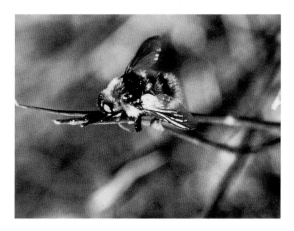

Fig. 5.112   The hairy body of adult warble (bot) flies makes them look more like bees than flies. The presence of adult warble flies, like this *Hypoderma bovis*, is distressing to potential hosts, which will actively try to avoid the flies. Photo courtesy of Dr. Philip Scholl, Agricultural Research Service, USDA, and Dr. Jerry Weintraub, Agriculture Canada.

ARTHROPODS

PARASITE: ***Cuterebra* spp.** (Figs. 5.113–5.115)

Common name: Rodent bot fly.

Taxonomy: Insect (order Diptera).

Host: Rodents and rabbits are the principal hosts. Dogs, cats, and rarely humans may also be infected.

Geographic Distribution: Western Hemisphere.

Location on Host: Larvae are found in subcutaneous cysts in various locations. In dogs and cats, they are seen most often on the head and neck.

Life Cycle: Adult flies lay eggs around rodent holes. Larvae crawl onto animals and enter through facial orifices. Following migration to subcutaneous sites, the *Cuterebra* larva forms a visible nodule with an external breathing hole. After completing development, the larva emerges and pupates on the ground.

Laboratory Diagnosis: *Cuterebra* larvae can be preliminarily identified by location on the host. Confirmation requires examination of larval spiracular plates.

Clinical Importance: The presence of one or two bots in most hosts is not associated with clinical problems. However, abnormal migration to the nervous system or other tissues occasionally occurs, resulting in disease.

ARTHROPODS

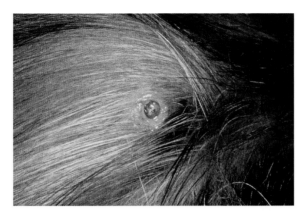

Fig. 5.113   Bot larvae (*Cuterebra* sp.) spiracles visible through patent opening into dermal cyst in an infested cat.

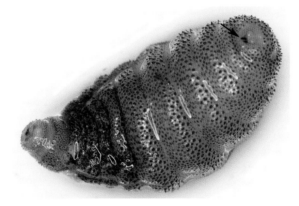

Fig. 5.114   *Cuterebra* larvae are about 2.5 cm in length and covered with spines when fully developed. Spiracles are present on the posterior end (left) and paired hooks are evident on the anterior end (arrow).

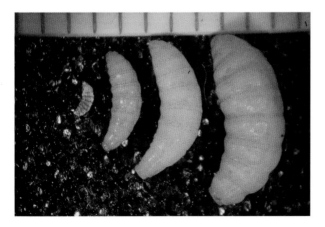

Fig. 5.115   Veterinary practitioners occasionally remove young *Cuterebra* larvae from animals and, because of their small size and white color, may have difficulty recognizing them as *Cuterebra*. Starting at the left, this figure shows larvae at 6, 8, 10, and 13 days after infestation of the host. Photo courtesy of Dr. Philip Scholl, Agricultural Research Service, USDA.

PARASITE: ***Dermatobia hominis*** (Fig. 5.116)

Common name: Human bot fly.

Taxonomy: Insect (order Diptera).

Host: Cattle, humans, dogs, other domestic and wild animals.

Geographic Distribution: Central and South America.

Location on Host: Various subcutaneous sites.

Life Cycle: Adult female *Dermatobia* glue clusters of eggs to various muscid flies and mosquitoes. When these organisms visit a host, the *Dermatobia* larvae are deposited and enter the subcutaneous tissue, where each larva develops in a nodule with a hole in the skin through which respiration occurs. Larvae leave the host to pupate.

Laboratory Diagnosis: Identification of larvae is based on shape and pattern of the spiracles.

Clinical Importance: Although best known as a human parasite, *D. hominis* is primarily a cattle pest.

ARTHROPODS

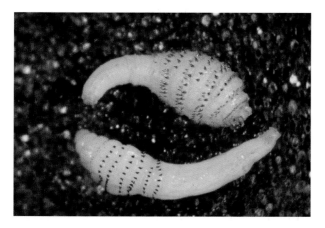

Fig. 5.116   *Dermatobia hominis* bots are often seen in the second-instar larval stage. At this stage, they have a distinctive narrow, spineless posterior end that becomes less prominent as they continue development. Photo courtesy of Dr. Philip Scholl, Agricultural Research Service, USDA.

ARTHROPODS

PARASITE: ***Gasterophilus* spp.** (Figs. 5.117–5.120)

Common name: Stomach bot.

Taxonomy: Insect (order Diptera). Species include *G. intestinalis*, *G. nasalis*, *G. haemorrhoidalis*, and *G. pecorum*.

Host: Horses and other equids.

Geographic Distribution: Worldwide.

Location on Host: Equine stomach (*G. intestinalis*), small intestine (*G. nasalis*), or rectum (*G. haemorrhoidalis*). Developing stages may be found in the oral cavity.

Life Cycle: Most *Gasterophilus* spp. deposit eggs on the legs or face of horses. After hatching, larvae enter through the mouth and spend a period of development in the tongue and gums before moving to the stomach. After a period of 8–11 months in the stomach, bots pass out in the feces and pupate on the ground.

Laboratory Diagnosis: Bots are usually identified by presence in the stomach or intestine at necropsy, but they may also be seen in the feces at different stages of development following treatment of the host with macrocyclic lactone anthelmintics. They can be recognized as bots by their barrel shape and rows of spines. Eggs (nits) may be evident attached to the hairs of the legs or face.

Clinical Importance: Horses appear to tolerate small to moderate burdens of bots. In rare instances, humans in close contact with horses are infested and develop a transient dermatitis usually occurring on the face.

ARTHROPODS

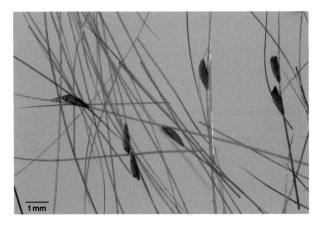

Fig. 5.117   Eggs (nits) of *Gasterophilus* adhered to horse hair. Photo courtesy of Dr. Heather Walden, College of Veterinary Medicine, University of Florida, Gainesville, FL.

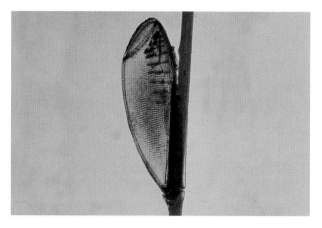

Fig. 5.118 Eggs of *Gasterophilus intestinalis*, the most common equine bot species, can be seen attached to the hairs of the forelegs. Photo courtesy of Dr. Jeffrey F. Williams, Vanson HaloSource, Inc., Redmond, WA.

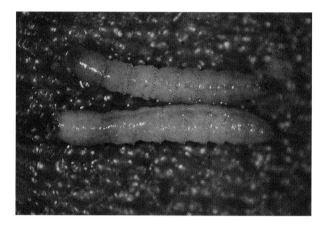

Fig. 5.119 Second-instar *Gasterophilus* larvae. Following treatment with a macrocyclic lactone anthelmintic or other effective drug, young *Gasterophilus* larvae may also be present in manure. Although the less mature larvae lack the barrel shape of mature bots, they still show the distinctive rows of spines around each segment. Photo courtesy of Dr. Philip Scholl, Agricultural Research Service, USDA.

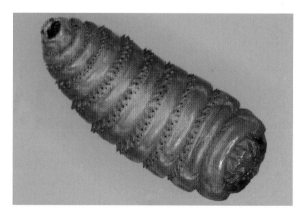

Fig. 5.120 Equine stomach bot, *Gasterophilus*. Species can be distinguished based on patterns of spines on the body, but species identification is unnecessary for control and treatment of the parasite. Photo courtesy of Dr. Manigandan Lejeune, Animal Health Diagnostic Center, Cornell University, Ithaca, NY.

ARTHROPODS

PARASITE: ***Hypoderma bovis, H. lineatum*** (Figs. 5.121 and 5.122)

Common name: Cattle grub, ox warble.

Taxonomy: Insect (order Diptera).

Host: Cattle are the normal hosts; horses and goats are occasionally infested. Other species of *Hypoderma* parasitize deer and reindeer, and *Przhevalskiana silenus* is a similar parasite of goats in the Mediterranean region.

Geographic Distribution: North America, Europe, Asia.

Location on Host: Visible nodules with an external opening appear on the backs of infested animals.

Life Cycle: Adult flies deposit eggs on cattle. After hatching, larvae penetrate through the skin and migrate to sites either along the esophagus (*H. lineatum*) or in the tissue surrounding the spinal cord (*H. bovis*). After a period of development lasting several months, the larvae migrate to the host's back and form subcutaneous nodules with a breathing hole. After several more months of development, larvae emerge, pupate on the ground, and adult flies are formed.

Laboratory Diagnosis: Diagnosis can usually be made based on parasite location in the host and history.

Clinical Importance: Damage from *Hypoderma* comes from several sources. Adult fly activity associated with oviposition worries cattle and may interfere with grazing; migrating larvae cause necrotic tracks in muscle tissue and the hide is damaged for leather production. In addition, if larvae die while along the esophagus or spinal cord, serious inflammatory reactions can lead to bloat or paralysis.

PARASITE: ***Oestrus ovis*** (Fig. 5.123), ***Rhinoestrus* spp.**

Common name: Nasal bot.

Taxonomy: Insects (order Diptera).

Host: *Oestrus ovis* larvae are found in sheep and goats. *Rhinoestrus* larvae are found in horses. Other species parasitize deer and camels (e.g., *Cephalopina titillator*).

Geographic Distribution: *Oestrus ovis* is found worldwide. *Rhinoestrus* infestation occurs in Africa, Europe, and Asia.

Location on Host: Nasal passages and sinuses.

Life Cycle: Adult female flies deposit larvae in or near the nasal passages. Larvae develop in nasal passages and sinuses. When development is complete, they fall out of the nose and pupate on the ground.

Laboratory Diagnosis: Nasal bots are not usually presented for identification because of their location, but they are sometimes found by owners in water troughs or on the ground after they exit the host. Specific identification is made by examination of the spiracular plates.

Clinical Importance: Although infested animals show increased levels of nasal discharge, small or moderate numbers of bots are usually well tolerated. Sheep will attempt to avoid ovipositing female flies by keeping their muzzles near the ground or under available shelter (buildings, cars, one another, etc.). Bots occasionally wander to abnormal sites, where they may cause serious disease.

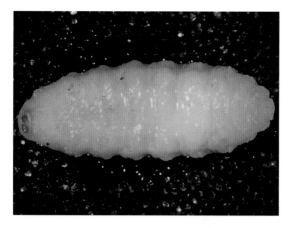

Fig. 5.121 Early third-instar cattle grub, *Hypoderma lineatum*. Grubs or warbles can be distinguished from fly maggots by their barrel-shaped bodies and typical location in the host. Photo courtesy of Dr. Philip Scholl, Agricultural Research Service, USDA.

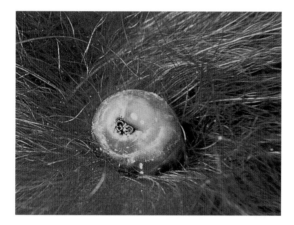

Fig. 5.122 *Hypoderma* sp. grub emerging from its subcutaneous location on the back of the bovine host. Photo courtesy of Dr. Philip Scholl, Agricultural Research Service, USDA.

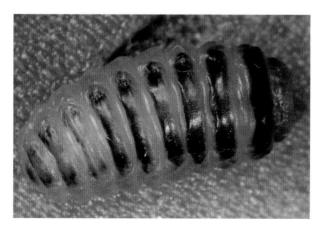

Fig. 5.123 Ovine nasal bot, *Oestrus ovis*. These bots are occasionally seen by producers when they leave the small ruminant host to pupate or following treatment. Photo courtesy of Dr. Philip Scholl, Agricultural Research Service, USDA.

ARTHROPODS

PARASITE: **Fly Strike or Blow Flies** (Figs. 5.124–5.127)

Taxonomy: Insects (order Diptera). Many of the maggots causing fly strike belong to the families Calliphoridae (blow flies) and Sarcophagidae (flesh flies).

Host: Various, not host-specific.

Geographic Distribution: Worldwide.

Location on Host: Various, wherever there is blood or other body secretion that attracts female flies.

Life Cycle: Larvae of most of the flies in this group are not obligatory parasites. Adults are attracted by the odors of decaying organic material and deposit their eggs on carrion. Wounds or skin on animals soiled with blood or feces may also attract the flies. Larvae feed primarily on necrotic material, and when development is completed, they leave the host and pupate in the environment.

Laboratory Diagnosis: Recognition of maggots on animals is sufficient for diagnosis of fly strike. Specific identification of fly larvae requires examination of larval spiracles.

Clinical Importance: "Fly blown" animals can be seriously affected by fly larvae. The presence of large numbers of maggots may produce tissue destruction, toxemia, and even death.

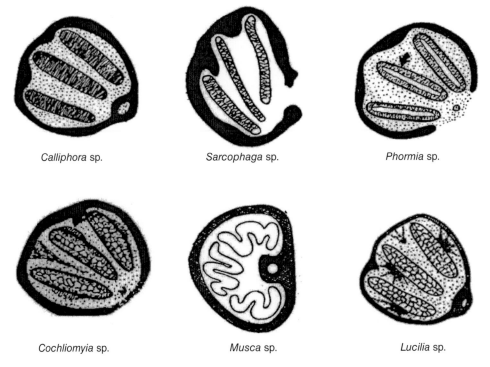

Calliphora sp.   *Sarcophaga* sp.   *Phormia* sp.

Cochliomyia sp.   *Musca* sp.   *Lucilia* sp.

Fig. 5.124   Posterior spiracles of maggots associated with fly strike. Adapted from Pictorial Keys to Arthropods, Centers for Disease Control and Prevention, 1969.

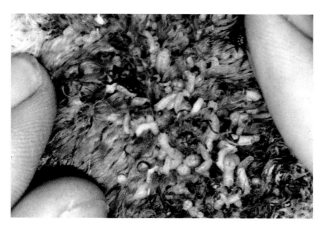

Fig. 5.125 A case of ovine "fly strike" or "fly blow" in which an animal has become infested with fly maggots. In most cases, these flies are not true parasites and would be equally attracted to carrion. Sheep are particularly susceptible to fly strike in warm weather if wool is persistently wet or becomes soiled with blood or feces. Photo courtesy of Dr. Dwight Bowman, College of Veterinary Medicine, Cornell University, Ithaca, NY.

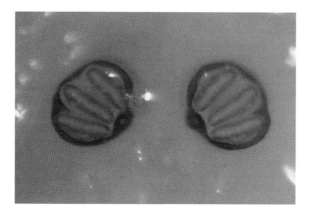

Fig. 5.126 Posterior spiracles of *Lucilia* spp. larva. Photo courtesy of Kellee Sundstrom, Oklahoma State University, Stillwater, OK.

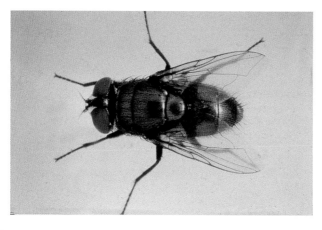

Fig. 5.127 *Lucilia* spp. is one of the genera of blow flies that cause facultative myiasis (fly strike). Blow flies are typically metallic blue, green, or bronze in color. *Lucilia* spp. infestations of sheep are a source of significant economic loss to the Australian sheep industry. Photo courtesy of Dr. Nick Sangster, Charles Sturt University, NSW and Ms. Sally Pope, University of Sydney, NSW, Australia.

ARTHROPODS

PARASITE: ***Cochliomyia hominivorax, Chrysomya bezziana*** (Figs. 5.128–5.130)

Common name: Screwworm.

Taxonomy: Insects (order Diptera). Screwworms belong to the blow fly family (Calliphoridae). Several species of sarcophagid flies are also obligatory parasites but are of less importance.

Host: Wild and domestic animals, humans.

Geographic Distribution: *Cochliomyia hominivorax*, the New World screwworm, is found in South America. The Old World screwworm, *Chrysomya bezziana*, occurs in Africa, India, and Southeast Asia.

Location on Host: Various, often on body openings or the edges of wounds.

Life Cycle: Adult female flies deposit eggs on the host. Larvae feed invasively on living tissue. Following completion of development, larvae fall to the ground and pupate. Adults emerge and mate. The entire life cycle can be completed in as little as 24 days.

Laboratory Diagnosis: Examination of larval spiracles is important for larval identification. The larvae also have two posterior tracheal trunks, which look like dark lines extending anteriorly from the posterior end. Although screwworm has been eradicated from the United States, reintroduction is possible. If screwworm infestation is suspected, larvae should be collected in 70% alcohol and submitted to federal or state veterinarians for identification.

Clinical Importance: Screwworm infestation is a serious disease that can rapidly lead to the death of the host. The parasite was eradicated from the United States in the 1960s through a sterile-male release program. This program has now been successful in removing the fly from Mexico and Central America, with only occasional outbreaks still reported.

ARTHROPODS

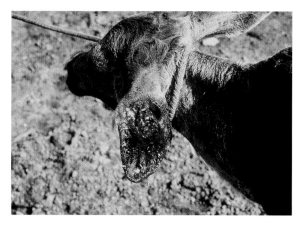

Fig. 5.128   Screwworm infestation on the ear of a calf. If untreated, these infestations are often fatal. Photo courtesy of Dr. Donald B. Thomas, USDA Subtropical Agriculture Research Laboratory, Weslaco, TX.

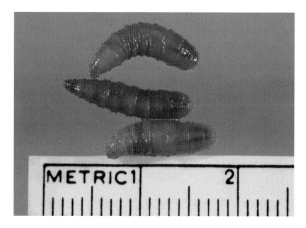

Fig. 5.129   Screwworm maggots. If screwworm infestation is suspected in the United States, larvae should be submitted in 70% alcohol to state or federal veterinarians.

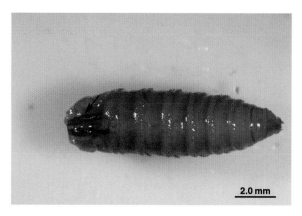

Fig. 5.130   *Cochliomyia* sp. larvae showing pigmented tracheal trunks (*arrow*). If screwworm infestation is suspected in the United States, larvae should be submitted in 70% alcohol to state or federal veterinarians. Photo courtesy of Kellee Sundstrom, Oklahoma State University, Stillwater, OK.

ARTHROPODS

PARASITE: **Louse Flies, including *Melophagus ovinus* (Figs. 5.131–5.133)**

Common name: Sheep ked, louse fly.

Taxonomy: Insects (order Diptera).

Host: Sheep and goats are parasitized by *M. ovinus*, the sheep ked. Louse flies may be found on a variety of animals. Examples include *Hippobosca variegata* on horses, cattle, and camels; *Lipoptena* spp. on wild ruminants; *Hippobosca longipennis* on dogs; and *Pseudolynchia* spp. on birds.

Distribution: Worldwide, although in North America, only the sheep ked and the pigeon fly (*Pseudolynchia*) are found on domestic animals.

Location on Host: Various.

Life Cycle: In some species, winged adult flies are temporary parasites while feeding; in others, louse flies lose their wings after finding a host and become permanent parasites. The sheep ked, *Melophagus*, has no functional wings and is transmitted only by direct contact of hosts. Adult female sheep keds deposit larvae that pupate immediately on the skin of the host.

Laboratory Diagnosis: Identification is based on adult flies. Hippoboscid flies generally have a rather flat, leathery appearance compared with other flies. Ked feces, which resemble flea feces, may be found on the host.

Clinical Importance: Sheep keds can cause significant damage to the skin, making it unsuitable for leather production, and can also reduce the value of the sheep fleece. Biting activity of flies causes pain and irritation.

ARTHROPODS

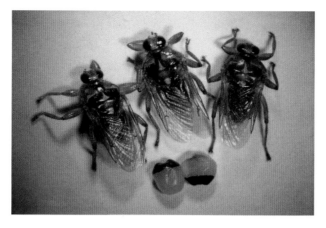

Fig. 5.131   Typical hippoboscid louse flies showing the flattened appearance of the body with relatively large legs and wings. Some species of hippoboscid flies retain their wings, others lose their wings after finding a host, and still others are wingless throughout their development. Photo courtesy of Dr. Alvin Gajadhar, Centre for Animal Parasitology, CFIA, Saskatoon, Saskatchewan, Canada.

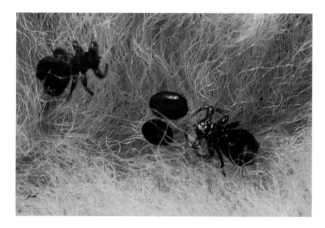

Fig. 5.132   Adult and pupal stages of the sheep ked, *Melophagus*. Although sometimes mistaken for ticks, these organisms are insects with six legs and three main body parts. Ked excrement, which resembles flea feces, can also be found on the host and is helpful in diagnosis. Photo courtesy of Dr. Jeffrey F. Williams, Vanson HaloSource, Inc., Redmond, WA.

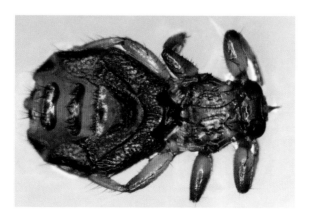

Fig. 5.133   Adult *Lipoptena cervi* from a moose. Alopecia is reported in moose due to massive *L. cervi* infestations. Photo courtesy of Dr. Manigandan Lejeune, Animal Health Diagnostic Center, Cornell University, Ithaca, NY.

ARTHROPODS

PARASITE: **Biting Flies** (Figs. 5.134–5.141)

Common names: Horse fly, deer fly, mosquito, black fly, sand fly, tsetse fly, horn fly, stable fly, midge, and so on.

Taxonomy: Insects (order Diptera). Biting flies belong to many families within the order.

Host: Domestic and wild animals and humans.

Geographic Distribution: Worldwide.

Location on Host: Various, although many biting flies have predilection sites.

Life Cycle: Like other Diptera, biting flies lay eggs that hatch into larvae. Pupation follows a period of larval development, followed by the emergence of adult flies. In some biting fly species, like the mosquito, only the females are blood feeders. In other species, adults of both sexes feed on blood.

Laboratory Diagnosis: Although detailed descriptions of biting flies are not within the scope of this book, some generalizations can be made that allow basic identification (see figures).

Clinical Importance: Biting flies have enormous importance in veterinary medicine and public health because of their role as disease vectors. In addition, the activity of biting flies causes irritation, and their bites can lead to allergic dermatitis and, in some cases of massive fly attacks, toxemia, and death.

ARTHROPODS

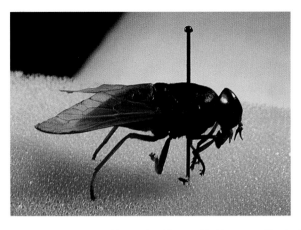

Fig. 5.134   Tabanid flies. These large biting flies are familiar worldwide. Horse flies (*Tabanus* spp., pictured) may reach 2.5 cm in length. Photo courtesy of Dr. Jeffrey F. Williams, Vanson HaloSource, Inc., Redmond, WA.

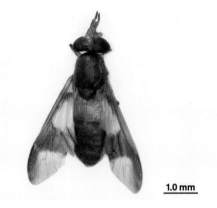

1.0 mm

Fig. 5.135   Deer flies, *Chrysops*, also belong to the tabanid group but are smaller and have distinct bands on their wings. Photo courtesy of Kellee Sundstrom, Oklahoma State University, Stillwater, OK.

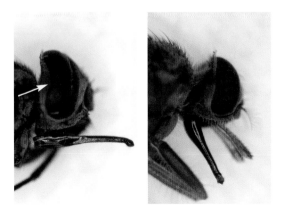

Fig. 5.136   Head and mouthparts of *Stomoxys calcitrans*, the stable fly (*left*), and *Haematobia irritans*, the horn fly (*right*). The mouthparts of *Stomoxys* project from the head at a right angle and the lateral aspect of the eye has a concave shape (*arrow*). Photos courtesy of Kellee Sundstrom, Oklahoma State University, Stillwater, OK.

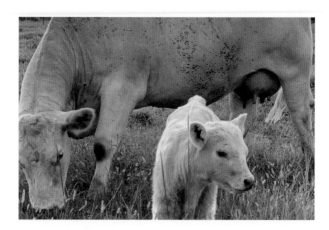

Fig. 5.137   Horn flies, *Haematobia irritans*, are a major pest of cattle throughout the world. Horn flies often cluster on the backs and sides of cattle, heads pointing toward the ground. If disturbed, they fly a short distance into the air and rapidly settle on the host again. Photo courtesy of Kellee Sundstrom, Oklahoma State University, Stillwater, OK.

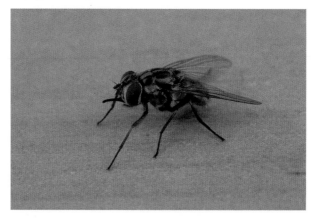

Fig. 5.138   The stable fly, *Stomoxys calcitrans*, is approximately the size of a house fly but is a major blood-feeding pest of cattle and, sometimes, domestic dogs. Photo courtesy of Dr. Lyle Buss, Entomology and Nematology Department, University of Florida, Gainesville, FL.

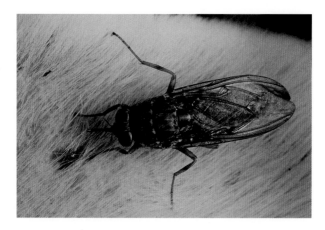

Fig. 5.139   *Glossina*, the tsetse fly, is the vector of trypanosomiasis in domestic animals and humans in Africa. Species reach up to 14 mm in length. Like stable flies, the mouthparts of the fly project forward from the head, but the wings of tsetse flies lie across the back like scissors. Photo courtesy of Dr. Andrew Peregrine, Ontario Veterinary College, University of Guelph, Guelph, Ontario, Canada.

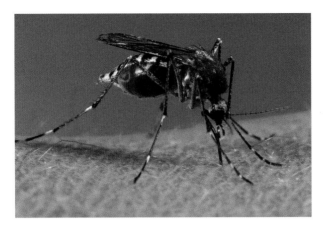

Fig. 5.140   Mosquitoes are common in many regions. Mosquito larvae develop in or near water. These delicate flies with long legs have mouthparts that are at least twice as long as the head. Photo from Agricultural Research Service, USDA.

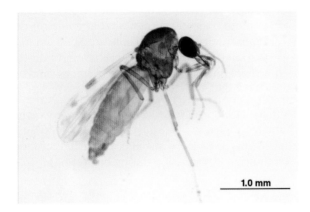

1.0 mm

Fig. 5.141   *Culicoides* (midges or no-see-ums) are very small biting flies (rarely larger than 2 mm) with patterned wings. Species are found worldwide. Photo courtesy of Kellee Sundstrom, Oklahoma State University, Stillwater, OK.

Other Insects

PARASITE: **Triatomine or reduviid bugs** (Fig. 5.142)

Common name: Kissing bugs, conenose bugs, assassin bugs, chinches.

Taxonomy: Insect (order Hemiptera, family Reduviidae).

Host: Humans, wildlife, and domestic animals.

Geographic Distribution: Several different species of triatomine bugs are found in forested and dry areas in the southern United States, Mexico, Central America, and South America.

Location on Host: Hide in dark crevices during day, emerging at night to feed.

Life Cycle: Kissing bugs visit the host at night to feed and spend daylight hours in cracks and crevices in human or animal environments. Eggs are laid in the environment.

Laboratory Diagnosis: Identification of immature or adult instars of triatomine bugs from the environment around animals or people, including kennels, chicken coops, and other housing. There are more than 100 species of triatomines in the Americas; common genera include *Triatoma* and *Rhodnius*. Adults are 1.5–3 cm in length and size of most stages increases with blood feeding. Some beetles and non-triatomine reduviid bugs may be confused with kissing bugs, including wheel bugs, corsairs, and leaf-footed bugs.

Clinical Importance: Kissing bugs serve as vector of *Trypanosoma cruzi,* the agent of Chagas disease, to humans, dogs, and other hosts. Over 50% of kissing bugs collected in Texas are infected with *T. cruzi*. Dogs become infected when they ingest the kissing bug as well as through stercorarian transmission during bug feeding.

ARTHROPODS

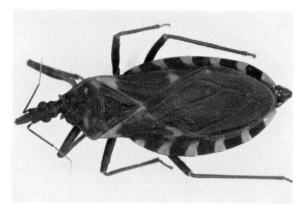

Fig. 5.142   Adult triatomine bug, *Triatoma sanguisuga*, an important vector of *Trypanosoma cruzi* in the southcentral United States. Photo courtesy of Megan Lineberry, Oklahoma State University, Stillwater, OK.

PARASITE: *Cimex lectularis, C. hemipterus, C. adjunctus* (Fig. 5.143–5.145)

Common name: Bedbug.

Taxonomy: Insect (order Hemiptera).

Host: Humans and domestic animals. Other members of the genus parasitize birds and bats.

Geographic Distribution: Worldwide with *C. lectularis* in temperate and *C. hemipterus* in tropical areas.

Location on Host: Bedbugs do not have specific predilection sites on the host.

Life Cycle: Five nymphal instars with the sixth stage being sexually mature, dimorphic males and females. All motile stags of bedbugs visit the host only at night to feed and spend daylight hours in cracks and crevices in human or animal environments. Eggs are laid in the environment.

Laboratory Diagnosis: Identification of reddish-brown, dorsoventrally flattened, wingless insects. Adults are 5–7 mm in length. In human infestations, bedbug feces may be seen in the bed.

Clinical Importance: Bedbugs are most important as human parasites, but they will also attack domestic animals. In the United States, bedbugs have recently become more common human parasites as the use of broad-spectrum pesticides for other insect pests has declined. The role of bedbugs as vectors for pathogens is uncertain. There is some laboratory data suggesting *Trypanosoma cruzi* may be transmitted by bedbugs. However, the epidemiological data to support vector competency and establish this transmission as a naturally occurring phenomenon is lacking.

ARTHROPODS

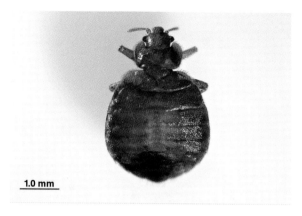

Fig. 5.143   Adult bedbug, *Cimex lectularis*. Photo courtesy of Megan Lineberry, Oklahoma State University, Stillwater, OK.

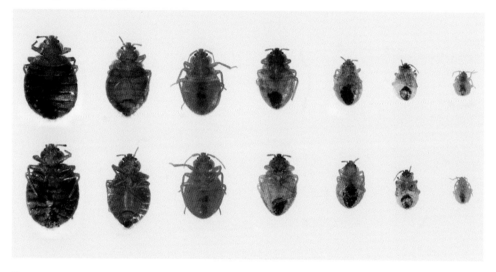

Fig. 5.144   Dorsal (*top row*) and ventral (*bottom row*) adult and nymphal bedbugs, *Cimex lectularis*. Females are slightly larger with rounded abdomens (*far left*). Males are smaller with a pointed abdomen (*second from left*). Each motile stage of *Cimex* spp. must take a blood meal before molting to the next stage. Photo courtesy of Megan Lineberry, Oklahoma State University, Stillwater, OK.

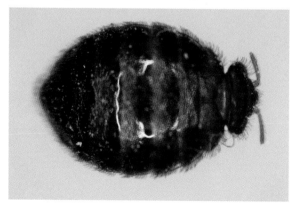

Fig. 5.145   *Cimex adjunctus*, the eastern bat bug, can be mistaken for *C. lectularis*. However, bat bugs are found in cracks and crevices of bat roosting areas, and the hairs on the thorax of a bat bug are longer than those of a bed bug. Photo courtesy of Dr. Manigandan Lejeune, Animal Health Diagnostic Center, Cornell University, Ithaca, NY.

ARTHROPODS

CHAPTER 6

Parasites of Fish

Stephen A. Smith

Fish can serve as definitive, intermediate, or paratenic (transport) hosts in the life cycle of many species of protozoan, metazoan, and crustacean parasites. Most of these parasites can be readily identified grossly or microscopically, and as with mammalian parasites, the correct identification and an understanding of their life cycle are important in the prevention or management of an outbreak of disease due to parasites.

Protozoan parasites probably cause more disease in both ornamental and cultured fish than any other group of parasites. An example of a common protozoan disease in fish is white spot disease, or "ich," caused by *Ichthyophthirius multifiliis* in freshwater fish or by *Cryptocaryon irritans* in marine species. Other protozoan parasites that commonly occur on fish include *Tetrahymena* spp., *Trichodina* spp., *Trichophyra* spp., *Amyloodinium* spp. and *Ichthyobodo* spp.

Metazoan parasites can be found as larval or adult forms in almost every tissue of fish. Most can be grossly identified as monogeneans, digenetic trematodes, nematodes, cestodes, acanthocephalans, or crustaceans, but specific identification generally involves special staining techniques or clearing of specimens.

Examples of common fish helminths include monogeneans on the gills and skin; larval digenetic trematodes (metacercariae) in the eyes, skin, musculature, and abdominal cavity; larval cestodes and nematodes in the visceral organs and abdominal cavity; and an assortment of adult trematodes, nematodes, cestodes, and acanthocephalans in the lumen of the gastrointestinal tract. In addition, a number of arthropod parasites and leeches can be found occurring on or attached to the skin and fins of fish.

TECHNIQUES FOR RECOVERY OF ECTOPARASITES

A variety of nonlethal techniques that include skin, fin, and gill biopsies have been developed for the diagnosis of the common external parasites of fish. Most of these biopsy techniques can be performed on live fish without the use of anesthesia, although light sedation often simplifies the procedure and makes it less stressful for the fish.

Veterinary Clinical Parasitology, Ninth Edition. Anne M. Zajac, Gary A. Conboy, Susan E. Little, and Mason V. Reichard.

FISH

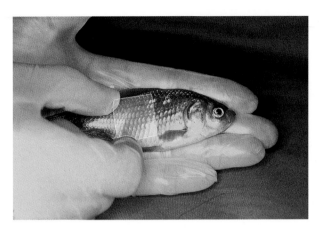

Fig. 6.1   Collection of mucus sample via a skin biopsy from the side of a fish for external-parasite examination.

Skin Biopsy (Mucus Smear)

The skin is the primary target organ for many of the external fish parasites. Therefore, a biopsy of the skin (Fig. 6.1) is one of the most useful and common samples for diagnosing ectoparasitic problems. This biopsy is performed by gently scraping a small area on the surface of the fish with a scalpel blade or the edge of a microscope coverslip in a cranial to caudal direction. Care should be taken to use only a minimal amount of pressure to obtain this superficial scraping, since damage to the skin may result in secondary bacterial and fungal infections or osmoregulatory imbalance in the fish.

The mucus from the skin scraping should be transferred immediately to a drop of aquarium, tank, or pond water (either fresh or salt water, depending on the species of fish, but *not* city tap water or distilled water) on a glass microscope slide and a coverslip carefully applied. This wet mount should then be examined under the compound microscope for the presence of free-swimming, attached, or encysted protozoan or metazoan parasites.

Fin Biopsy (Fin Snip)

A fin biopsy (Fig. 6.2) is obtained by snipping a small piece of tissue from the peripheral edge of one of the fins. This procedure is more traumatic to the fish than a skin biopsy, since a physical wound is produced. The fin snip should be transferred immediately to a drop of aquarium, tank, or pond water on a glass microscope slide, spread to its full extent, and a coverslip carefully applied. This wet mount should then be examined under the compound microscope for the presence of protozoan or metazoan parasites.

Gill Biopsy (Gill Snip)

A gill biopsy (Fig. 6.3) is obtained by inserting the tip of a pair of fine scissors into the branchial cavity behind the operculum (gill cover) and cutting off the distal ends of several of the primary gill lamellae attached to the gill arch. Since only the tips of the primary lamellae are removed, minimal bleeding should occur. The gill tissue should be transferred immediately to a drop of aquarium, tank, or pond water on a glass

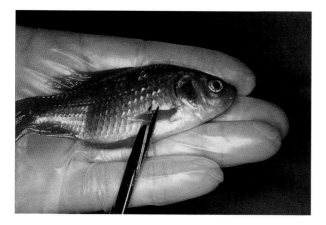

Fig. 6.2 Collection of a fin biopsy by clipping a small portion of the distal tip of the pectoral fin.

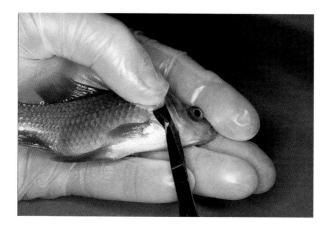

Fig. 6.3 Collection of a gill biopsy by lifting the operculum (gill chamber cover) and removing the distal tips of several filaments (lamellae) of the gill.

microscope slide; the individual lamellae separated; and a coverslip carefully applied. This wet mount should then be examined under the compound microscope for the presence of protozoan or metazoan parasites.

RECOVERY OF ENDOPARASITES

Examination of fish feces for the presence of internal parasites is accomplished with the same techniques as those used for mammals and birds. A fresh fecal sample is collected with a pipette either from the bottom of the aquarium or as it hangs from the vent of the fish. If an appropriate sample cannot be acquired from the environment or if examination of a specific individual is desired, the application of gentle pressure on the sides of a netted fish often produces the desired sample. The fecal specimen is then processed by standard flotation, sedimentation, or direct smear techniques and evaluated for the presence of parasite eggs and larvae. Though specific parasite identification is generally impossible, fecal examination does provide useful information about the types of parasites (nematodes, trematodes, cestodes, acanthocephalans) that may be present in a fish.

PARASITES OF FISH

PARASITE: *Ichthyophthirius multifiliis* (Figs. 6.4 and 6.5)

Common name: "Ich" or freshwater white spot disease.

Taxonomy: Protozoa (ciliate).

Geographic Distribution: Freshwater fish worldwide.

Location in Host: Within the surface epithelial layer of the skin, fins, and gills.

Life Cycle: This parasite has a direct life cycle, with free-swimming, ciliated tomites (theronts) in the water invading the skin, fins, and gills of fish. The tomites penetrate into the epithelial tissues and form large, feeding trophozoites (trophonts) that eventually excyst from the host and enter the water, where each develops into a cyst. The cyst stage then undergoes multiple divisions, producing numerous infective tomites that are released to the environment to infect other fishes.

Laboratory Diagnosis: This large, holotrich ciliate has a characteristic C-shaped macronucleus and is detected in wet mounts of skin biopsies and gill and fin snips.

Size:	Trophozoite in tissue	up to 1 mm in diameter
	Tomite in water	25–50 × 15–22 μm

Clinical Importance: The parasite causes small, raised, white lesions on skin, fins, and gill tissue. Penetration into and excystation out of the epithelial tissue by the parasite causes loss of integrity of external tissues and results in disruption of normal homeostatic osmoregulatory processes.

PARASITE: *Cryptocaryon irritans* (Fig. 6.6)

Common name: Marine white spot disease.

Taxonomy: Protozoa (ciliate).

Geographic Distribution: Marine and brackish water fishes worldwide.

Location in Host: Within the surface epithelial layer of the skin, fins, and gills.

Life Cycle: The life cycle is similar to that of freshwater *Icthyopththirius multifiliis*: free-swimming, ciliated tomites in the water invade the skin, fins, and gills, penetrate into the epithelial tissues, and form large, feeding trophozoites that eventually excyst from the host into the water and develop into cysts. The cyst stage then undergoes multiple divisions, producing numerous infective tomites that are released to the environment to infect other fishes.

Laboratory Diagnosis: This holotrich ciliate, which does *not* have a C-shaped nucleus like *I. multifiliis*, is detected in wet mounts of skin biopsies and gill and fin snips.

Size:	Trophozoite in tissues	up to 1 mm in diameter
	Tomite in water	25–50 × 15–22 μm

Clinical Importance: *Cryptocaryon irritans* causes small, raised, white lesions on the skin, fins, and gill tissue. Penetration into and excystation out of host epithelial tissue by the parasite causes loss of integrity of external tissues and results in disruption of normal homeostatic osmoregulatory processes.

FISH

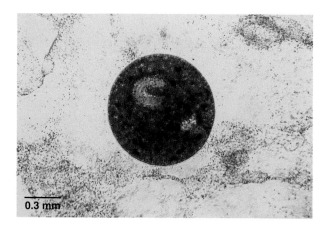

Fig. 6.4 *Ichthyophthirius multifiliis* trophozoite. This ciliate, which produces small, raised, white lesions on the skin, fins, and gills of fish, is commonly called "ich" or "white spot disease." This freshwater parasite varies in size, ranging from 100 to 1000 μm, depending on the stage of maturation, available nutrition, and host species.

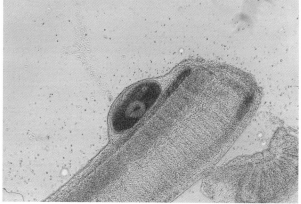

Fig. 6.5 Encysted trophozoite of *Ichthyophthirius multifiliis* embedded in the epithelial tissues of a gill filament of a goldfish (*Carassius auratus*).

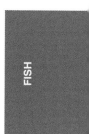

FISH

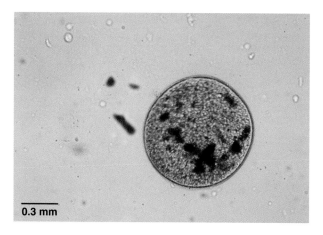

Fig. 6.6 *Cryptocaryon irritans* trophozoite. This ciliated parasite, which has a similar life cycle to *Ichthyophthirius multifiliis*, occurs in marine fish species.

Parasite: ***Tetrahymena* spp.** (Fig. 6.7)

Taxonomy: Protozoa (ciliate). Species include *T. corlissi* and *T. pyriformis*.

Geographic Distribution: Freshwater fish worldwide.

Location in Host: Trophozoites are generally found on surface epithelial layers of the skin and fins but may occasionally be found in deeper skin tissues, muscle, and abdominal organs.

Life Cycle: This parasite forms reproductive cysts in the freshwater environment in which two to eight infective tomites are produced.

Laboratory Diagnosis: Small, cylindrical- to pyriform-shaped ciliates can be found in wet mounts of skin biopsies.

Size: Trophozoite 55×30 μm

Clinical Importance: This facultative parasite can become histophagous and invade the skin, muscle, and internal organs causing osmoregulatory problems and body system dysfunction.

Parasite: ***Uronema* spp., including *U. marinum*** (Fig. 6.8)

Taxonomy: Protozoa (ciliate).

Geographic Distribution: Marine and brackish water fishes worldwide.

Location in Host: Surface epithelial layers of skin and fins of marine fish, but may also invade deeper skin tissues, muscle, and abdominal organs.

Life Cycle: This parasite (similar to freshwater *Tetrahymena* spp.) forms reproductive cysts in the marine environment in which several infective tomites are produced.

Laboratory Diagnosis: Small, cylindrical- to pyriform-shaped ciliates can be found in wet mounts of skin biopsies.

Size: Trophozoite 50×30 μm

Clinical Importance: This facultative, histophagous parasite (similar to freshwater *Tetrahymena* spp.) can invade the skin, muscle, and internal organs, causing osmoregulatory problems and body system dysfunction.

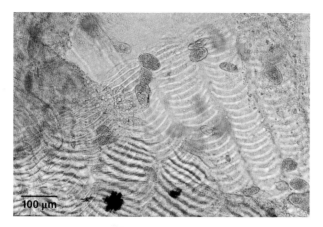

Fig. 6.7   Trophozoites of *Tetrahymena* spp. in a skin biopsy of a hybrid striped bass (*Morone saxatilis* × *M. chrysops*). This small ciliate also infects many species of ornamental aquarium fish.

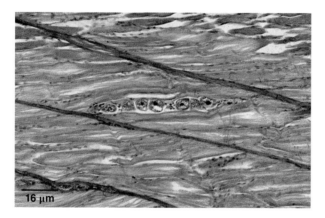

Fig. 6.8   Tissue section showing numerous trophozoites of *Uronema* spp. invading the deeper tissues of a summer flounder (*Paralichthys dentatus*) species. This marine organism causes pathology similar to that of *Tetrahymena* spp. of freshwater species of fish.

FISH

Parasite: ***Epistylis* spp.** (Fig. 6.9)

Taxonomy: Protozoa (ciliate). Species include *E. colisarum* and *E. lwoffi*.

Geographic Distribution: Freshwater fish worldwide.

Location in Host: Attached to surface epithelial layers of the skin and fins.

Life Cycle: This sessile, peritrichous ciliate divides by binary fission along the longitudinal axis, producing two daughter cells.

Laboratory Diagnosis: This colonial parasite is detected in wet mounts of the skin and is identified by its conical or elongated cylindrical body, branched noncontractile stalk, and epistomal disk for attachment.

   Size: 150–300 × 40–60 µm

Clinical Importance: The epistomal disk used for attachment to the host causes a localized skin lesion and mechanical disruption of the normal osmoregulatory process of the skin. Generally, fish develop skin lesions only in heavy infestations.

Parasite: ***Trichodina* spp.** (Fig. 6.10)

Taxonomy: Protozoa (ciliate). Related genera include *Trichodinella* spp., *Hemitrichodina* spp., *Dipartiella* spp., *Paratrichodina* spp., and *Tripartiella* spp.

Geographic Distribution: Freshwater, brackish, and marine fish worldwide.

Location in Host: Generally on the external surface of the skin, fins, and gills, though a few species are parasitic in the urinary tract of fish.

Life Cycle: This peritrichous ciliate divides by binary fission, producing two daughter cells.

Laboratory Diagnosis: This flattened, circular, ciliated protozoan is detected in wet mounts of skin biopsies and gill and fin snips and is identified by its prominent internal denticular (toothlike) ring and its ventrally located concave adhesive disk.

   Size: Variable, 150–300 × 40–60 µm

Clinical Importance: These organisms are usually ectocommensal but can become ectoparasitic when environmental and host conditions are suitable. This mobile scrub-brush-like parasite may cause localized to generalized skin lesions and disruption of the normal respiratory process of the gill and osmoregulatory processes of the skin. Generally, the parasite is only a problem in heavy infestations of the skin and gill.

FISH

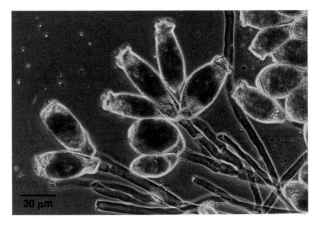

Fig. 6.9   *Epistylis* sp. is a colonial ciliate that has a conical or elongated cylindrical body, a noncontractile stalk, and an epistomal disk for attachment to the host. The parasite generally causes only localized skin lesions.

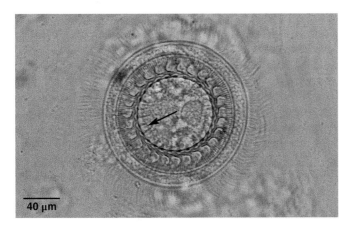

Fig. 6.10   *Trichodina* sp. from a skin biopsy of a tropical freshwater oscar (*Astronotus ocellatus*). These flattened ciliates have a prominent circular, denticular ring (*arrow*), upon which specific identification is based.

PARASITE: *Trichophyra* **spp.** (Fig. 6.11)

Taxonomy: Protozoa (ciliate).

Geographic Distribution: Freshwater fish worldwide.

Location in Host: Attached to epithelial surfaces of the skin, fins, and gills.

Life Cycle: This parasite reproduces by endogenous budding.

Laboratory Diagnosis: The parasite can be observed in wet mounts of skin biopsies and gill snips and is diagnosed by its numerous suctorial tentacles.

> Size: 30–50 μm

Clinical Importance: This small, sedentary parasite is generally only a problem in heavy infestations, where this pincushion-like ciliate attaches to the skin, fin, and gill tissues and causes irritation and localized lesions that disrupt normal respiratory and osmoregulatory processes of the fish.

PARASITE: *Amyloodinium ocellatum* (Figs. 6.12 and 6.13).

> Common name: Velvet disease or rust disease.

Taxonomy: Protozoa (flagellate). Other genera include *Oodinium* spp. and *Piscinoodinium* spp.

Geographic Distribution: Freshwater, marine, and brackish fish worldwide.

Location in Host: Attached to epithelial tissues of the skin, fins, and gills.

Life Cycle: The trophozoite attaches to the host via an attachment disk with filiform projections that penetrate into the epithelial tissue of the host. The trophozoite detaches from the host and forms an encysted tomont that divides and produces up to 256 free-swimming, infective dinospores that are released into the water.

Laboratory Diagnosis: Large, cylindrical dinoflagellates may be seen in wet mounts of gill snips where the organism is attached to the lamellae of the gill tissue.

Size:	Trophozoite attached to tissues	up to 150–200 μm in length
	Dinospores in water	12–15 μm in diameter

Clinical Importance: This ectoparasite primarily causes irritation of the gill, resulting in hyperplasia of the epithelial tissues and fusion of gill lamellae. Outbreaks may be fatal in heavily infected fish, especially in fish that are weakened or stressed by other conditions.

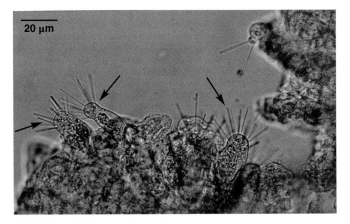

Fig. 6.11   *Trichophyra* sp. on a gill biopsy of a channel catfish (*Ictalurus punctatus*). This freshwater ciliate parasite has a "pincushion" appearance (*arrow*) and is often found on the skin and gills of pond-reared fish.

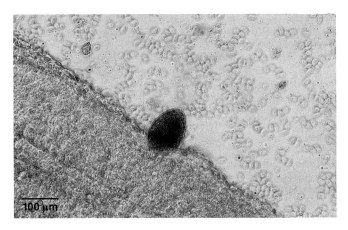

Fig. 6.12   *Amyloodinium ocellatum* on the gill tissue of a striped bass (*Morone saxatilis*). This organism is the cause of "velvet" or "rust" in ornamental marine species of fish. *Oodinium* sp. is a similar parasite in freshwater fish.

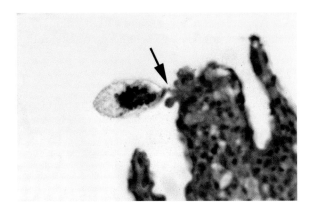

Fig. 6.13   Histopathology of *Amyloodinium ocellatum* attached to the gill tissue of a striped bass (*Morone saxatilis*) showing the basilar site of rhizoid penetration (*arrow*) into the epithelial cells of the gill.

FISH

PARASITE: *Ichthyobodo (= Costia) necator* (Fig. 6.14)

Taxonomy: Protozoa (flagellate).

Geographic Distribution: Freshwater fish worldwide.

Location in Host: Attached to epithelial tissues of the skin, fins, and gills.

Life Cycle: The attached feeding stage alternates with a free-swimming nonfeeding stage and reproduces by simple transverse division.

Laboratory Diagnosis: This very small flagellate with two unequal flagella extending from its posteriolateral groove is detected in wet mounts of skin biopsies and gill snips. The parasite is diagnosed by its small size and characteristic rapid erratic movements through the water.

> Size: Trophozoite   10–20 × 5–10 μm

Clinical Importance: This often-overlooked parasite is extremely pathogenic in young fish and older fish with lowered resistance. *Icthyobodo* causes irritation of the skin and gill tissue, resulting in hyperplasia of the epithelial tissues and fusion of gill lamellae.

PARASITE: *Myxobolus* spp., including *M. cerebralis* (Fig. 6.15)

Taxonomy: Cnidaria (Myxosporea). Fish are parasitized by numerous myxosporean genera and species including *Ceratomyxa* spp., *Kudoa* spp., *Sphaeromyxa* spp., *Myxidium* spp., and *Henneguya* spp.

Geographic Distribution: Freshwater, brackish, and marine fish worldwide.

Location in Host: Generally the epithelial tissues of the gills, skin, or intestine, but may also invade the muscle, cartilage, and other internal organs.

Life Cycle: The myxospore stage of this parasite develops in an annelid or polychaete worm to produce an actinospore stage that either penetrates or is eaten by the definitive fish host. The sporoplasm stage then develops and produces a polysporic cyst in the target tissue of the fish.

Laboratory Diagnosis: Variable-sized cysts found within wet mounts of various tissues contain spores with ellipsoidal, rounded, or spindle-shaped smooth valves.

> Size: Spore   7–10 μm in diameter

Clinical Importance: Infection of salmonids with *M. cerebralis* may cause loss of melanophore control in the skin resulting in black-colored tails in very young fish, or skeletal deformities due to cartilage destruction in older fish. This protozoan is a significant pathogen of wild and cultured trout populations. Other myxosporean species may cause white cysts within the skin, gill, or muscle tissue.

FISH

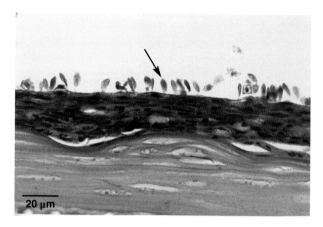

Fig. 6.14 *Ichthyobodo necator*, attached to the skin (*arrow*), is an extremely pathogenic flagellate parasite of freshwater fish that is often overlooked due to its small size.

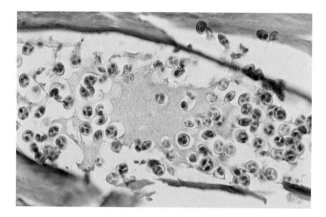

Fig. 6.15 Myxospores of *Myxobolus* sp. (a myxosporean parasite) in cartilaginous tissues of a rainbow trout (*Oncorhynchus mykiss*). Note the two polar capsules within the myxospore.

PARASITE: ***Henneguya* spp., including *H. ictaluri*** (Fig. 6.16)

Taxonomy: Cnidaria (Myxosporea). Myxosporean fish parasites include numerous genera and species; see *Myxobolus* spp.

Geographic Distribution: Freshwater, brackish, and marine fish worldwide.

Location in Host: Generally the epithelial tissues of the gills and skin, but may also invade muscle and internal organs.

Life Cycle: The myxospore stage of this parasite develops in an annelid or polychaete worm to produce an actinospore stage that either penetrates or is eaten by the definitive fish host. The sporoplasm stage then develops and produces a polysporic cyst in the target tissue of the fish.

Laboratory Diagnosis: Variable-sized cysts found within wet mounts of gill or other tissues containing spores with ellipsoidal, rounded, or spindle-shaped smooth valves, with or without caudal appendages.

Size: Spore   19 × 4.5 μm, with two caudal appendages of 45 μm each

Clinical Importance: *Henneguya ictaluri* causes a hyperplastic reaction in the epithelial cells of the gills, causing severe branchitis with respiratory compromise, and is a significant pathogen of the commercial catfish industry.

PARASITE: **Monogeneans** (Fig. 6.17)

Taxonomy: Monogenea (Monopistocotylea). Including the genera *Gyrodactylus* spp., *Dactylogyrus* spp., and *Neobenedenia* spp.

Geographic Distribution: Freshwater, brackish, and marine fish worldwide.

Location in Host: Attached to external surface of the skin, fins, and gills.

Life Cycle: Monogeneans complete their viviparous or ovoviviparous life cycle on one host. Larvae are morphologically similar to adults.

Laboratory Diagnosis: These small- to medium-sized flatworms have a posterior attachment organ, or opisthaptor, that may have hooks, anchors, clamps, or suckers. Monogeneans can be detected in wet mounts of gill snips or skin biopsies.

Size: Up to 5 mm in length

Clinical Importance: These parasitic flatworms cause local damage at the site of attachment and also through their feeding activity on the external surfaces of the fish.

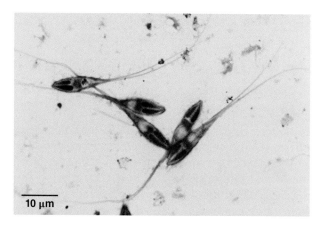

Fig. 6.16 Giemsa-stained myxospores of the myxosporean parasite *Henneguya* sp. from a ruptured cyst in the gill filament of a freshwater channel catfish (*Ictalurus punctatus*). Note the two anterior polar capsules within the spore and forked caudal appendages.

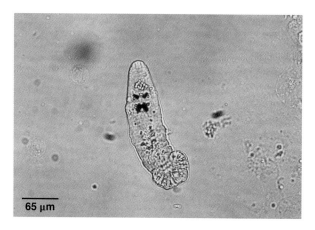

Fig. 6.17 Adult monogenean from a skin biopsy of a rainbow trout (*Oncorhynchus mykiss*). These external parasites have hooks, anchors, clamps, or suckers for attachment to the skin, fins, and gills.

FISH

Parasite: **Larval flukes** (Fig. 6.18)

Taxonomy: Trematode (Digenea).

Geographic Distribution: Freshwater, brackish, and marine fish worldwide.

Location in Host: Encysted metacercaria can be found in various tissues of the fish, including the skin, gills, muscle, eyes, brain, and visceral organs.

Life Cycle: Digenetic trematodes require at least one intermediate host, commonly a snail or other mollusk, to complete their life cycle. Eggs are deposited in the water by the definitive host (mammal, bird, or fish), which hatch, and release free-swimming miracidia that enter a first intermediate snail host. The developing parasites emerge into the water from the snail as free-swimming cercariae that penetrate the tissues of a second intermediate host, commonly a fish. The parasites then become encysted metacercariae and do not develop further until ingested by the appropriate carnivorous host (e.g., fish-eating bird, fish, or mammal) where the parasite becomes a mature adult.

Laboratory Diagnosis: Larval trematodes are generally visible grossly within the fish tissue.

Size: Metacercaria   Variable, up to several millimeters

Clinical Importance: These parasites are often unsightly in tissues, but generally are of minimal significance unless large numbers of metacercariae interfere with organ function.

Parasite: *Argulus* sp. (Fig. 6.19)

        Common name: Fish louse.

Taxonomy: Arthropod (Crustacea, Branchiura).

Geographic Distribution: Freshwater, brackish, and marine fish worldwide.

Location in Host: Generally on the external surfaces of the skin and fins.

Life Cycle: Eggs, which are laid in water, release free-swimming copepod larvae that attach to suitable fish hosts and metamorphose several times before reaching the adult stage.

Laboratory Diagnosis: These grossly visible dorsoventrally flattened, oval parasites have two prominent sucking disks, two dark-colored eyespots, and a centrally located piercing stylet.

Size: 3–5 mm

Clinical Importance: This crustacean causes damage by piercing the external tissues of the host and ingesting cellular fluids, and often causing a severe localized reaction at the site of stylet penetration. These parasitic arthropods may be important vectors in the transmission of certain viral, bacterial, and protozoan fish diseases.

FISH

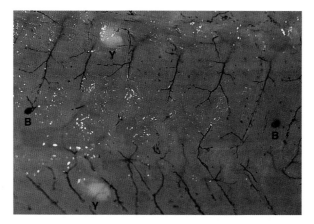

Fig. 6.18 Encysted metacercariae of two different species of digenetic trematodes in the muscle of a bluegill (*Lepomis macrochirus*). The smaller organism (B) is commonly called "black spot disease" (*Neascus* sp.), and the larger, paler one (Y) is commonly called a "yellow grub" (*Clinostomum* sp.). Both are larval stages that will not complete metamorphosis until ingested by a carnivorous definitive host.

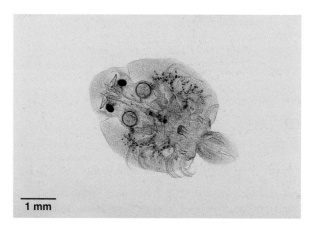

1 mm

Fig. 6.19 *Argulus* sp. from a goldfish (*Carassius auratus*), commonly known as a "fish louse." This ectoparasitic crustacean can be found on the skin and fins of freshwater fish. Other species can be found on brackish and marine species of fish.

PARASITE: *Lepeophtheirus* spp., *Caligus* spp. (Fig. 6.20)

Common name: Sea louse.

Taxonomy: Arthropod (Crustacea, Copepoda).

Geographic Distribution: Marine fish worldwide.

Location in Host: Generally on the external surfaces of the skin and fins.

Life Cycle: Attached female lice release eggs into the water where the eggs hatch releasing free-swimming nauplii larvae. The copepod metamorphoses through multiple free-swimming and then attached larval stages (copepodid and chalimus) to become parasitic adults feeding on the mucus, skin, and blood of the fish.

Laboratory Diagnosis: These grossly visible parasites have a large cephalothorax that acts like a suction organ for holding the louse on the fish. Females, which are larger than males, often have two long egg sacs trailing from their body.

Size: 5–8 mm

Clinical Importance: This crustacean causes physical, enzymatic, and inflammatory damage at the site of attachment and feeding resulting in hemorrhagic ulcerative skin lesions. These parasitic arthropods may also be important vectors for certain viral fish diseases.

PARASITE: *Ergasilus* spp. (Fig. 6.21)

Common name: Gill louse.

Taxonomy: Arthropod (Crustacea, Copepoda).

Geographic Distribution: Freshwater, brackish, and marine fish worldwide.

Location in Host: Most commonly found attached to the gills, rarely the skin and fins.

Life Cycle: Females release eggs into the water that hatch and release free-swimming larvae. The copepod metamorphoses through numerous free-swimming stages to become either free-living males or attached parasitic females feeding on the mucus and skin of the fish.

Laboratory Diagnosis: These parasites have a large modified prehensile antennal segment for grasping gill filaments of the fish. Gravid females commonly have two egg sacs trailing from their body.

Size: 4–6 mm

Clinical Importance: This crustacean causes traumatic crushing damage at the site of attachment to the gill filaments of the host resulting in focal devitalized gill tissue.

FISH

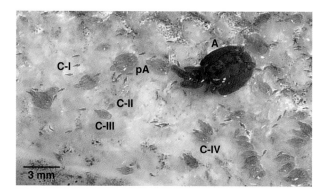

Fig. 6.20   *Lepeophtheirus salmonis.* Sea lice on the skin of an Atlantic salmon (*Salmo salar*). This copepod has several free-swimming stages known as nauplii that molt into an infectious copepodid stage. Once on the fish, the copepodid molts into parasitic chalimus stages (C-I through C-IV), then a pre-adult stage (pA) before becoming a reproductive adult (A = female adult). Photo courtesy of Dr. Larry Hammell, Atlantic Veterinary College, University of Prince Edward Island, Charlottetown, PEI, Canada.

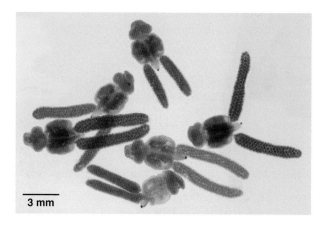

Fig. 6.21   *Ergasilus* spp. Adult female copepod parasites removed from the oral cavity of a freshwater striped bass (*Morone saxatilis*) where they were firmly attached to the gill filaments. Each parasite has a cephalothorax with modified grasping appendages, a central abdomen, and two elongated egg sacs.

FISH

PARASITE: ***Lernaea* spp.** (Fig. 6.22)

Common name: Anchor worm.

Taxonomy: Arthropod (Crustacea, Copepoda).

Geographic Distribution: Freshwater fish worldwide.

Location in Host: Most commonly found attached to the skin and fins.

Life Cycle: Females release eggs into the water that hatch and release free-swimming larvae. The copepod metamorphoses through several free-swimming stages with mating occurring during the last copepodid stage. After mating, the female attaches to the skin of the fish and transforms into an unsegmented wormlike parasite. The anterior end becomes modified into an anchor-like holdfast organ buried in the skin, while the posterior end hangs free in the water.

Laboratory Diagnosis: These parasites have a large anchor-like anterior end and a long unsegmented body. Females commonly have two egg sacs trailing from their body.

Size: 4–6 mm

Clinical Importance: This crustacean induces a localized, hyperplastic inflammatory reaction at the site where the parasite is embedded in the tissue.

PARASITE: **Leeches** (Fig. 6.23)

Taxonomy: Phylum Annelida (subclass Hirudinea).

Geographic Distribution: Freshwater, brackish, and marine fish worldwide.

Location in Host: Attached to external tissues of the skin, fins, and gills.

Life Cycle: Leeches are hermaphroditic and reproduce by reciprocal fertilization.

Laboratory Diagnosis: These grossly visible flat to cylindrical wormlike parasites have a varying number of body divisions and generally both anterior and posterior suckers.

Size: Variable, up to several centimeters in length

Clinical Importance: Besides the physical damage caused by attachment and blood-sucking activities, leeches are vectors for a variety of fish pathogens, including viruses, bacteria, and hemoparasites.

FISH

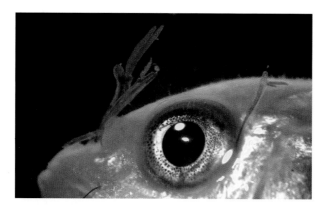

Fig. 6.22   *Lernaea* spp. This parasitic copepod, commonly known as an anchor worm, has several free-swimming larval stages before becoming infective to the host. After mating, the male generally dies, while the female burrows into the flesh of the fish. The anterior end of the parasite develops into an anchor-like adaptation that becomes embedded in the tissues of the fish, while the posterior end becomes modified into an unsegmented, wormlike body with two egg sacs that hang from the fish's body. Photo courtesy of Dr. Roy P. E. Yanong, Tropical Aquaculture Laboratory, University of Florida, Ruskin, FL.

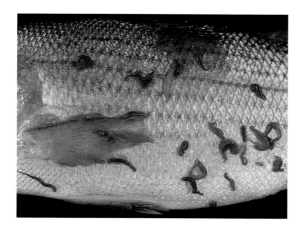

Fig. 6.23   Leeches of an unidentified species attached to the skin of a cultured hybrid striped bass (*Morone saxatilis* × *M. chrysops*). These parasites can cause anemia in fish, as well as act as vectors of hemoparasites and other pathogens.

PARASITE: **Thorny-headed worm** (Fig. 6.24)

Taxonomy: Phylum Acanthocephala.

Geographic Distribution: Freshwater, brackish, and marine fish worldwide.

Location in Host: Lumen of the posterior intestinal tract.

Life Cycle: These parasites have an indirect life cycle, with usually a crustacean intermediate host.

Laboratory Diagnosis: Eggs are observed on standard fecal flotation or direct smear.

   Size: 50–65 × 30–40 μm

Clinical Importance: These parasites generally do not cause any clinical signs in fish. Rarely, a severe infestation will result in perforation of the intestinal tract, with subsequent peritonitis.

PARASITE: **Nematode Parasites** (Figs. 6.25 and 6.26)

Taxonomy: Nematode.

Geographic Distribution: Freshwater, brackish, and marine fish worldwide.

Location in Host: Lumen of the intestinal tract.

Life Cycle: Both direct and indirect life cycles have been reported.

Laboratory Diagnosis: A variety of nematode-type eggs may be observed on standard fecal flotation or direct smear.

   Size: Variable

Clinical Importance: Adult nematodes generally do not cause significant clinical signs in fish. A severe infestation sometimes will result in mechanical blockage of the intestinal tract and/or chronic weight loss.

FISH

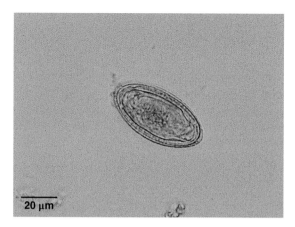

Fig. 6.24 Egg of an acanthocephalan parasite from a black crappie (*Pomoxis nigromaculatus*).

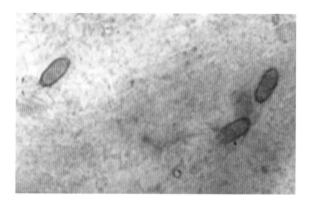

Fig. 6.25 Eggs of *Capillaria* sp. from a freshwater angelfish (*Pterophyllum scalare*).

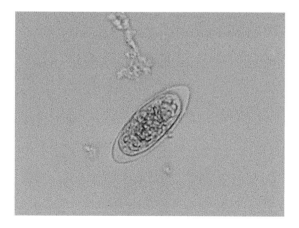

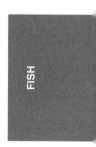

FISH

Fig. 6.26 Unidentified nematode egg from a largemouth bass (*Micropterus salmoides*).

CHAPTER 7

Treatment of Veterinary Parasites

INTRODUCTION

A wide variety of safe, effective parasiticides can eliminate infections and infestations or prevent development or exacerbation of parasitic disease. Despite the availability of these powerful treatments, parasite control continues to be an unmet need for many domestic animals due to lack of use or incomplete knowledge on efficacy. Choosing the parasiticide treatment most appropriate for a particular clinical situation requires careful assessment of risk factors as well as veterinary expertise regarding individual patient, herd, or flock characteristics and needs. Rarely is one treatment or a single protocol the best option for all patients, even when general concerns about the type of parasitic disease of greatest risk are similar. In this chapter we summarize information about anthelmintics, ectoparasiticides, and antiprotozoals currently available to veterinarians. Only products approved by FDA, EPA, or similar regulatory agencies and that have been confirmed to be safe and efficacious will be discussed here; availability of some approved products or formulations may be limited. Products covered in this chapter are largely restricted to those available in the United States and Canada. Veterinarians should be familiar with and consult current regulatory-approved label information prior to prescribing or recommending any specific product.

ANTHELMINTICS

Effective control of helminths involves more than just selection of a safe, effective anthelmintic. Effective parasite management programs must incorporate likelihood of environmental contamination and thus risk of re-infection, seasonality of transmission, age and immune status of animals, and zoonotic risk of allowing infections to persist. Selection of the best anthelmintic for a given clinical situation is often based on factors other than efficacy, including safety, application route, persistence, and knowledge about resistance. Traditionally, anthelmintics were administered in liquid oral formulations either directly or via nasogastric tube. However, many anthelmintics are

Veterinary Clinical Parasitology, Ninth Edition. Anne M. Zajac, Gary A. Conboy, Susan E. Little, and Mason V. Reichard.
© 2021 John Wiley & Sons, Inc. Published 2021 by John Wiley & Sons, Inc.
Companion website: www.wiley.com/go/zajac/parasitology

Table 7.1. Common administration routes for anthelmintics

Application route	Examples	Species available for
Oral		
Tablets/chewable	Milbemycin oxime +/- praziquantel	Cats, dogs
	Ivermectin +/- pyrantel +/- praziquantel	Cats, dogs
	Pyrantel/praziquantel +/- febantel	Cats, dogs
Paste	Fenbendazole, ivermectin, moxidectin, oxibendazole, pyrantel pamoate	Horses
	Fenbendazole	[a]Cattle
Liquid	Albendazole, closantel, fenbendazole, ivermectin, levamisole, moxidectin, oxfendazole	[a]Cattle, [a]sheep, [a]goats
Water additive	Fenbendazole	[a]Pigs
Feed additive	Fenbendazole, morantel tartrate	[a]Cattle
	Dichlorvos, fenbendazole, ivermectin, levamisole, piperazine, pyrantel tartrate	[a]Pigs
Block / mineral	Fenbendazole	[a]Cattle
Pellets	Fenbendazole, pyrantel tartrate	Horses
Injectable	Melarsomine dihydrochloride	Dogs
	Moxidectin	Dogs
	Doramectin, ivermectin	[a]Cattle, [a]pigs
	Levamisole, moxidectin	[a]Cattle
	Eprinomectin extended release parasiticide	[a]Cattle
	Praziquantel	Cats, dogs
Transdermal	Moxidectin, selamectin	Cats, dogs
	Emodepside/praziquantel	Cats
	Eprinomectin/praziquantel	Cats
	Doramectin, eprinomectin, ivermectin, moxidectin	[a]Cattle

[a] Products listed not approved for use in all food animals; always consult label prior to administering.

now given with the feed, injected, or as a transdermal product that is administered topically and absorbed systemically (Table 7.1).

Anthelmintics also differ in the degree to which they persist in the animal after administration, with some products being cleared within 24 hours and others lasting and remaining efficacious as long as 6 months. Persistency is often desired to reduce the number of times animals must be treated but can affect withdrawal times (Table 7.2) and influence selection for resistance. With use of any antiparasitic drug treatment, including anthelmintics, selection for resistance will occur. Anthelmintic resistance has reduced the utility of these drugs in certain clinical situations. Accordingly, recognizing resistance when it occurs and developing appropriate strategies to protect animal health in the face of diminished anthelmintic efficacy are important clinical skills. Resistance to parasiticides is discussed further below.

Specific Anthelmintics

Macrocyclic lactones, also referred to as avermectin/milbemycin compounds, constitute some of the safest, most effective, and most widely used anthelmintics ever developed. First marketed in the early 1980s, the class now includes **abamectin, doramectin, eprinomectin, ivermectin, milbemycin oxime, moxidectin**, and **selamectin**. These compounds cause flaccid paralysis by impeding glutamate-gated chloride channels; removal

Table 7.2. **Examples of withdrawal times for selected anthelmintics**

Anthelmintic	Species treated	[a]Withdrawal times
Albendazole	Beef cattle	27 d oral liquid
	Goats, sheep	7 d oral liquid
Dichlorvos	Pigs	0 d feed additive
Doramectin	Pigs	24 d injectable
	Beef cattle	35 d injectable; 45 d pour-on
	Dairy cattle	Injectable only in heifers <20 mo. of age
Eprinomectin	Beef cattle	0 d pour-on; 48 d injectable
	Dairy cattle	0 d pour-on; injectable only in heifers <20 mo. of age
Fenbendazole	Pigs	0 d feed additive
	Beef cattle	8 d oral liquid, paste; 11 d molasses block; 13 d flaked meal, free-choice mineral, pellets; 16 d protein block
	Dairy cattle	0 d oral liquid, flaked meal, free-choice mineral, paste, pellets
	Goats	6 d oral liquid
Ivermectin	Pigs	5 d feed additive; 18 d injectable
	Beef cattle	35 d injectable; 48 d pour-on
	Dairy cattle	Injectable only in heifers <20 mo. of age
	Sheep	11 d oral liquid
Levamisole	Pigs	3 d water or feed additive
	Beef cattle	2 d bolus, oral liquid, feed additive; 7 d injectable; 9 d pour-on
	Sheep	3 d oral liquid
Morantel tartrate	Beef cattle	14 d feed additive
	Dairy cattle	0 d feed additive
Moxidectin	Beef cattle	0 d pour-on; 21 d injectable
	Dairy cattle	0 d pour-on; injectable only in heifers <20 mo. of age
	Sheep	7 d oral liquid
Oxfendazole	Beef cattle	7 d oral liquid
Piperazine	Pigs	21 d water or feed additive
Pyrantel tartrate	Pigs	24 h feed additive

[a] Withdrawal times listed are according to FDA-approved labels and may vary by formulation; always consult label prior to administering. Food Animal Residue Avoidance Databank (FARAD; http://www.farad.org/) withdrawal times may differ from those on the FDA-approved label.

of gastrointestinal parasites follows via peristalsis and stages in tissues are cleared by the immune system. Although the specific efficacy of individual compounds differs and formulations influence spectrum of activity, in general, members of this class are effective against a diverse array of nematodes and arthropods. All available formulations are safe when administered according to label directions. However, extralabel use of high doses can result in toxicity, particularly in collies and other dogs that carry the MDR1 mutation and in certain exotic animals, including chelonians and some other reptiles.

Originally developed as plant fungicides, the benzimidazoles have been used as anthelmintics since the early 1960s. Key members of this class still used in veterinary medicine include **albendazole, fenbendazole, flubendazole, mebendazole, oxfendazole, oxibendazole, ricobendazole**, and **triclabendazole** as well as **febantel**, a pro-benzimidazole. The benzimidazoles bind tubulin, preventing formation of microtubules necessary for cellular function, including energy metabolism. Depending on the compound considered, efficacy has been demonstrated against a wide variety of nematodes as well as some platyhelminths and *Giardia* sp. Although generally safe, some members of this class, notably albendazole and febantel, are potentially teratogenic when administered early in pregnancy.

The tetrahydropyrimidines have been used as anthelmintics since the 1970s and include the popular dewormer **pyrantel**, which is available in several different salt forms, as well as **morantel tartrate**. After administration, these drugs remain in the gastrointestinal lumen and thus are not effective against tissues stages of helminths. Pyrimidines are acetylcholine agonists that lead to spastic paralysis and subsequent expulsion of parasites. Efficacy has been documented against a variety of nematodes as well as equine tapeworms. The safety profile of this class is excellent even at elevated doses.

Levamisole is an imidazothiazole that also acts as a nicotinic acetylcholine agonist; levamisole has a narrow safety margin and overdosing can lead to nicotinic-type symptoms, particularly when animals are dehydrated or stressed. Other anthelmintics that bind to acetylcholine receptors include **monepantel**, an amino-acetonitrile derivative, and **derquantel**, a semi-synthetic spiroindole. Both compounds lead to paralysis of gastrointestinal nematodes and are marketed for sheep in some areas. **Emodepside** is a cyclic depsipeptide anthelmintic developed for treating hookworms and ascarids in cats and dogs. The drug paralyzes nematodes upon binding to lactrophilin-like receptors. **Closantel** is a salicylanilide effective against adult and immature *Fasciola hepatica*, some nematodes, and larval stages of some arthropods. This compound is a potent oxidative phosphorylase uncoupler and toxicity has been reported in ruminants at both standard and elevated doses.

Melarsomine dihydrochloride is an arsenical compound with a narrow therapeutic index used to treat infection with adult *Dirofilaria immitis* in dogs. The arsenic salt reacts with sulfhydryl enzymes resulting in parasite death. Injections are administered deep in the epaxial muscle and both injection site reactions and systemic reactions can occur. Reactions are most common in dogs with high numbers of *D. immitis*. Due to toxicity concerns, melarsomine dihydrochloride should not be used in dogs with reduced liver function or in cats. Less commonly used dewormers effective against nematodes include **piperazine**, which disrupts GABA neurotransmitters in ascarids leading to neuromuscular blockade; **dichlorvos**, an organophosphate labeled against gastrointestinal nematodes in swine; and **hygromycin B**, an antibiotic fed to poultry and swine that also controls intestinal nematodes.

Some anthelmintics are only effective against cestodes or trematodes, including the isoquinolones **praziquantel** and **epsiprantel**, and the benzene sulfonamide **clorsulon**. The isoquinolones act by increasing membrane permeability to calcium resulting in destruction of the tegument and parasite paralysis and have wide efficacy against a number of intestinal and tissue stages of cestodes and trematodes. Safety of these compounds is excellent; high doses can be used extralabel when necessary. Clorsulon is primarily used against *Fasciola hepatica* in cattle but availability is limited in many countries. Combination anthelmintics also are available. For example, a macrocyclic lactone, benzimidazole, or tetrahydropyrimidine with broad spectrum nematode efficacy may be combined with an isoquinolone effective against cestodes. These formulations provide efficacy against a broader spectrum of helminths and facilitate ease of use. In some areas, multiple anthelmintic groups with similar spectrums of action are combined to enhance efficacy against resistant nematodes.

Selection for resistance occurs within a population of parasites as anthelmintics are used. Examples of anthelmintic resistance include resistance to benzimidazoles in equine small strongyles and ruminant trichostrongyles; resistance to macrocyclic lactones in *Dirofilaria immitis*, equine ascarids, and ruminant trichostrongyles; and resistance to pyrantel in canine hookworms and equine small strongyles. Strategies to delay selection for resistance focus on maximizing **refugia**, the portion of the parasite population not exposed to an anthelmintic and thus not subject to selection pressure, along with pasture and animal management strategies that reduce the need for anthelmintic use.

ECTOPARASITICIDES

Arthropod pests and disease vectors are controlled by environmental management, animal treatment, or a combination of both strategies. As with anthelmintics, treatment decisions may be influenced by seasonal activity, production loss, and potential for zoonotic risk. Selection of an appropriate compound is influenced by persistence, route of application, safety, and resistance. Traditionally, control of arthropod pests was achieved by topical application of short-acting compounds. However, in addition to topical application, many modern systemic insecticides and acaricides may be administered orally, transdermally, or by injection, and efficacy persists for weeks to months after treatment (Table 7.3, Table 7.4). Products should only be used in accordance with regulatory requirements. In the United States, it is a violation of federal law to use EPA-registered pesticides in a manner inconsistent with the label. Pesticides approved by EPA for one host (e.g., cattle, dogs) should not be used in another host (e.g., horses, cats).

Isoxazolines have persistent efficacy against fleas, ticks, and other arthropods. First introduced in 2014, members of the class include **afoxolaner**, **fluralaner**, **lotilaner**, and **sarolaner**. The compounds are administered by the oral or transdermal route and provide systemic control against fleas, ticks, and mites in dogs and cats for 4–12 weeks following a single administration. Efficacy is achieved through inhibition of arthropod GABA/glutamate-gated chloride channels. While isoxazolines are considered safe and effective, the class has been associated with adverse reactions, including muscle tremors, ataxia, and seizures, in some pets and should not be used in patients with a history of seizures.

Fipronil, a phenylpyrazole developed in the mid-1990s, is a GABA chloride channel antagonist effective against fleas, lice, mites, and ticks. Although safe for dogs and cats, fipronil should not be applied to rabbits. Macrocyclic lactones (see earlier) also have efficacy against a variety of arthropods. Specific claims vary with individual formulations, but members of this class may be effective against fleas, flies, lice, mites, and ticks with injectable, oral, otic, topical, and transdermal formulations available. **Indoxacarb** is an oxadiazine insecticide that, once ingested and metabolized by insects, blocks insect voltage-gated sodium ion channels. Indoxacarb has efficacy against eggs, larvae, and adult fleas; some formulations are combined with permethrin and thus should not be applied to cats (see below).

Neonicotinoids were first developed in 1991 and are widely used to control plant pests and fleas; members of this class include **imidacloprid**, **dinotefuran**, and **nitenpyram**. Neonicotinoids are agonists of insect nicotinic acetylcholine receptors (nAChR) and have rapid efficacy against fleas and other insects. **Spinosad** is a macrolide that, similar to neonicotinoids, activates nAChR but at a unique site, leading to paralysis and death of fleas and other arthropods. These compounds have high affinity for insect receptors making them very safe for use in mammals and birds. Topical neonicotinoids are often formulated in combination with pyrethroids (see below) for efficacy against ticks, as

Table 7.3. Common administration routes for insecticides and acaricides used in small animals and primary arthropods targeted

Application route	Examples	[a]Compounds used	Primary target for control
Environmental	Premise spray, fogger	Pyrethrins/pyrethroids	Fleas, flies, ticks on premise
		Methoprene, pyriproxyfen	Fleas (immature stages)
Topical	On-animal spray, wipe, powder	Fipronil, pyrethrins/pyrethroids	Fleas, ticks on dogs, cats
		Dinotefuran	Fleas on dogs, cats
	Shampoo	Pyrethrins/pyrethroids	Fleas, ticks on dogs, cats
		Methoprene, pyriproxyfen	Fleas (immature stages) on dogs, cats
	Dip	Pyrethroids	Fleas, ticks on dogs
	Collar	Amitraz	Ticks on dogs
		Deltamethrin	Fleas, ticks, flies on dogs
		Imidacloprid/flumethrin	Fleas, ticks on dogs, cats
		Methoprene, pyriproxyfen	Fleas (immature stages) on dogs, cats
	Spot-on	Dinotefuran, fipronil, imidacloprid, indoxacarb, pyrethroids	Fleas on dogs, cats
		Methoprene, pyriproxyfen	Fleas (immature stages) on dogs, cats
		Fipronil, pyrethroids	Fleas, ticks on dogs
		Permethrin	Flies on dogs
		Spinetoram	Fleas on cats
Systemic	Oral	Nitenpyram, spinosad	Fleas on dogs, cats
		Afoxolaner, fluralaner, lotilaner, sarolaner	Fleas, ticks on dogs
		Lufenuron	Fleas (immature stages) on dogs
	Transdermal	Moxidectin, selamectin	Fleas, mites, ticks on dogs, cats
		Fluralaner, sarolaner	Fleas, ticks on dogs, cats

[a] All types of compounds listed may not be approved or safe for use in all breeds or species; always consult label prior to administering.

well as **insect growth regulators** like **methoprene** or **pyriproxyfen**, juvenile hormone mimics that limit development of fleas in the environment. **Lufenuron** and **diflubenzuron** are examples of insect development inhibitors that disrupt chitin synthesis and prevent development of immature fleas. While neonicotinoids have an excellent safety profile when used alone, products combined with permethrin should not be applied to cats.

Pyrethrins are natural botanical compounds first isolated from *Chrysanthemum cinerariaefolium* in the 1960s and provide short-acting control of arthropods; several generations of synthetic pyrethroids with higher potency, longer photostability, and more persistent efficacy have since been developed. Examples of pyrethroids used in veterinary medicine include **betacyfluthrin**, **cypermethrin**, **cyphenothrin**, **deltamethrin**, **esfenvalerate**, **flumethrin**, **lambdacyhalothrin**, and **permethrin**; **etofenprox** is a related compound with similar activity. These chemicals disrupt sodium- and potassium-mediated neurotransmission in arthropods, and formulations often include **piperonyl butoxide** as a synergist to inhibit arthropod oxidation of the compounds, thus increasing activity. Pyrethrins and pyrethroids are effective against both insects and ticks, with

Table 7.4. Common administration routes for insecticides and acaricides used in large animals and primary arthropods targeted

Application route	Examples	[a]Compounds used	Primary target for control
Environmental	Premise spray, fogger	Pyrethrins/pyrethroids, organophosphates, spinosad	Flies on premise
	Granule	Imidacloprid, indoxacarb, pyrethroids, spinosad	Flies on premise
	Fly strip	Organophosphates, pyrethroids	Flies on premise
Topical	On-animal spray	Amitraz	Lice, ticks on cattle, pigs
	On-animal spray, wipe, dust	Pyrethrins/pyrethroids, organophosphates	Flies, lice on cattle, horses
	Back rubber	Pyrethroids, organophosphates	Flies, lice, ticks on cattle
	Ear tag	Abamectin, pyrethroids, organophosphates	Flies, lice, ticks on cattle
Systemic	Oral	Cyromazine, diflubenzuron	Flies (immature stages) on horses
		Cyromazine, methoprene	Flies (immature stages) on cattle
		Macrocyclic lactones	Lice on cattle; grubs/bots in cattle, horses
	Injectable	Macrocyclic lactones	Lice, mites on cattle, pigs; grubs, in cattle
	Transdermal	Macrocyclic lactones	Flies, lice, grubs, mites on cattle

[a] All types of compounds listed may not be approved or safe for use in all breeds or species; always consult label prior to administering.

persistency of different formulations varying from as short as 1 day (pyrethrins) to as long as 6 or 8 months (deltamethrin and flumethrin/imidacloprid collars for dogs and dogs and cats, respectively). Products are intended for application to the environment or directly to animals, and on-animal formulations often repel and kill insects and ticks. Pyrethrins have an excellent safety profile and can be used in all ages of animals. When label directions are followed, pyrethroids are also safe but caution must be taken to avoid applying highly concentrated formulations of some pyrethroids, most notably permethrin, to cats.

Organophosphates (e.g., **coumaphos, diazinon, dichlorvos, phosmet, pirimiphos,** and **tetrachlorvinphos**) were first developed as insecticides in the 1930s and 1940s; carbamates (e.g., **carbaryl, propoxur**) followed in the 1950s. Organophosphates and carbamates inhibit acetylcholine esterase (AChE) by binding to the enzyme irreversibly or reversibly, respectively. Present use includes flea and tick collars, powders, sprays, and dips for small animals; ear tags, sprays, dusts, and rub-ons for fly, tick, mite, or lice control on cattle; and adhesive fly strips or sprays for environmental arthropod control; the compounds may be used alone or in combination with pyrethroids. Mammalian toxicity with organophosphates and carbamates results in some combination of diarrhea, urination, miosis, bronchospasm, bradycardia, emesis, lacrimation, and salivation, referred to by the mnemonic "DUMBBELS"; atropine is used to block overstimulation due to either class while 2-PAM is used only in organophosphate toxicity to reactivate inhibited AChE. Lean animals are particularly susceptible to cholinesterase inhibition, and use of these compounds should be avoided in young animals, cats, sighthounds (e.g., whippets, greyhounds), Brahman cattle, and some other cattle breeds (e.g., Charolais, Gelbvieh, Simmental). Due to human safety concerns, on-animal use of organophosphates and carbamates is often avoided, particularly in animals likely to be handled by people (e.g., dogs, cats, horses). **Amitraz** is a formamidine approved for use in dogs, pigs, and cattle that acts as a monoamine oxidase inhibitor. Dog products are labeled against mites and ticks; food animal products are labeled against lice, mites, and ticks. Due to safety concerns, amitraz should not be used in cats or horses.

PROTOZOAL TREATMENT

Protozoal infections of animals are treated with a variety of different drugs, many of which are not label-approved for that application. For some infections, such as coccidia, environmental sanitation to limit infection is as important as effective treatment at preventing disease. Not all compounds are readily available in all countries. Care must be taken in food animals to avoid residues that can create human health risk. Safety concerns exist with some of the antiprotozoal treatments discussed.

Some benzimidazoles (e.g., **albendazole**, **fenbendazole**) and pro-benzimidazoles (**febantel**) have efficacy against *Giardia* sp. by preventing microtubule formation. Fenbendazole is label-approved to treat dogs for giardiasis in Europe and is safe to use in pregnancy; fenbendazole is also safe in cats. Febantel is teratogenic but also effective against *Giardia* sp. Both compounds must be administered for at least 3 consecutive days with fenbendazole treatment often continued for a week or more. Albendazole may cause aplastic anemia in some canine and feline patients and, because alternatives are available, should not be used for protozoal treatment in dogs and cats. **Imidocarb** inhibits nucleic acid metabolism in some apicomplexan protozoa and has been used to treat babesiosis, hepatozoonosis, and cytauxzoonosis, although atovaqone and azithromycin combination therapy is preferred for *Babesia gibsoni and Cytauxzoon felis*. Pretreatment with glycopyrrolate or atropine is recommended in debilitated or young animals.

Antibiotics with efficacy against protozoa include **clindamycin**, the nitroimidazoles (e.g., **metronidazole**, **ronidazole**, **benznidazole**), and the **sulfonamides**. Clindamycin is a lincosamide antibiotic used to treat clinical toxoplasmosis in cats and dogs. Although metronidazole is somewhat effective against *Giardia* sp., fenbendazole (see earlier) is considered both safer and more effective for treating canine giardiasis; side effects reported with metronidazole include weakness, ataxia, tremors, and seizures. Ronidazole is used in cats with diarrhea due to *Tritrichomonas foetus*. Treated cats may develop neurologic signs. Benznidazole is used for treating dogs with Chagas disease due to *Trypanosoma cruzi*. The nitroimidazoles are not FDA-approved for use in any veterinary species and should not be used in food animals.

Sulfonamides are antibiotics available since the 1930s that are commonly used as coccidiostats. Common sulfonamides include **sulfadiazine**, **sulfadimethoxine**, **sulfamerazine**, **sulfamethazine**, **sulfamethoxazole**, and **sulfaquinoxaline** and act as competitive inhibitors of folic acid synthesis, impairing pathogen growth and metabolism. These compounds are often combined with potentiators such as **ormetoprim**, **pyrimethamine**, or **trimethoprim** that inhibit a subsequent step in folic acid synthesis. Sulfonamides are also used to treat equine protozoal myeloencephalitis. Adverse effects associated with this class include crystalluria and keratoconjunctivitis sicca, as well as hypersensitivity reactions, hepatic necrosis, and anemia. Resistance to sulfonamides is common among *Eimeria* spp.

A number of other compounds also are used as coccidiostats. Of these, only **amprolium** also is approved for treatment of coccidiosis in cattle and chickens in the United States. Amprolium competitively inhibits thiamine; neurotoxicity can occur due to overdose and is treated with thiamine supplementation. **Toltrazuril, ponazuril**, and **diclazuril** are triazine antiprotozoals that are very effective against coccidia and some other apicomplexan parasites. Toltrazuril is approved for treatment of coccidiosis in cattle and sheep in many areas of the world, while ponazuril and diclazuril are approved to treat equine protozoal myeloencephalitis in horses. Ponazuril is commonly used extralabel for coccidiosis in dogs, cats, rabbits, bearded dragons, and camelids, and for *Hepatozoon americanum* in dogs. Diclazuril is an approved coccidiostat in poultry. **Clopidol** and **decoquinate** are quinolone or quinolone-like coccidiostats effective against coccidia sporozoites. **Nicarbazin** and **robenidine** are synthetic coccidiostats used in chickens. Ionophore coccidiostats have been used since the early 1970s and include **lasalocid, monensin, narasin, salinomycin**, and **semduramicin**. Ionophores are primarily used as growth promoters but also have efficacy as coccidiostats by inhibiting mitochondrial function. These compounds are widely used in cattle, small ruminants, and poultry but can be fatal when inadvertently fed to horses or birds other than chickens.

NON-TRADITIONAL TREATMENTS

Alternative parasite treatment strategies are occasionally promoted, but only products approved by FDA, EPA, or similar regulatory agencies have been confirmed to be safe and efficacious. Feeding some types of high-tannin forage and administering copper oxide wire particles (COWP) to small ruminants support control of *Haemonchus contortus*, but should be used with care to avoid adverse effects. Boric acid can be used to desiccate larval stages of fleas in the environment. Supplementing fiber and probiotics has been shown to support resolution of clinical disease in dogs with diarrhea due to giardiasis when combined with an effective antiprotozoal agent. Garlic products, herbal dewormers, pumpkin seed, papaya seed, apple cider vinegar, vitamin supplements, peppermint oil, brewer's yeast, and other home remedies have not been shown to be effective parasite control strategies.

Diagnostic Dilemmas

Presented below are seven challenging cases in diagnostic parasitology. Case scenarios are based on information and specimens provided to the veterinary diagnostician. The answers to these diagnostic dilemmas are available on the accompanying website www.wiley.com/go/zajac/parasitology to this volume.

Diagnostic Dilemma 1

A 2.5-year-old neutered male, indoor/outdoor American bulldog family pet presented in Scranton, PA for an annual wellness exam. The dog had been dewormed monthly and was currently on prevention for heartworm, intestinal helminths, fleas, and ticks. During preparation of the fecal flotation, the veterinary technician noted a small (~5 mm) organism in the fecal material and suspected it might be a worm of some kind. What is the identification of this specimen?

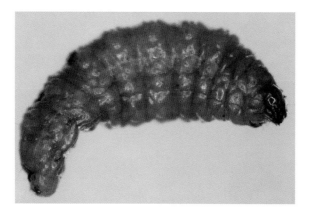

Fig. 8.1   Specimen observed in the fecal material of a dog. The specimen was approximately 5 mm in length. Photo courtesy of Dr. Manigandan Lejeune, Animal Health Diagnostic Center, Cornell University, Ithaca, NY.

Veterinary Clinical Parasitology, Ninth Edition. Anne M. Zajac, Gary A. Conboy, Susan E. Little, and Mason V. Reichard.
© 2021 John Wiley & Sons, Inc. Published 2021 by John Wiley & Sons, Inc.
Companion website: www.wiley.com/go/zajac/parasitology

Diagnostic Dilemma 2

A 4-year-old mixed breed neutered male dog was presented in Jonesboro, Arkansas for annual physical examination and vaccination. The dog was not on heartworm preventive and had an intermittent cough. A blood sample was negative for heartworm antigen on a well-validated commercial test. Numerous microfilariae were found on microscopic examination of a saline wet mount. Whole blood was submitted for Knott's test, which confirmed the presence of *Dirofilaria immitis* microfilariae based on morphologic appearance, size, and nuclear staining (Figs. 8.2, 8.3).

What is the most likely explanation for a negative heartworm antigen test in the face of numerous *Dirofilaria immitis* microfilariae in this dog?

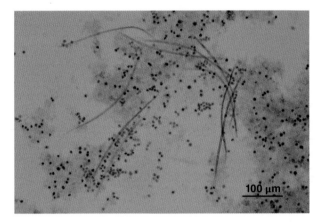

Fig. 8.2   *Dirofilaria immitis* microfilariae recovered on Knott's test from an infected dog. The identification of *D. immitis* is supported by the presence of numerous microfilariae in the sample (see Table 3.2).

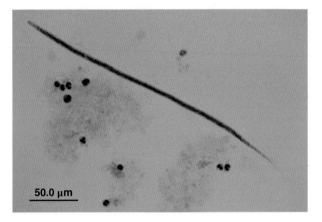

Fig. 8.3   Higher magnification view of a single *Dirofilaria immitis* microfilaria. Although individual microfilaria will shrink in formalin over time, when first prepared, *D. immitis* microfilaria recovered on a Knott's test usually measure 295–325 μm long by 5–7.5 μm wide.

Diagnostic Dilemma 3

A horse owner with 6 pleasure horses read about anthelmintic resistance and was curious to know if the dewormer in use on the farm was still effective since it had been used exclusively for several years. The owner collected a fecal sample from each horse, dewormed them and dropped the samples off at your hospital for quantitative egg counts. A month later, the owner collected a second set of samples and had those evaluated as well. The results are shown in the table below. The minimum detection limit of the modified McMaster test used to perform the egg counts was 25 eggs/gram. How effective was the deworming treatment?

Horse	Pretreatment egg count	Posttreatment egg count
Madison	200	<25 (none seen)
Finn	500	100
Chessie	100	<25 (none seen)
Simon	<25 (none seen)	25
Thea	350	75
Sammy	175	100

Diagnostic Dilemma 4

A 6-year-old spayed female German shorthaired pointer used for hunting in Virginia presented for a persistent cough. Results of centrifugal fecal flotation included nematode larvae that could not be identified because of distortion by flotation solution. A Baermann test was performed and several live nematode larvae, approximately 350 μm long, were recovered (Fig. 8.4). What is the identification of these larvae?

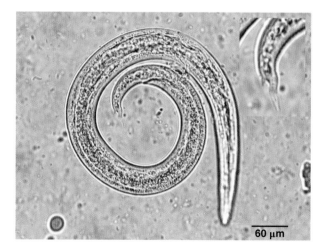

Fig. 8.4   Nematode larva, approximately 350 μm long, recovered from the feces of a dog presented for chronic cough. The inset shows a higher magnification of the tail of the larva. Photo courtesy of Dr. Meriam Saleh, Virginia-Maryland College of Veterinary Medicine, Blacksburg VA.

Diagnostic Dilemma 5

The owner of a 1-year-old intact female Chesapeake Bay retriever submitted a fecal sample from the dog after noticing small (7–10 mm) whitish oval to rectangular-shaped structures passed in the dog's feces (Figs. 8.5, 8.6). The client lived on a hobby farm and the dog had freedom to roam over a fairly large area on the property.

What is the identification of these structures?

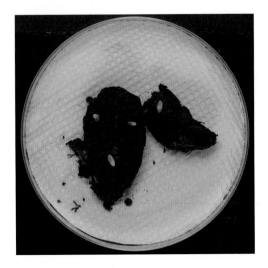

Fig. 8.5   Fecal sample from a clinically normal Chesapeake Bay retriever.

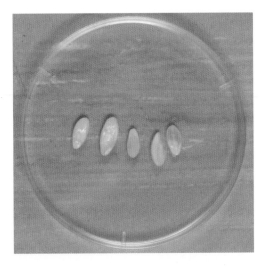

Fig. 8.6   Closer view of 7–10 mm white objects present in the fecal sample.

Diagnostic Dilemma 6

A 2-year-old intact male, indoor–outdoor domestic shorthair cat was presented to a veterinary practice in Battle Creek, Michigan for lethargy and inappetance. An abscess was identified on the right rear leg and a bite wound secondary to fighting was suspected. The wound was cleaned and flushed and a course of antibiotics instituted. During physical examination, a partially engorged tick was identified and removed from the neck. Although not associated with the primary complaint (abscess due to fighting), the owner asked if the tick might have transmitted any infections to the cat.

The tick was examined dorsally and ventrally (Figs. 8.7, 8.8).

What tick genus and species is this? What disease agents might it transmit?

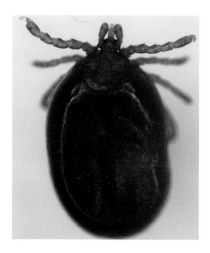

Fig. 8.7   Dorsal view of tick removed from a cat. Photo provided courtesy of Dr. Katie Clow, Ontario Veterinary College, University of Guelph, Guelph, Ontario, Canada.

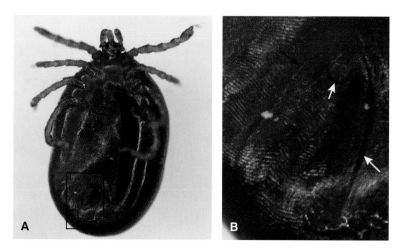

A   B

Fig. 8.8   (A) Ventral view of tick removed from a cat. (B) Higher magnification of area outlined in black showing the presence of an anal groove (black arrows) arching anterior to the anus (white arrow). Photo provided courtesy of Dr. Katie Clow, Ontario Veterinary College, University of Guelph, Guelph, Ontario, Canada.

Diagnostic Dilemma 7

An approximately 25-year-old, castrated male Arab horse spit a worm from his mouth. The owner submitted the worm for identification. No other abnormalities were observed with this horse.

The worm was approximately 10 cm in length and appeared to be a fragment consisting of only the mid-body section of an adult female nematode (Fig. 8.9). There were many eggs (about 30 × 60 µm) in the uterus of the female worm fragment (Fig. 8.10).

What further testing could be done and what is the diagnosis?

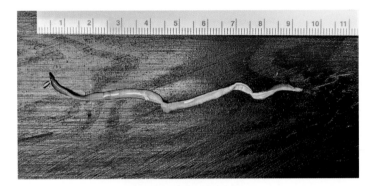

Fig. 8.9   Fragment of an adult worm expelled from the mouth of a horse. Figure courtesy of Dr. Yoko Nagamori, College of Veterinary Medicine, Oklahoma State University, Stillwater, OK.

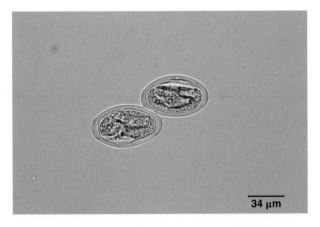

Fig. 8.10   Eggs recovered from the fragment of female worm from a horse. Figure courtesy of Dr. Yoko Nagamori, College of Veterinary Medicine, Oklahoma State University, Stillwater, OK.

BIBLIOGRAPHY

American Association of Equine Practitioners. 2019. AAEP Internal Parasite Control Guidelines. Accessed May 2020. https://aaep.org/guidelines/internal-parasite-control-guidelines

Atkinson, C. T., Thomas, N. J., and Hunter, D. B. 2008. Parasitic Disease of Wild Birds. Wiley-Blackwell, Ames, IA.

Baker, D. G. 2007. Flynn's Parasites of Laboratory Animals, 2nd ed. Blackwell Publishing, Ames, IA.

Barnard, S. M., and Upton, S. J. 1996. A Veterinary Guide to the Parasites of Reptiles: Protozoa. Krieger Publishing Co., Malabar, FL.

Bowman, D. D. 2021. Georgis' Parasitology for Veterinarians, 11th ed. Elsevier Saunders, St. Louis, MO.

Bowman, D. D., Hendrix, C. M., Lindsay, D. S., and Barr, S. C. 2002. Feline Clinical Parasitology. Iowa State University Press, Ames, IA.

Clyde, V. L., and Patton, S. 1996. Diagnosis, treatment and control of common parasites in companion and avian birds. Semin. Avian Exot. Pet Med. 5:75–84.

Coles, G. C., Bauer, C., Borgsteede, F. H. M., Geerts, S., Klei, T. R., Taylor, M. A., and Waller, P. J. 1992. World Association for the Advancement of Veterinary Parasitology (W.A.A.V.P.) methods for the detection of anthelmintic resistance in nematodes of veterinary importance. Vet. Parasitol. 44:35–44.

Coles, G. C., Jackson, F., Pomroy, W. E., Prichard, R. K., von Samson-Himmelstjerna, G., Silvestre, A., Taylor, M. A., and Vercruysse, J. 2006. The detection of anthelmintic resistance in nematodes of veterinary importance. Vet. Parasitol. 136:167–185.

Day, M. J. 2015. Introduction to antigen and antibody assays. Top. Companion Anim. Med. 30:128–131.

Deplazes, P., Eckert J., Mathis, A., von Samson-Himmelstjerna, G., and Zahner, H. 2016. Parasitology in Veterinary Medicine. Wageningen Academic Publishers, Wageningen, the Netherlands.

Egwang, T. G., and Slocombe, J. O. D. 1982. Evaluation of the Cornell-Wisconsin centrifugation flotation technique for recovering trichostrongylid eggs from bovine feces. Can. J. Comp. Med. 46:133–137.

Environmental Health Services, Centers for Disease Control and Prevention. 2019. Pictorial Keys to Arthropods, Reptiles, Birds, and Mammals of Public Health Significance. Accessed October 2019. https://www.cdc.gov/nceh/ehs/publications/pictorial_keys.htm

Foreyt, W. J. 1997. Veterinary Parasitology Reference Manual. Iowa State University Press, Ames, IA.

Fowler, M. E. 2010. Medicine and Surgery of Camelids, 3rd ed. Wiley-Blackwell, Ames, IA.

Garcia, L. S. 2016. Diagnostic Medical Parasitology, 6th ed. ASM Press, Washington, DC.

Georgi, J. R., and Georgi, M. E. 1992. Canine Clinical Parasitology. Lea & Febiger, Philadelphia, PA.

Greiner, E. C., and Ritchie, B. W. 1994. Parasites. In: Avian Medicine: Principles and Application, ed. B. W. Ritchie, G. J. Harrison, and L. R. Harrison, 1007–1029. Wingers Publishing, Lake Worth, FL.

Hendricks, C. M. 2002. Laboratory Procedures for Veterinary Technicians, 4th ed. Mosby, St. Louis, MO.

Veterinary Clinical Parasitology, Ninth Edition. Anne M. Zajac, Gary A. Conboy, Susan E. Little, and Mason V. Reichard.
© 2021 John Wiley & Sons, Inc. Published 2021 by John Wiley & Sons, Inc.
Companion website: www.wiley.com/go/zajac/parasitology

Hoffman, G. L. 1999. Parasites of North American Freshwater Fishes. Cornell University Press, Ithaca, NY.

Jacobs, D. E. 1986. A Colour Atlas of Equine Parasites. Gower Medical Publishing, London.

Jacobson, E. R. 2007. Infectious Diseases and Pathology of Reptiles. CRC Press, Boca Raton, FL.

Kaplan, R. M. 2020. Biology, epidemiology, diagnosis and management of anthelmintic resistance in gastrointestinal nematodes of livestock. Vet. Clin. North Am. Food Anim. Pract. 36:17–30.

Kassai, T. 1999. Veterinary Helminthology. Butterworth-Heinemann, Oxford.

Kaufmann, J. 1996. Parasitic Infections of Domestic Animals. Birkhäuser, Boston, MA.

Kennedy, M. J., Mackinnon, J. D., and Higgs, G. W. 1998. Veterinary Parasitology: Laboratory Procedures. Alberta Agriculture, Food and Rural Development Publishing Branch, Edmonton.

Klingenberg, R. J. 2016. Understanding Reptile Parasites, 2nd ed. Advanced Vivarium Systems, Irvine, CA.

Levine, N. D. 1980. Nematode Parasites of Domestic Animals and Man, 2nd ed. Burgess Publishing, Minneapolis, MN.

Little, S., Saleh, M., Wohltjen, M., and Nagamori, Y. 2018. Prime detection of *Dirofilaria immitis*: understanding the influence of blocked antigen on heartworm test performance. Parasit. Vectors. 11:186.

Lom J., and Dykova, I. 1992. Protozoan Parasites of Fishes. Developments in Aquaculture and Fisheries Science, Volume 26. Elsevier, Amsterdam.

Ministry of Agriculture, Fisheries and Food. 1986. Manual of Veterinary Parasitological Laboratory Techniques. Reference Book 418. Her Majesty's Stationery Office, London.

Mullen, G., and Durden, L. 2018. Medical and Veterinary Entomology, 3rd ed. Academic Press, New York.

Neimester, R., Logan, A. L., Gerber, B., Egleton, J. H., and Kleger, B. 1987. Hemo-De as substitute for ethyl acetate in formalin-ethyl acetate concentration technique. J. Clin. Microbiol. 25:425–426.

Nielsen, M. K., and Reinemeyer, C. R. 2018. Handbook of Equine Parasite Control, 2nd ed. Wiley Blackwell, Hoboken, NJ.

O'Farrell, B. 2015. Lateral Flow Technology for Field-Based Applications—Basics and Advanced Developments. Top. Companion Anim. Med. 30:139–147.

Owen, D. G. 1992. Parasites of Laboratory Animals. Royal Society of Medicine Services, London.

Roberts, R. J. 2001. The parasitology of teleosts. In: Fish Pathology, 3rd ed., ed. R. J. Roberts, 254–296. W. B. Saunders, Philadelphia, PA.

Samuel, W. M., Pybus, M. J., and Kocan, A. A. 2001. Parasitic Diseases of Wild Mammals, 2nd ed. Iowa State University Press, Ames, IA.

Smith, S. A. 1996. Parasites of birds of prey: their diagnosis and treatment. Semin. Avian Exot. Pet Med. 5:97–105.

Smith, S. A. 2002. Non-lethal clinical techniques used in the diagnosis of fish diseases. J. Am. Vet. Med. Assoc. 220:1203–1206.

Smith, S. A., and Noga, E. J. 1992. General parasitology of fish. In: Fish Medicine, ed. M. K. Stoskopf, 131–148. W. B. Saunders, Philadelphia, PA.

Smith, S. A., and Roberts, H. E. 2009. Chapter 8: Parasites of fishes. In: Fundamentals of Ornamental Fish Health, ed. H. E. Roberts, 102–112. Wiley-Blackwell, Hoboken, NJ.

Sonenshine, D. E., and Roe, R. M. 2014. Biology of Ticks, 2nd ed. Oxford University Press, New York.

Soulsby, E. J. L. 1965. Textbook of Veterinary Clinical Parasitology. F. A. Davis Co., Philadelphia, PA.

Taira, N., Ando, Y., and Williams, J. C. 2003. A Color Atlas of Clinical Helminthology of Domestic Animals. Elsevier Science, Amsterdam.

Taylor, M. A., Coop, R. L., and Wall, R. L. 2015. Veterinary Parasitology, 4th ed. Wiley Blackwell, Ames, IA.

Telford, S. R. Jr. 2009. Haemoparasites of the Reptilia. CRC Press, Boca Raton, FL.

Thienpont, D., Rochette, F., and Vanparijs, O. F. J. 1979. Diagnosing Helminthiasis through Coprological Examination. Janssen Research Foundation, Beerse, Belgium.

Timsit, E., Leguillette, R., White, B. J., Larson, R. L., and Buczinski, S. 2018. Likelihood ratios: an intuitive tool for incorporating diagnostic test results into decision-making. J. Am. Vet. Med. Assoc. 252(11):1362–1366.

U.S. Department of Agriculture. 1976. Ticks of Veterinary Importance. Agriculture Handbook 485. U.S. Government Printing Office, Washington, DC.

Valkiūnas, G. 2005. Avian Malaria Parasites and other Haemosporidia. CRC Press, Boca Raton, FL.

van Wyk, J., and Mayhew, E. 2013. Morphological identification of parasitic nematode infective larvae of small ruminants and cattle: a practical lab guide. Onderstepoort J. Vet. Res. 80:539–553.

Verocai, G. G., Chaudhry, U. N., and Lejeune, M. 2020. Diagnostic methods for detecting internal parasites of livestock. Vet. Clin. North Am. Food Anim. 36:125–143.

Wall, R., and Shearer, D. 2001. Veterinary Ectoparasites: Biology, Pathology and Control. Blackwell Science, London.

Weiss, D. J., and Wardrop, K. J. 2010. Schalm's Veterinary Hematology, 6th ed. Wiley-Blackwell, Ames, IA.

Williams, R. E., Hall, R. D., Broce, A. B., and Scholl, P. J. 1985. Livestock Entomology. John Wiley & Sons, New York.

Wilson, S. C., and Carpenter, J. W. 1996. Endoparasitic disease of reptiles. Semin. Avian Exot. Pet Med. 5:64–74.

Woo, P. T. K. (ed.). 2006. Fish Diseases and Disorders, Volume 1: Protozoan and Metazoan Infections, 816. CABI Publishing, Oxfordshire, UK.

INDEX

Page references given in *italics* indicate figures or tables.

abamectin, *98*, 372, *377*
Acanthocheilonema spp.
   A. dracunculoides, 210, *211*
   A. reconditum, 210, *211*, 224, *225*
acaricides. *see* ectoparasiticides
Acuaria spp., 166
Adelina spp., 23
Aelurostrongylus abstrusus, 24, 26, 28,
   43–45, *74*, *75*
afoxolaner, 375, *376*
African blue louse, 302
African Coast fever, 230
African tampan, 298
Alaria spp., *42–45*
albendazole, *98*, *372*, 373, *373*, 378
alpaca. *see* ruminants and camelids
Amblyomma spp., *279*, 281, 282, *283–285*,
   286
   A. americanum, 216, *280*, 282, *283*
   A. cajennense, 282, *284*
   A. hebraeum, 282
   A. maculatum, 213, *280*, 282, *284*
   A. variegatum, 282, *285*
American dog tick, *280*, 290
American Heartworm Society, 209–210
Amidostomum spp., 164
   A. anseri, 164
amitraz, *376*, *377*, 378
amprolium, *98*, 379
Amyloodinium ocellatum, 347, 356, *357*
Anaplasma spp., 245, 290, 292, 294
anaplasmosis, 278
anchor worm, 366, *367*
Ancylostoma spp., *42–45*, 56, *57*, 64, *67*
   A. braziliense, 56
   A. caninum, *3*, 56

A. ceylanicum, 56
A. tubaeforme, 56, *57*
eggs, *17*, *42*, 56, *57*, *64*, *67*
Angiostrongylus vasorum, 24, 28, 76, *77*
annelids, 193, 366, *367*
Anocenter nitens, 290, *291*
Anoplocephala spp., *126*, 138, *139*
   A. magna, 138
   A. perfoliata, *3*, *127*, 138
anthelmintics, 371–375, *372*, *373*
   administration routes for, *372*
   anthelmintic efficacy testing (FECRT),
      36–39
   for dogs and cats, *44*, *46*
   for horses, *127*
   persistency, 372
   resistance to, 372, 374–375
   for ruminants and camelids, *98*
   for swine, *141*
   withdrawal times, *373*
antibiotics, as protozoal treatment, 378
antibody detection, 239, 241
antibody titer, 241–242
antigen detection, 239
Antricola spp., *281*
Aonchotheca spp., 68, *69*, 96, *97*, 112, *113*
   A. bovis, 112
   A. longipes, 112
   A. putorii, *43*, 68, *69*
Aponomma spp., *281*
Argas spp., *281*, 298, *299*
   A. persicus, 298
   A. reflexus, 298
Argulus sp., 362, *363*
arsenicals, 374
Ascaridia spp., 162, *163*

Veterinary Clinical Parasitology, Ninth Edition. Anne M. Zajac, Gary A. Conboy, Susan E. Little,
and Mason V. Reichard.
© 2021 John Wiley & Sons, Inc. Published 2021 by John Wiley & Sons, Inc.
Companion website: www.wiley.com/go/zajac/parasitology